PRESSURE ULCERS

Guidelines for Prevention and Nursing Management

Second Edition

PRESSURE ULCERS

Guidelines for Prevention and Nursing Management

Second Edition

JoAnn Maklebust, MSN, RN, CS, CNP
Clinical Nurse Specialist/Case Manager
Harper Hospital/Detroit Medical Center
Detroit, Michigan

Mary Y. Sieggreen, MSN, RN, CS, CNP
Clinical Nurse Specialist/Case Manager
Harper Hospital/Detroit Medical Center
Detroit, Michigan

Springhouse Corporation
Springhouse, Pennsylvania

STAFF

Senior Publisher
Minnie B. Rose, RN, BSN, MEd

Clinical Consultant
Patricia Dwyer Schull, RN, MSN

Art Director
John Hubbard

Senior Associate Art Director
Stephanie Peters

Designers
Amy Litz, Lorraine Lostracco, Mary Ludwicki

Associate Acquisitions Editors
Louise Quinn, Betsy K. Snyder

Editorial Assistants
Stephanie Franchetti, Jeanne Napier

Manufacturing
Deborah Meiris (director), T.A. Landis, Andreas Hess

For information, write Springhouse Corporation, 1111 Bethlehem Pike, P.O. Box 908, Springhouse, PA 19477-0908.
Printed in the United States of America.

PU2-030396

A member of the Reed Elsevier plc group

Library of Congress Cataloging-in-Publication Data
Maklebust, JoAnn.
  Pressure ulcers: guidelines for prevention and nursing management / JoAnn Maklebust, Mary Sieggreen. — 2nd ed.
    p. cm.
Includes bibliographical references and index.
1. Bedsores—Prevention. 2. Bedsores—Nursing. I. Sieggreen, Mary. II. Title.
[DNLM: 1. Decubitus Ulcer—prevention & control. 2. Decubitus Ulcer—nursing. 3. Wound Healing. WR 598 M235p 1996]
RL675.M35 1996
616.5'45—dc20
DNLM/DLC   95-594
ISBN 0-87434-836-6 (alk. paper)   CIP

DEDICATION

To Tom and Dwight, who are always there;
to David, Doug, Rick, Marisa, and Marcy, who are
ever forgiving; to Vaughn, Margaret, Bill, and Carolyn,
who are the spirit behind us; and to Tyler, who is
the promise of the future.

CONTENTS

FOREWORD

The first edition of *Pressure Ulcers: Guidelines for Prevention and Nursing Management,* published in 1991, was based on the most up-to-date research and knowledge base then available. It is difficult to believe that a period of four years could add so much more to our knowledge base about a problem that has plagued humankind for millennia. However, in that interim, the Agency for Health Care Policy and Research (AHCPR) published two significant clinical guidelines: *Pressure Ulcers in Adults: Prediction and Prevention* and *Treatment of Pressure Ulcers.*

Both of these publications synthesized the relevant existent research on the pressure ulcer problem. Representatives from the National Pressure Ulcer Advisory Panel (NPUAP)—an interdisciplinary body of 15 expert professionals whose mission is to provide leadership, recommendations, guidance, and action toward pressure ulcer prevention and management—served on the two AHCPR panels that created the clinical guidelines mentioned above. JoAnn Maklebust served on both groups and participated in the preparation of the publications of each organization. She and her co-author, Mary Sieggreen, are both recognized throughout the country for their clinical knowledge, practical expertise, and unwavering dedication to pressure ulcer prevention and management.

Some readers of *Pressure Ulcers: Guidelines for Prevention and Nursing Management, Second Edition* may believe that they already have a strong knowledge base and a good command of the literature about pressure ulcers. These readers are in for a surprise. Among other topics added to the second edition, the authors discuss the current Staging system advocated by both the AHCPR and the NPUAP and the problems created by some health care personnel who continue to use the system inappropriately. Maklebust and Sieggreen also point out anatomic skin differences among races, the relevance of which to pressure ulcer susceptibility is not yet apparent.

Other equally interesting and important topics include closed pressure ulcers, the role of infection in the production of pressure ulcers, the errors inherent in using simple surface and volume measurements to determine the progress of healing, the decreased effectiveness of foam mattresses with duration of use over time, continuous quality improvement, and benchmarking. In short, this new second edition will elucidate many aspects of pressure ulcer care that may have caused confusion in the past and will provide an informative overview of other areas where definitive answers have yet to emerge.

Nurses in all care settings—hospitals, long-term care facilities, outpatient clinics, and homes—will not find a more informative or comprehensive guide to the recognition and management of pressure ulcers. The authors have distilled the volume of literature into a practical book that the reader can use to form the basis for devising an action plan appropriate to any practice setting. *Pressure Ulcers: Guidelines for Prevention and Nursing Management, Second Edition* will serve as a much-needed resource for health providers who work daily to manage one of the largest and most troublesome clinical problems faced by health professionals.

Mary L. Shannon, EdD, RN
Founding Member, National Pressure Ulcer Advisory Panel
Professor and Chair, Adult Health Nursing
School of Nursing
University of Texas at Galveston
Galveston, Texas

PREFACE

Pressure ulcer management consumes a large percentage of nursing time and is financially and emotionally costly to the patient. There is little to guide the bedside practitioner in providing safe, economic, and effective care for patients with pressure ulcers. Scientific rationales for pressure ulcer management are often lacking in the health care literature. Recently, however, the Agency for Health Care Policy and Research (AHCPR) released two guidelines with recommendations for the prevention and treatment of pressure ulcers. *Pressure Ulcers: Guidelines for Prevention and Nursing Management, Second Edition* will provide clinicians with a scientific basis for decision-making in the application of the AHCPR recommendations.

This text is the result of many years of work by clinicians and researchers at both Harper and Grace Hospitals in the Detroit Medical Center. Our original interest in pressure ulcers was stimulated by the lack of standards for pressure ulcer care and by a seemingly disorganized attempt to educate the staff about pressure ulcer management. As Clinical Nurse Specialists, we were consultants to the nursing staff providing care for patients with multiple complex problems. We received many requests to assist in planning care for chronic wound management, and we found that each patient care unit had a different favorite remedy for pressure ulcers. In our attempt to study the etiology of pressure ulcers and the scientific basis for treatment, we carefully researched the problem and then assumed accountability for investigating the management of pressure ulcers. This investigation led us to formal research on the topic, and we have published many reports to share our findings. However, these reports are scattered among several journals and often inaccessible to staff nurses. Thus we decided to combine our findings with the findings of others who were studying pressure ulcers, and our original book evolved.

This second edition of *Pressure Ulcers: Guidelines for Prevention and Nursing Management* is a major update. Two new chapters have been added, and nursing care plans and policies and procedures have been updated to include the latest developments in caring for patients with pressure ulcers. The expanded content enhances the book's usefulness to caregivers in extended care facilities as well as in home care settings.

The book consists of 13 chapters and 16 appendices. Chapter 1 describes normal anatomy and physiology of the skin. Chapter 2 discusses the problem of pressure ulcers as a major health problem, and Chapter 3 covers the etiology and pathophysiology of the development of pressure ulcers. Chapter 4 details factors necessary for normal wound healing. Chapter 5 explains proper assessment of pressure ulcers. Together, Chapters 1 to 5 provide a background for understanding the problem of pressure ulcers, identifying their far-reaching consequences and a scientific basis for treatment.

Chapter 6 presents the most common risk factors and prevention techniques for pressure ulcers. Chapter 7 presents the latest thinking in treatment, including pressure ulcers in the case management system. Chapter 8 details a nursing care plan tailored to specific nursing diagnoses associated with pressure ulcers. Chapter 9 provides the nurse with step-by-step how-to policies and procedures that have been developed and implemented successfully for the care of pressure ulcers. Chapter 10 reviews continuity of care, and Chapter 11 explores patient education. Chapter 12 deals with continuous quality improvement (CQI), including data collection, audits, and methods necessary to develop a successful quality assurance program for pressure ulcers. Chapter 13 looks to the future of pressure ulcers as a major health problem and how it will be dealt with by nurses and other health care providers. Finally, numerous appendices include the most widely accepted pressure ulcer assessment tools, the most important skin and wound care decision-making flow charts, and completed documentation forms related to nursing care of pressure ulcers.

We hope that our work will be used by bedside caregivers to improve the quality of care for patients who are at risk for pressure ulcers and for patients who already have pressure ulceration.

Pressure ulcers are more than physical wounds. In our quest for scientific understanding, compassion and empathy must not be lost. Nothing stirs one to action more than seeing a part of oneself reflected in the suffering of others. The story on pages 14 and 15 helps to place in perspective the true significance of pressure ulcers — a human condition.

JoAnn Maklebust
Mary Sieggreen

ACKNOWLEDGMENTS

We gratefully acknowledge the ongoing work of the Pressure Ulcer Committee of Harper Hospital and offer a special thank you to those members of the committee who worked with us to develop the decision flow charts: Mary Berry, Mary Brugger, Barbara Horvath, Antoinette Tessier, and Michelle Matthews.

CHAPTER 1

Anatomy and Physiology of Skin

Human skin is a large organ comprising a sheetlike investment of the whole body. The appearance and texture of the skin are influenced by regional variations in blood flow, distribution of glandular structures, and varying degrees of hairiness.[1] Smooth, unblemished, healthy skin tells much about its wearer. As the most readily accessible body system, the skin is a sensitive indicator of both physical and emotional status. Unscarred, disease-free, flexible skin is desirable for both functional and cosmetic reasons. Functionally, the skin must adapt to all the body contours and conform to all the body movements. Cosmetically, the psychosocial aspect of skin appearance is extremely important to a person's well-being, especially in our beauty-conscious society. Because skin is the most visible organ system, altered skin integrity can, unfortunately, be a ready means for social discrimination.

The skin, also known as the cutis or integument, weighs from 6 to 8 pounds. It is the largest organ of the human body, covering more than 20 square feet in an average-size adult.[2] The skin is not a uniform organ; its appearance and thickness vary according to anatomical site. Skin thickness ranges from 1/50 of an inch over the eyelids to 1/3 of an inch on the palms of the hands and the soles of the feet.[2,3] Specialized skin cells form appendages that harden sufficiently to form nails and elongate to form hair. The pH of skin normally ranges from 4.5 to 5.5. This is the so-called protective acid mantle of the skin that serves to maintain the normal skin flora. The power and complexity of the skin are illustrated in Figure 1.1.

The skin has multiple functions. It provides an interface between the body and its environment, protecting the inner tissues from invasion. It transmits a range

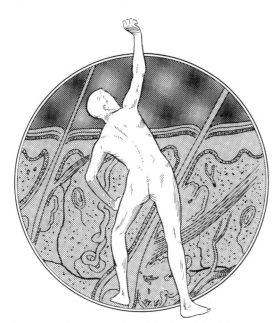

Figure 1.1 The power and complexity of the skin

Table 1.1
Skin Assessment Factors

Function	Focus	Findings
Temperature regulation	Palpate skin surface, including extremities; observe color.	A warm flesh pink tone is normal. Hot suggests increased blood flow as a result of the body's response to inflammation or infection, and the surface usually is red or purplish in color. Cool or cold is usually due to decreased blood flow to the surface as a result of impaired circulation from internal or external factors; color is usually white or pallor.
Sensory communicator	Check temperature, tactile, and two-point discrimination on various parts of the body.	Normally, one should be able to distinguish degrees of temperature, sharpness, dullness, and pressure sensations against skin surface. Diminished sensation may be generalized or affect only a part of the body, such as lower extremities.
Storage of water and fat	Observe skin tone (turgor and tension) and body build.	Skin should normally be smooth and resilient. Dehydration is present if skin is very wrinkled, withered, and/or dry. Edema may cause the skin to be taut and shiny. Bony prominences will be very pronounced on low-body-weight persons; obesity may result in extra folds where skin surfaces approximate, causing friction and irritation to the skin.
Absorption and excretion	Observe skin surface for texture and moisture.	Skin texture among individuals varies from dry to oily, depending on the amount of body secretions. Skin usually becomes more dry with advancing age; excessive perspiration may be due to environmental factors or elevated body temperature.
Protection	Observe for breaks in skin integrity.	Normally, there should be no eruptions of the skin surface.
Physical beauty	Observe texture, color, and general appearance of the skin.	Blemishes, rashes, lesions, and discolored areas on the skin surface are warning signs of irritation or trauma.

of sensations, such as touch, pressure, and pain. The skin regulates body temperature and, while aiding in excretion, also prevents excessive loss of body fluids.[4,5] Assessment of the skin should consider each of these vital functions. A guide to facilitate skin assessment can be found in Table 1.1.[6]

Anatomically, the skin consists of the epidermal, dermal, and subcutaneous layers of tissue (Figure 1.2). The epidermis and the dermis make up the true skin. However, the subcutaneous tissue often is included as part of skin anatomy. The three distinct layers of skin have different structures and cell types. Each individual skin layer also has its own function, yet all these functions are interrelated.[1,2,3,7]

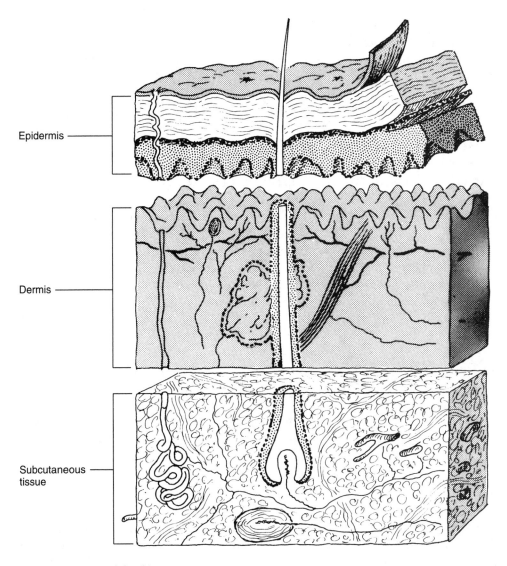

Epidermis

Dermis

Subcutaneous
tissue

Figure 1.2 Layers of the skin

Epidermis

The epidermis, or cuticle, is thin, avascular, and divided into five of its own distinct layers. The outer horny layer, or stratum corneum, is composed of anucleated, flattened, nonviable, desiccated cells. The stratum corneum, containing mostly keratinocyte cells, is the major chemical and mechanical barrier of the body. Keratinocytes produce keratin, the principal constituent of the epidermis. Keratin is a protective protein that provides the waterproof covering for the body. Dead keratinized cells on the body surface are constantly being replaced by new cells pushing to the top. The surface layer of cells is shed, and a new epidermis is formed about every four to six weeks. This normal shedding of the keratin layer of skin is a defense mechanism against infection.[1,2,3,8]

The second major cell type in the epidermis is the melanocyte. Melanocytes are found in the germinative cell layer of the epidermis. Melanocytes release granules of pigment called melanin that provides yellow, brown, and black skin tones. All individuals have approximately the same number of melanocytes, although melanocytes are reported to be larger and more heterogeneous in aging skin. Darkly pigmented skin results from both increased size and function of the melanocyte. Melanin, produced at a steady rate, assists in protecting the body from damage to cellular DNA from solar radiation. Ultraviolet light increases skin pigmentation through two pathways: photooxidation of preformed melanin and delayed new melanin production through the process of tanning.

The third major component of the epidermis, the Langerhans cells, is found between the keratinized cells in the stratum spinosum. Langerhans cells participate in immunologic responses by functioning in antigen recognition and processing. They act as macrophages that ingest potential antigenic compounds to prevent the body from allergic reaction.[1-7] Langerhans cells are particularly susceptible to destruction by ultraviolet irradiation, which may be important in the pathogenesis of sunlight-induced skin malignancy.

Epidermal layers

The epidermis consists of five layers, as shown in Figure 1.3. Starting from the innermost layer, they are as follows[8]:

1. The *stratum germinativum,* or basal strata, is a single layer of cells forming the base of the epidermis. It is the only layer with the ability to regenerate or undergo mitosis to form new cells. Tissues that do not regenerate are repaired by scar formation.

2. The *stratum spinosum* is made up of several layers of spinelike extensions of the basal layer. This layer may be included as part of the basal layer, but it does not have the ability to regenerate.

3. The *stratum granulosum* contains Langerhans cells, which are dispersed throughout the granular section. They play a primary role in immune reactions and affect the inflammatory phase of allergic contact dermatitis.

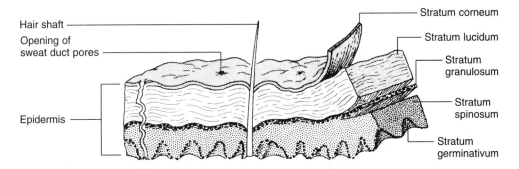

Figure 1.3 The epidermal skin layers

4. The *stratum lucidum* is a packed, translucent line of flat cells found only on the palms and soles. Thin skin has no stratum lucidum.

5. The *stratum corneum,* or horny layer, is the tough, outer strata of the epidermis. The acid mantle of the stratum corneum helps to maintain the ecology of the skin and retards certain fungal and bacterial growth. The protective protein, keratin, provides the water-repellent covering of the body.

Dermal-epidermal junction

Between the epidermis and dermis is the *basement membrane,* an undulating junction that both separates and attaches the epidermis and the dermis. The configuration of the dermal-epidermal junction provides structural support and allows exchange of fluids and cells between the skin layers. The epidermis has an irregular surface, with downward fingerlike projections known as rete ridges or pegs. These pegs of epidermis interface with upward projections of the papillary dermis, as shown in Figure 1.4. Together, the two surfaces resemble the inner surface of a waffle iron. The two opposing surface projections anchor the epidermis to the dermis and help prevent the epidermis from sliding back and forth on the dermis. With aging, this dermal-epidermal junction tends to flatten, with the area of contact between the epidermis and dermis decreasing by one-third. This places older adults at risk for skin tears from dermal-epidermal separation.[5]

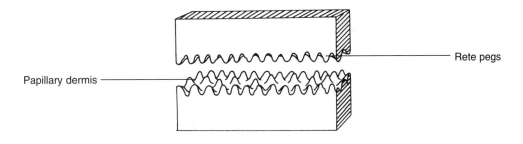

Figure 1.4 The dermal-epidermal junction

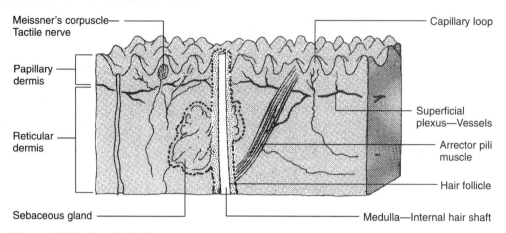

Figure 1.5 The dermal skin layer

Dermis

The dermis, or corium, lies directly beneath the epidermis. It supplies support and nutrition to the epidermis. The dermis is a strong, structural, extracellular matrix composed of collagen and elastic fibers that provide the skin with mechanical strength. It is composed of two layers of connective tissue containing blood vessels, nerves, and integumentary appendages: hair, nails and skin glands (Figure 1.5). Fibroblasts are the most important cells of the dermis. Fibroblasts produce collagen, a protein that gives the skin strength. Fibroblasts also synthesize the elastic fibers that help the skin stretch. Additionally, they produce ground substance that serves as a cushion and lubricant.[8] Dermal fibroblasts possess a finite replicative capacity of 50 to 100 doublings, and then cease replicating in response to growth factors.

The layers of the dermis are described as follows[8]:

1. The *papillary dermis*, or outer layer, is formed of collagen and reticular fibers important for healing. Also present are capillaries providing nourishment for the metabolic activity needed by the epidermis and appendages.

2. The *reticular dermis*, or inner layer, is formed of thick networks of collagen bundles that anchor the skin to the subcutaneous tissue. The thick fibers allow for increased elasticity.

Subcutaneous tissue

The hypodermis, also called the subcutis or subcutaneous tissue, is made up of dense connective and adipose tissue. Anatomically, it often is considered a part of the skin (Figure 1.6). It houses major vessels, lymphatics, and nerves; acts as a heat insulator; and provides a nutritional depot that is used during illness or starvation. The subcutaneous fat also acts as a mechanical shock absorber. This cushioning effect of the fatty tissue facilitates mobility of the skin over the underlying structures.[8] The distribution of the subcutaneous fat tissue depends on age, heredity, and gender.

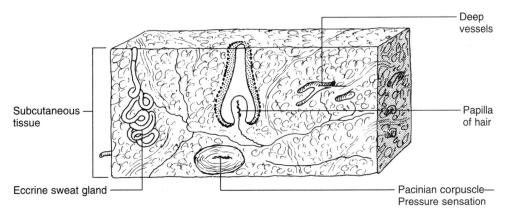

Figure 1.6 The subcutaneous skin layer

Fascia

Below the subcutaneous layer is dense, firm, membranous connective tissue that covers muscles, nerves, and blood vessels. This is called fascia, and it varies in thickness and strength throughout the body. There are two divisions, superficial and deep. The superficial fascia, directly beneath the skin, connects the skin to subadjacent parts, facilitating movement. The deep fascia, which is less elastic, forms sheath- or envelope-like coverings for muscles, blood vessels, and nerves.[8]

Blood flow to soft tissue

Blood supply to the skin comes from cutaneous branches of the subcutaneous musculocutaneous arteries. With the exception of the perforating muscular vessels, most of the cutaneous circulation is microcirculation. This microcirculation of blood supplies oxygen and nutrients directly to surrounding fibroblasts and to basal keratinocytes by diffusion across the basement membrane.[3]

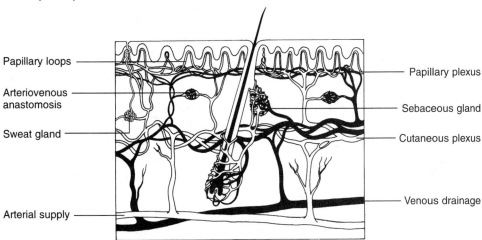

Figure 1.7 The cutaneous blood supply

It is important to understand the relationship between anatomy and physiology of the cutaneous blood supply and pressure ulcers. The blood supply to the skin originates in the underlying muscles, as shown in Figure 1.7. The cutaneous vasculature consists of (a) arteries that supply the blood to the skin, (b) capillary beds, and (c) veins that drain the blood from the skin. The blood pressure at the arteriolar end of the capillaries is approximately 32 mm Hg. The pressure at the venous end of the capillaries is approximately 12 mm Hg. Therefore, the average blood pressure in the capillaries is about 20 mm Hg, which is very low compared with the blood pressure in the larger arteries.[9]

The vasculature of the dermis is the most expansive of any organ system. The main purpose of the vast blood supply to the skin is to regulate body temperature. The skin does not use all of its blood supply to nourish the tissue and, in fact, is oversupplied with blood when compared to its metabolic needs. This is not true of muscle and subcutaneous fat. Muscle and fatty tissue do not tolerate ischemia or hypoxia. Studies have shown repeatedly that muscle and subcutaneous tissues are more susceptible to the effects of pressure than the dermis and epidermis.[9,10] Pressure ulcers usually result from a prolonged failure of capillary blood supply as a consequence of externally applied pressure.[10]

Skin colors and ethnic variations

Human skin comes in a variety of colors. There are basic similarities in structure and function of all skin types, but the subtleties in variation can lead to different skin care needs and assessment skills. The majority of the material presented in the literature deals with black skin.[11,12,13]

Melanocytes are pigment-forming cells. The variation in melanin pigmentation is the most obvious difference between light and dark skin tones. Interestingly, in black-skinned and white-skinned individuals, there is no variation in the number of melanocytes, only in their activity and size. In blacks, the melanosomes, or melanin granules, are larger, dispersed singly inside the keratinocytes, and not easily degraded, and the melanocytes are more active. Melanin is not reabsorbed by the surrounding cells, and the pigment reaches the stratum corneum. This was demonstrated by washing clean, black skin and seeing the dark horny layers on the washcloth. In whites, the melanin does not get past the first few layers of the epidermis.[11,12,13]

Another established difference between black and white skin is the structure of the stratum corneum, the outer layer of the epidermis. While thickness of the stratum corneum is the same for both blacks and whites, in blacks it is more compact and has more cell layers. For this reason, black skin resists chemical irritation and offers a more effective barrier against external stimuli. Black skin is generally smooth and dry. As the epidermis flakes off the underlying dark skin, it gives it an "ashy" look. Application of petrolatum jelly or lotion helps to eliminate flaky skin.[11]

Soap should be used sparingly on dry skin. Use of lanolin-based lotion is preferable to either water-based or perfumed lotion. Lanolin acts as a lubricant, while water-based and perfumed lotions dry the skin.[11]

Obvious change in skin color will not be easily recognized in individuals whose normal skin color is dark. Black skin may have such high melanin content that the deep color makes it difficult to discern changes. Bennett has studied the problem of assessing darkly pigmented skin and has developed a shading strip to facilitate accurate assessment.[14] When assessing dark-skinned individuals, it is important to have good lighting in order to accurately assess pressure-related skin changes. If erythema is suspected in black-skinned persons, it can be assessed by palpation of the area for increased warmth, a feeling of tightness, and areas of hardness under the skin.[14,15,16] Because it is more sensitive than the palm of the hand, the dorsal surface of the fingers should be used for palpation of the area in question.

Hypopigmentation frequently accompanies healing of superficial injuries of dark skin. When the outer layer heals, it often requires time for the melanin to reach the stratum corneum. Vitiligo, or partial loss of pigmentation, can occur in all races, but dark-skinned persons are more frequently affected. Post-injury hypopigmentation often leads to more anxiety than the primary cutaneous lesion. The etiology of post-inflammatory hypopigmentation is unknown, but it is thought to be familial and may be associated with diabetes mellitus, pernicious anemia, hypothyroidism, and hyperthyroidism. The most commonly affected sites are the face and eyes, the chest, the axilla, the groin, and the dorsal aspects of the hands. The white patches are sensitive to ultraviolet rays and burn easily if exposed to sunlight. There are few skin changes with vitiligo except for the complete absence of melanocytes.

Another problem occurring more frequently in dark-skinned people is keloid formation. Keloids have been reported in all races, but they are more common in dark-skinned individuals. Males and females are equally affected. Keloids are dense collagenous growths that usually follow an injury. They are easily distinguished by claw-like projections but may be confused with hypertrophic scarring. Keloid tissue tends to be pruritic and may be very painful or tender. Treatment is difficult because keloids recur and may even enlarge after surgical attempts at correction. Intralesional injection of corticosteroid solution has had varied degrees of success. More recently, carbon dioxide laser has been used with good results. Keloid formation can occur without injury and also may be familial.[12,13]

Changes associated with aging skin

Dramatic changes in the skin occur with aging. Sweat glands diminish in number. There is atrophy and thinning of both the epithelial and fatty layers of tissue, as shown in Figure 1.8. In older individuals, there is little subcutaneous fat on the legs or forearms. This may be the case even if abundant abdominal or hip fat is present. One result of the general loss of fat from the subcutaneous tissue is the relative prominence of the bony protuberances of the thorax, scapula, trochanters, and knees. The loss of this valuable padding contributes to pressure ulcer risk in the aged.[17]

Changes in skin appearance are due to a progressive destruction of the delicate

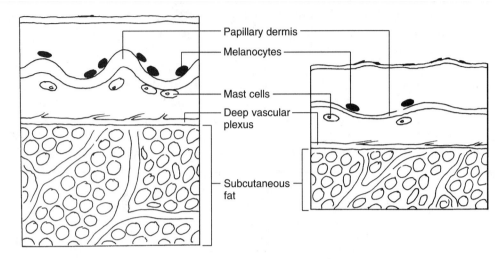

Figure 1.8 Skin changes associated with aging

architecture of dermal connective tissue.[17] Both collagen and elastin components of the dermis display degenerative changes. This results in shrinkage of collagen and elastic fibers. Collagen content of the skin has been shown to decrease during aging by approximately 1% per year throughout adult life. The net effect of all these changes is thin, dry, and inelastic skin. The attachment between the epidermis and the dermis weakens, resulting in a tendency for the epidermis to slide over the dermis. Minor friction and/or shearing forces can cause separation or tearing of the two layers, resulting in an injury known as skin tear.[18]

Older people are more likely to complain of dryness and itchiness of the skin. They also complain of being cold. Most likely, this is due to a loss of insulating subcutaneous fat. Among the cellular changes are a loss of melanocyte production. This results in graying of the hair, whitening of Caucasian skin, and pallor. A pale appearance or loss of ruddiness also may result from the decreased size of cutaneous blood vessels.[19,20,21]

In general, old people tend to lose their body hair. They also develop wrinkles that are permanent infoldings of the epithelium and subepithelium. Wrinkles are most noticeable on the face, in part because of repeated stress on the skin from facial expressions.

Exposure to the sun is the single most important factor in producing wrinkles of the skin. Sun damage is responsible for a large majority of age-related changes of the skin. In addition to environmental factors, heredity and hormonal fluctuations also contribute to skin changes in aged persons.[4,17,19,20,21]

Elderly people have thin, fragile skin that needs special care. Intermittent gentle cleansing with warm water usually is all that is needed for daily skin hygiene. During the cleansing and drying processes, care should be taken to minimize friction against the skin. Use of a soft cloth to pat the skin dry is recommended over rubbing with a towel. Forceful scrubbing and use of caustic agents and harsh cleansers are harmful and should be avoided.[15,18,20]

Summary

The skin is the largest organ of the body. It is composed of tissue that constantly grows and renews itself. The skin provides the interface between the body and the rest of the world. A basic clinical knowledge of the structure and function of human skin is important for pressure ulcer management. Actual or potential impaired skin integrity has important implications for a person's well-being. Loss of tissue integrity compromises the function of the skin. Injury to the integumentary system involves damage to some combination of the epidermis, dermis, and underlying tissue. Through careful understanding of skin function, thorough skin assessment, selection of appropriate interventions, and professional and public education, nurses can promote the maintenance of healthy skin and decrease the risk for pressure ulcers.[4,15,16,18,20]

References

1. Mehregan, A.H., and Hashimoto, K. *Pinkus' Guide to Dermatohistopathology,* 5th ed. Norwalk, Conn.: Appleton & Lange, 1991.

2. Mast, B.A. "The Skin," in Cohen, I.K., et al., eds. *Wound Healing: Biochemical and Clinical Aspects.* Philadelphia: W.B. Saunders Co., 1992.

3. Wysocki, A.B. "A Review of the Skin and Its Appendages," *Advances in Wound Care* 8(2): 53-70, February 1995.

4. Klein, L. "Maintenance of Healthy Skin," *Enterostomal Ther* 15(6): 227-231, June 1988.

5. Lynch, P.J. *Dermatology,* 3rd ed. House Officer Series. Baltimore: Williams & Wilkins, 1994.

6. Gosnell, D.J. "Assessment and Evaluation of Pressure Sores," *Nurs Clin North Am* 22(2): 401, February 1987.

7. Hill, M.J. *Skin Disorders.* St. Louis: Mosby-Yearbook, 1994.

8. Dains, J.E. "Integumentary System," in Bloom, W., and Fawcett, D.W., eds. *A Textbook of Histology,* 11th ed. Philadelphia: W.B. Saunders Co., 1986.

9. Maklebust, J. "Pressure Ulcers: Etiology and Prevention," *Nurs Clin North America* 22(2): 359-377, February 1987.

10. Parish, L.C., et al. *The Decubitus Ulcer.* New York: Masson Publishing Co., 1983.

11. Jackson, F. "The ABCs of Black Hair and Skin Care," *Today's Professional Nurse* (1): 6-18, January-February, 1990.

12. Laude, A.T., and Russo, R.M. *Dermatologic Disorders in Black Children and Adolescents.* Medical Examination Publishing Co., Inc., 1983.

13. Basset, A., et al. *Dermatology of Black Skin.* Translated by Oxford University Press, 1986.

14. Bennett, M.A. "A Shading Strip to Facilitate Assessment of Darkly Pigmented Skin." Personal communication, 1995.

15. Panel for the Prediction and Prevention of Pressure Ulcers in Adults. *Pressure Ulcers in Adults: Prediction and Prevention.* Clinical Practice Guideline No. 3. AHCPR Publication No. 92-0047. Rockville, Md.: U.S. Department of Health and Human Services, Agency for Health Care Policy and Research, May 1992.

16. Bergstrom, N., et al. *Treatment of Pressure Ulcers.* Clinical Practice Guideline No. 15. AHCPR Publication No. 95-0652. Rockville, Md.: U.S. Department of Health and Human Services, Agency for Health Care Policy and Research, December 1994.

17. West, M.D. "The Cellular and Molecular Biology of Skin Aging," *Archives of Dermatology* 130: 87-95, 1994.

18. Payne, R.L., and Martin, M.L. "Skin Tears: The Epidemiology and Management of Skin Tears in Older Adults," *Ostomy/Wound Management* 26(1): 26-37, January 1990.

19. Marks, R. "Structure and Function of Aged Skin" in *Skin Diseases in Old Age.* Philadelphia: J.P. Lippincott Co., 1987.

20. Rossman, I. "Human Aging Changes," in Burnside, I.M., ed. *Nursing and the Aged.* New York: McGraw-Hill, 1981.

21. Gilchrist, B.A. *Skin and Aging Processes.* Boca Raton, Fla.: CRC Press, 1984.

CHAPTER 2

Approaching the Pressure Ulcer Problem

Common terms used for tissue destruction resulting from prolonged pressure are "bedsore," "decubitus ulcer," "pressure sore," and "pressure ulcer." The terms "decubitus ulcer" and "bedsore" originated from the observation that ulcers frequently developed in persons who were bedridden. However, individuals need not be lying down or bedridden to develop tissue ulcerations related to pressure. Ulcers can form with the patient in any constantly maintained position. Because the primary cause is pressure, the term "pressure ulcer" most accurately describes both the lesion and the etiology. "Pressure ulcer" is the term used in this text.

Clinicians frequently use the term "decubiti" when more than one decubitus ulcer is present. This is incorrect grammatical use of the word. The term "decubitus" is a fourth declension Latin noun, and the plural form ends in "-us" just as the singular form. The plural of "decubitus" is "decubitus." There is no such word as "decubiti."[1]

The size of the problem

The prevalence and incidence of pressure ulcers vary among populations. The variability is indicative of methodological problems in interpreting the data. To address this problem, the National Pressure Ulcer Advisory Panel sponsored a pressure ulcer consensus development conference in 1989. At that meeting, the following problems in calculating accurate incidence and prevalence rates were identified:

• Studies often confused incidence (new cases developing over time) and prevalence (a cross-section of all patients with pressure ulcers in a facility on a particular day).
• Study populations varied.
• Sources of information varied from direct observation of patients to chart reviews of discharged patients.
• Investigators determined pressure ulcer stages differently.[2]

Despite the problems determining accurate statistics, pressure ulcers are recognized as a national health concern.

In 1989, pressure ulcer prevalence in U.S. hospital settings ranged from 3.5%[3] to 29%[4] on any given day. More recently, Meehan conducted two extensive surveys of acute care facilities. In 1990, she found a 9.2% pressure ulcer prevalence rate among 148 hospitals,[5] and in 1994 she reported an 11.1% prevalence rate among 177 hospitals.[6] Prevalence rates reported in the literature vary, depending on whether Stage I ulcers are defined as superficial breaks in the epidermis or reddened areas of unbroken skin. Some reports did not include reddened areas as Stage I pressure ulcers, whereas other reports included them.

Although incidence rates are difficult to determine, it is estimated that from 2.7%[7] to 29.5%[8] of patients in acute care facilities develop new ulcers during their hospital stay. Allman[9] reported a 29.9% incidence rate among elderly bedridden and chairbound patients at his acute care hospital.

The reported prevalence of pressure ulcers in nursing homes is not higher than in acute care hospitals, although nursing home patients may be more "at-risk." Long-term care facilities have a reported prevalence rate ranging from 2.4%[10] to 23%.[11] In 1989, Langemo and associates[11] found a prevalence rate of 23%, and Young[12] found a prevalence rate of 23.6% in two different long-term care settings. The National Health Survey of Nursing Homes in the United States reported that 2.6% of female residents and 2.9% of male residents had pressure ulcers.[13] The survey also reported that, of the patients who had pressure ulcers, 18% developed them in the nursing home setting. Other studies have shown that approximately 60% of nursing home patients with pressure ulcers developed them while hospitalized. According to McKnight, 70% of 200 long-term care nursing directors responding to a pressure ulcer prevalence survey stated that fewer than 5% of the residents had pressure ulcers and, of those who did, half were admitted from acute care in that condition.[14]

The National Health Survey of Nursing Homes also reported that, of patients who had pressure ulcers, 18% developed them at home.[13] While it is more difficult to obtain information on patients at home, there are reports of a 12.9% pressure ulcer prevalence rate and a 4.3% incidence rate.[15] These figures represent pressure ulcer patients being followed by health care professionals. The total number of patients at home who have pressure ulcers is unknown.

The cost of pressure ulcers

It is impossible to predict the total national cost of pressure ulcers because the precise incidence and prevalence is not known. However, Miller and Drozier estimated that the total national cost of pressure ulcer treatment exceeds $1.335 billion.[16] The wide variance in estimates of treatment costs reported in the literature may be related to inconsistencies or inaccuracies in data collection on ulcer assessment and management costs.[2] Cost estimates to heal one pressure ulcer range from $14,000 to $40,000.[17,18,19] A single pressure ulcer can lengthen a patient's stay by a factor of 3.5 to 5.[20] One study[21] compared the cost of product utilization for prevention of pressure ulcers in an "at-risk" population with treatment costs for patients with pressure ulcers. It was found that the daily ulcer treatment cost was 2.5 times the cost of prevention in the at-risk group, indicating that prevention is less expensive than treatment. Xakellis et al.[22] studied the actual cost of pressure ulcer prevention. Not surprisingly, the cost increased as the patient's risk level increased. Turning patients was the most expensive component of pressure ulcer prevention.

Of course, in addition to financial costs, there are a number of "intangible" costs, as stated by Alterescu:

▬ Table 2.1 On Deeper Reflection ▬

Mrs. Smith had been transferred to our geriatrics and chronic disease ward.... Her lengthy record looked painfully similar to so many others I had read during the first five months of my geriatrics fellowship. She was 87 years old. The chart listed her diagnoses as dementia, pressure sores, incontinence, diabetes, anemia, malnutrition, and multiple fractures. The history did not describe the fractures....

She was bedridden, responsive only to painful stimuli. A Foley catheter and a gastrostomy feeding tube were in place. Her albumin level was 1.5. She had been in this state for at least three months, as she had been in the transferring hospital for that long after being admitted there in a hypoglycemic coma. The head nurse informed me that Mrs. Smith was hypothermic.

"The temperature is 94.8 rectally," the...nurse said as I entered Mrs. Smith's room. She cried out, seemingly in pain, as the nurse turned her on her left side. The rest of her vital signs were surprisingly normal....She had many pressure sores, including large ones on both heels that were still covered by thick, black eschar.

"My name is Dr. Sachs, Mrs. Smith," I introduced myself. I placed a hopefully reassuring hand on the patient's shoulder. Her skin was cool and clammy. She cried out as I touched her. "I'm one of the doctors here on the floor," I said. "I'm going to examine you to see what we can do to help you feel better." I began to examine an open wound over her right trochanter.... The hip sore was two by three centimeters on the surface but was extensively undermined.

As I moved forward to look deeper into the sore, I thought I saw movement within the wound. I immediately felt repulsed and feared that there might be maggots in this poor woman's hip. I saw no organisms, the wound looked clean, and there was a strange clearness in the center of the crater. I took a deep breath and looked again at the ulcer. Once more I noted movement within the sore. This time the movement paralleled my own motions. I moved closer and peered deeper into the

"...the nurse who is emotionally drained because the pressure ulcer patient requires frequent, difficult dressing changes contributes to the nonfinancial cost of pressure ulcers. Other patients in the facility pay the penalty of receiving less nursing care, or waiting longer for certain services, when a person with a pressure ulcer requires treatment. If a facility is operating at capacity, there may be increased waiting times for ancillary services or admission because patients with pressure ulcers require services. Most importantly, irrespective of the financial costs to treat pressure ulcers, they are a source of anxiety and pain for the patient, the family, and the staff."[23]

Nurses and other health care professionals must not allow such "intangible" costs to be underestimated because, as Table 2.1 so vividly demonstrates, pressure ulcers are indeed more than physical wounds.

Separating fact from fiction

Health care practices must be grounded in science. All too often, there are "old wives' tales" and "lore" that permeate teachings of care of the ill. Pressure ulcer care is no exception. Common misconceptions about pressure ulcers may prevent caregivers from providing appropriate care. Frequent misconceptions include the notions that:
1. All pressure ulcers develop because of poor nursing care.
2. All pressure ulcers are preventable.

cavity. Right in the center, in the deepest portion of the wound, I saw my own reflection staring back at me.

Again I looked to convince myself that I was indeed seeing my own reflection, moving in the wound as I moved outside of it. I moved the opening in the skin back and forth to see more of the tissues below. As more was revealed, it dawned on me that I was seeing myself in Mrs. Smith's hip prosthesis, the shiny artificial head of her femur mirroring the image of my face.... I took one more look at myself and then left the room.

Seeing oneself in a pressure sore is a stark and frightening vision, disturbing on many levels. In addition to the grotesque wound and personal reflection, it seemed to mirror the topsy-turvy medical care given to many such patients. Mrs. Smith came from a hospital where she received mechanical ventilation for a respiratory arrest suffered when she was hypoglycemic. She had pleural effusions tapped and analyzed and innumerable laboratory tests performed. Yet she lay long enough without being turned for all the tissue between her skin and bones to necrotize.

It is sad that somewhere in the course of a dementing process Mrs. Smith lost many of the characteristics that most of us associate with meaningful adult life. It is sadder still that she received medical treatment that forgot about her as a human being.

...Debilitated and dependent patients need us to reach out and care for them most when we are starting to push them away. It is our distancing of ourselves from these people that is the true dehumanizing act.

Frequently, I have caught myself praying that I would not contract any of the horrible diseases I saw during residency. Now, mostly, I pray, "Please, dear Lord, do not let me die with pressure sores."
Greg A. Sachs, MD
Chicago

Used with permission from JAMA, vol. 259, p. 2145, April 8, 1988. Copyright 1988, American Medical Association.

3. All pressure ulcers are caused from pressure only.
4. Massaging reddened tissue helps prevent pressure ulcers.
5. The use of specialty equipment, such as air-fluidized beds, will prevent pressure ulcers independently and indefinitely.[24]

All pressure ulcers do not develop because of poor nursing care, although nurses are frequently blamed for the problem. Most pressure ulcers are preventable, but there are instances when, despite conscientious care, some ulcers may not be preventable. A patient who fell at home and maintained the same position for a prolonged period of time will have soft tissue ischemia over bony prominences that were subjected to pressure. The tissue breakdown may not become evident until the individual is hospitalized, but the original damage occurred from constantly maintained pressure following the fall at home. There are other situations where pressure ulcers are difficult to prevent. For example, individuals who are in a catabolic state are at increased risk for pressure ulceration when tissue breaks down. Because of poor nutrition or chronic disease, many of these patients suffer loss of pressure-absorbing soft tissue padding over the bone. In these patients, pressure ulcers may develop even when careful preventive measures are taken. LaPuma,[25] in discussing the ethics of pressure ulcers, questions why pressure ulcers are considered a sign of inadequate care. He points out that when the heart, lungs, or kidneys fail, it is not considered a sign of inadequate care. So why, he asks, should failure of the integument be treated as inadequate health care when it may be only a sign of physical decline and mortality?

Rarely does a pressure sore develop from pressure alone. More often, two causes (for example, pressure and shear) and frequently three (such as pressure, shear, and friction) combine to create pressure ulcers. If a sufficiently high level of shear is present, the pressure necessary to produce vascular occlusion is only half the amount than when shear is not present. It is difficult to create pressure without shear or shear without pressure. Consequently, most pressure ulcers are not caused from pressure only.[26]

Historically, nurses had been taught to massage reddened tissue over bony prominences. In recent years, massage has gone out of favor. Massaging reddened, hyperemic tissue may cause maceration and damage to the already ischemic tissue. The use of deep massage may angulate and tear the fragile vasculature. This could deprive the area of oxygen and nutrients. Massaging the hyperemic area may actually rupture capillaries that already are maximally dilated to compensate for temporary ischemia.[27,28]

Technological advances have resulted in specialty equipment to assist with pressure ulcer management. The use of specialty beds for pressure relief may assist the caregiver in preventing pressure ulcerations. However, the use of such equipment does not eliminate the need for vigilance and regular assessment of patients. High-tech equipment may give a caregiver a false sense of security. It is important to remember that any piece of equipment never substitutes for good nursing care. Equipment must only be used as part of the overall management plan to reduce the potential for tissue trauma.[29,30,31]

Science-based practice

A substantial amount of literature offers suggestions for nurses who are attempting to reduce or prevent pressure ulcers. The information in many articles is derived from experience, intuition, and common sense. Few reports are the result of systematic study. In the current and future health care environment of monetary limits and nursing shortages, it is helpful to be able to identify where one's energy and equipment dollars should be directed.

In an attempt to enhance the quality and decrease the cost of health care, the U.S. government established the Agency for Health Care Policy and Research (AHCPR) in 1989. One mission of the agency is to establish clinical practice guidelines to assist practitioners in prevention and treatment of various clinical conditions. In May 1992 and December 1994, the Agency for Health Care Policy and Research released Clinical Practice Guidelines for both prevention[32] and treatment[33] of pressure ulcers. These guidelines provide practitioners with current practice parameters based on a synthesis of research findings and expert opinion. Each guideline was developed by an interdisciplinary panel convened by the AHCPR. To support recommendations in the pressure ulcer guidelines, members of the guideline panels evaluated hundreds of abstracts from the National Library of Medicine and then developed scientific evidence tables and methodology ratings on articles of merit.[34]

The release of pressure ulcer clinical practice guidelines placed pressure ulcers in the limelight, making a significant impact on care of patients with pressure ulcers. The Joint Commission for Accreditation of Health Care Organizations (JCAHO) recommends use of the clinical practice guidelines, the Health Care Financing Administration (HCFA) is using the guidelines to create medical policy and reimbursement criteria, and surveyors of long-term care facilities are using the guidelines as quality criteria. The AHCPR guidelines for pressure ulcer prevention and treatment are meant to be living documents—that is, interested individuals and organizations must make them keep pace with science, research, and technology. There is much work to be done to generate new knowledge to fill scientific gaps found by the AHCPR Pressure Ulcer Guideline Panels.

Goals of care

"Pressure ulcers" may be an admitting medical diagnosis or a nursing diagnosis for a patient with other medical problems. In order to help patients determine goals of care, it is necessary to take into account the whole person. Nursing goals must be consistent with both patient and medical goals. For example, if there is no hope for recovery and a choice has been made to provide palliative care for a particular patient, the goal of care related to the pressure ulcer would be to provide comfort. A frequent, painful dressing change to debride a pressure ulcer would not be consistent with goals for a patient who was not expected to live long. However, for another patient who has developed a pressure ulcer, or for one whose medical treatment places him at risk for developing a pressure ulcer, the goal may include measures to reduce the risk and/or heal the ulcer. Decisions relating to treatment, therefore, reflect the goals of care.

Summary

When evaluating pressure ulcer management, nurses must consider all of the following:
- the goal of patient care
- physiological principles
- science-based interventions
- judicious use of products.

The real key to approaching the pressure ulcer problem is to focus on prevention. It is hoped that this text will heighten interest in nursing interventions aimed at prevention of pressure ulcers. For those patients who already have pressure ulcers, this text will provide a guide to effective management.

References

1. Arnold, H.L. "Decubitus: The Word," in Parish, L.C., et al., eds. *The Decubitus Ulcer*. New York: Masson Publishing USA, 1983.
2. National Pressure Ulcer Advisory Panel. "Pressure Ulcers: Incidence, Economics, and Risk Assessment. Consensus Development Conference Statement," *Decubitus* 2(2): 24-28, 1989.
3. Shannon, M.L., and Skorga, P. "Pressure Ulcer Prevalence in Two General Hospitals," *Decubitus* 2(4): 38-43, 1989.
4. Oot-Giromini, B., et al. "Pressure Ulcer Prevention Versus Treatment: Comparative Product Cost Study," *Decubitus* 2(3): 52-54, 1989.
5. Meehan, M. "Multisite Pressure Ulcer Prevalence Survey," *Decubitus* 3(4): 14-17, 1990.
6. Meehan, M. "National Pressure Ulcer Prevalence Survey," *Advances in Wound Care* 7(3): 27-38, 1994.
7. Gerson, L.W. "The Incidence of Decubitus Ulcers by Muscle Transposition: An Eight-Year Review," *Plastic and Reconstructive Surgery* 58(4): 201-204, 1975.
8. Clarke, M., and Kadhom, H.M. "The Nursing Prevention of Pressure Sores in Hospital and Community Patients," *Journal of Advanced Nursing* 13(3): 365-373, 1988.
9. Allman, R.M., et al. "Pressure Ulcer Risk Factors Among Hospitalized Patients with Activity Limitations," *JAMA* 273(11): 865-870, 1995.
10. Petersen, N.C., and Bittman, S. "The Epidemiology of Pressure Sores," *Scandinavian Journal of Plastic and Reconstructive Surgery* 5(1): 62-66, 1971.
11. Langemo, D.K., et al. "Incidence of Pressure Sores in Acute Care, Rehabilitation, Extended Care, Home Health and Hospice in One Locale," *Decubitus* 2(2): 42, 1989.
12. Young, L. "Pressure Ulcer Prevalence and Associated Patient Characteristics in One Long-Term Care Facility," *Decubitus* 2(2): 52, 1989.
13. National Center for Health Statistics. "Characteristics of Nursing Home Residents, Health Status, and Care Received: National Nursing Home Survey, United States, May-December 1977." DHHS publication no. (PHS) 81-1712. (Vital and Health Statistics; series 13; no. 51). Hyattsville, Md.: United States Department of Health and Human Services, 1981.
14. McKnight's Survey, "Data Watch: Pressure Sores," *McKnight's Long Term Care News* 26, 1992.
15. Hentzen, B., et al. "Prevalence and Incidence of Pressure Ulcers and Associated Risk Factors in a Rural-Based Home Health Population." Poster presentation at 17th Annual Midwest Nursing Research Society, Cleveland, Ohio, March 28-30, 1993.
16. Miller, H., and Delozier, J. *Cost Implications of the Pressure Ulcer Treatment Guideline*. Columbia, Md.: Center for Health Policy Studies. Contract No. 28-91-0070. 17 p. Sponsored by the Agency for Health Care Policy and Research, 1994.
17. Blom, M.F. "Dramatic Decrease in Decubitus Ulcers," *Geriatric Nursing* 6(2): 84-87, March-April, 1985.
18. Curtin, L. "Wound Management: Care and Cost—An Overview," *Nursing Management* 15(2): 22, 1984.
19. Frye, B.A. "A Coat of Many Colors: A Program to Reduce the Incidence of Hospital-Originated Pressure Sores," *Rehabilitation Nursing* 11(1): 24-25, 1986.
20. Allman, R.M., et al. "Pressure Sores in Hospitalized Patients," *Annals of Internal Medicine* 105: 337-342, 1986.
21. Oot-Giromini, B., et al. "Pressure Ulcer Prevention Versus Treatment: Comparative Product Cost Study," *Decubitus* 2(3): 52-54, 1989.
22. Xakellis, G.C., et al. "Cost of Pressure Ulcer Prevention in Long-Term Care," *Journal of the American Geriatrics Society* 43(5): 496-501, 1995.
23. Alterescu, V. "The Financial Costs of Inpatient Pressure Ulcers to an Acute Care Facility," *Decubitus* 2(3): 14-23, 1989.
24. Shannon, M.L. "Five Famous Fallacies About Pressure Sores," *Nursing84* 14(10): 34-41, 1984.
25. LaPuma, J. "The Ethics of Pressure Ulcers," *Decubitus* 4(2): 43-44, 1991.
26. Bennett, L., and Lee, B.Y. "Pressure Versus Shear in Pressure Sore Causation," in *Chronic Ulcers of the Skin*. New York: McGraw-Hill, 1985.
27. Dyson, R. "Bedsores—The Injuries Hospital Staff Inflict on Patients," *Nursing Mirror* 146(24): 30-32, 1978.
28. Ek, A.C., et al. "The Local Skin Blood Flow in Areas at Risk for Pressure Sores Treated with Massage," *Scandinavian Journal of Rehabilitation Medicine* 17(2): 81-86, 1985.
29. Stewart, T. "Materials Management and Decubitus Care," *J Healthcare Materiel Management* 1: 32-34, 1987.
30. Narsette, T.A., et al. "Pressure Sores," *Amer Fam Phys* 9: 135-139, 1983.
31. Maklebust, J. "Pressure Ulcers: Etiology and Prevention," *Nursing Clinics of North America* 22(2): 359-377, 1987.
32. Panel for the Prediction and Prevention of Pressure Ulcers in Adults. "Pressure Ulcers in Adults: Prediction and Prevention," Clinical Practice Guideline, No. 3. AHCPR Publication No. 92-0047. Rockville, Md.: U.S. Department of Health and Human Services, Agency for Health Care Policy and Research, May 1992.
33. Bergstrom, N., et al. "Treatment of Pressure Ulcers," Clinical Practice Guideline, No. 15. AHCPR Publication No. 95-0652. Rockville, Md.: U.S. Department of Health and Human Services, Agency for Health Care Policy and Research, December 1994.
34. Bergstrom, N., and Cuddigan, J., eds. *Treatment of Pressure Ulcers*. Clinical Practice Guideline, Guideline Technical Report No. 15. Rockville, Md.: U.S. Department of Health and Human Services, Public Health Service, Agency for Health Care Policy and Research. AHCPR Publication No. 95-xxxx. December 1994.

CHAPTER 3

Etiology and Pathophysiology of Pressure Ulcers

Pressure ulcers are the clinical manifestation of local tissue death. Cellular metabolism depends on blood vessels to carry nutrients to the tissues and to remove waste products. When the soft tissues are subjected to prolonged pressure and insufficient nutrients, cellular death occurs.[1-6] Pressure ulcers are defined as localized areas of cellular necrosis due to vascular insufficiency in an area under pressure.[7,8] Ulcers are found most frequently in soft tissue over bony prominences exposed to compressing surfaces. Unrelieved pressure applied to the skin surface exerts its greatest force near the bone.[1,2,5,9] There may be extensive damage to the tissue beneath the surface before the skin is broken. There are multiple interacting factors other than pressure that contribute to the mechanical destruction of soft tissue. These factors include shear,[10] friction,[11] excessive moisture, and possibly infection.[12,13] Each of these factors is discussed separately.

Pressure

Pressure, the amount of force exerted on a given area, is measured in millimeters of mercury (mm Hg). External pressure greater than capillary perfusion pressure will compress the vessels, leading to ischemia. Normal capillary filling pressure is approximately 32 mm Hg at the arteriolar end and 12 mm Hg at the venous end.[14,15] External pressure greater than 32 mm Hg may cause tissue damage by restricting blood flow to the area.[14,15] If pressure is applied to soft tissue for a long enough period, capillary vessels will collapse and thrombose.[1] The result is interference with oxygenation and nutrition of the involved tissues. Toxic metabolic byproducts accumulate in the tissue and lead to cell death.[16,17]

Body tissues have different tolerances for pressure and ischemia. Muscle tissue is more sensitive to compression than skin. In animal studies, Husain[1] demonstrated that external pressure applied for 2 hours to the skin produced ischemic changes in the underlying musculature. When the same amount of pressure was applied to the skin for 6 hours, complete muscle degeneration occurred. By the time the overlying skin is affected, the deeper muscle may be necrotic. It is suspected that ulcers of many bedridden patients are from pressure-induced muscle ischemia.

The force of pressure increases as the body surface area decreases.[6,16,18] For instance, the pressure exerted on the toe of a ballerina is 2,600 mm Hg, while the pressure against the skin when a person is floating in water is 20 mm Hg. The amount of pressure that soft tissue is subjected to while a person is lying and sitting was studied independently by Kosiak[2] and Lindan.[19] Pressures were about 70 mm Hg on the buttocks in the lying position and up to 300 mm Hg on the ischial tuberosities in the sitting position. These levels were sufficient to cause tissue ischemia. Pressure over bony prominences alters soft tissue and intravascular pressure relationships. If the external pressure exceeds venous capillary pressure, the vessels will leak with resultant edema. The edema impedes circulation, which leads to additional increases in pressure. Eventually, the interstitial pressure will equal or exceed the arterial pressure, resulting in hemorrhage into the tissue (nonblanchable erythema). The continued capillary occlusion, lack of oxygen and nutrients, and buildup of toxic wastes lead to necrosis of muscle, subcutaneous tissue, and, ultimately, necrosis of the dermis and epidermis. This irreversible ischemic response has been referred to as the "no reflow" phenomenon.[20]

The normal response to prolonged pressure is a change in body position before tissue ischemia occurs.[21] In pressure ulceration, this time-pressure relationship is critical. Kosiak demonstrated that there is an inverse relationship between the amount of pressure exerted and the amount of time before tissue damage occurs. Low pressure for long periods of time is believed to be more significant in producing pressure ulcers than higher pressure of short duration.[2] For example, constant pressure of 70 mm Hg for more than 2 hours can produce irreversible tissue damage. Conversely, pressure of 240 mm Hg sustained over a short duration may produce minimal changes in tissue. If the time-pressure threshold is reached or exceeded, tissue damage continues even after relief from compression.

Salcido[9] et al. studied the role of free radicals in pressure ulceration. Computer-controlled pressure was applied to skin over the greater trochanter of anesthetized rats for five 6-hour sessions. Ulceration developed first in the muscle rather than the dermis or epidermis. Recurrent pressure resulted in increasingly severe damage to the vascular system and parenchyma, consistent with an ischemia/reperfusion insult initiated through a free radical mechanism. In his study, infarction of the skin was a precursor to pressure ulcer formation.[9] The neutrophils, which accumulate at the border between viable and nonviable tissue, presumably generate free radicals and contribute to proteolytic digestion of the connective tissue. Production of oxygen free radicals may initiate a cascade of events that significantly contribute to pressure ulceration.

Repetition of pressure on vulnerable bony areas of the body is important and needs to be considered by clinicians. Husain[1] determined that tolerance to pressure and ischemia was drastically lowered by previous vascular insult. Although pressure ulceration can result from one period of sustained pressure, most pressure ulcers probably are secondary to repeated ischemic events without adequate time for recovery.

Pressure ulcers can develop over any bony prominence or any area of soft tissue subjected to prolonged pressure. Pressure points in the lying and sitting positions are shown in Figures 3.1 and 3.2. Pressure ulcers can occur over the sacrum, coccyx,

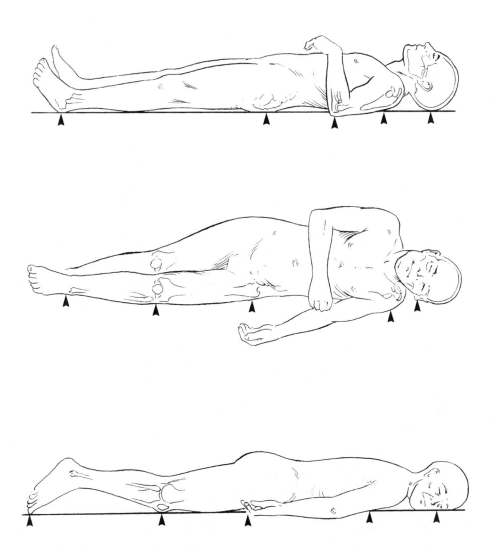

Figure 3.1 Pressure points in lying positions

ischial tuberosities, greater trochanters, elbows, heels, scapulae, occipital bone, sternum, ribs, iliac crests, patellae, lateral malleoli, and medial malleoli. Because of the presence of major bony prominences and unequal distribution of weight, the majority of pressure ulcers occur on the lower half of the body. Two-thirds of all pressure ulcers occur within the pelvic girdle. Figure 3.3 shows the most common locations of pressure ulcers.

Untreated contractures may be a cause of pressure ulceration.[22] At the very least, caregivers must consider any contractures as a possible cause of pressure necrosis. Because pressure is a primary cause of ulcers, assessment for pressure ulcer risk must include the way pressure is applied by dysfunctional alignment of the body and its

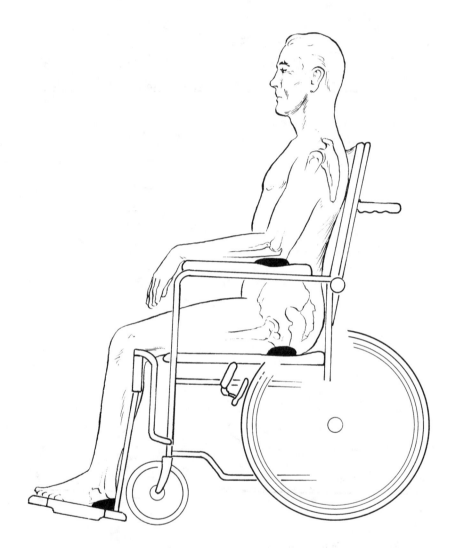

Figure 3.2 Pressure points in the sitting position

extremities. Pressure points may be found in areas other than bony prominences if contracted limbs press on one another. The pressure exerted against the mattress by a contracted limb may be greater than the degree of pressure exerted by a noncontracted limb. This exaggerated degree of pressure may increase the possibility of an ulcer developing in a short period of time. Pressure ulcers of the lower extremity may be preceded by a contracture of the leg or foot. The contracture, as well as the ulcer, must be considered when assessing the patient for tissue breakdown.[22]

One of the most overlooked factors in the development of pressure ulcers is thought to be sitting posture.[23] Preventive measures include limited use of the geri-

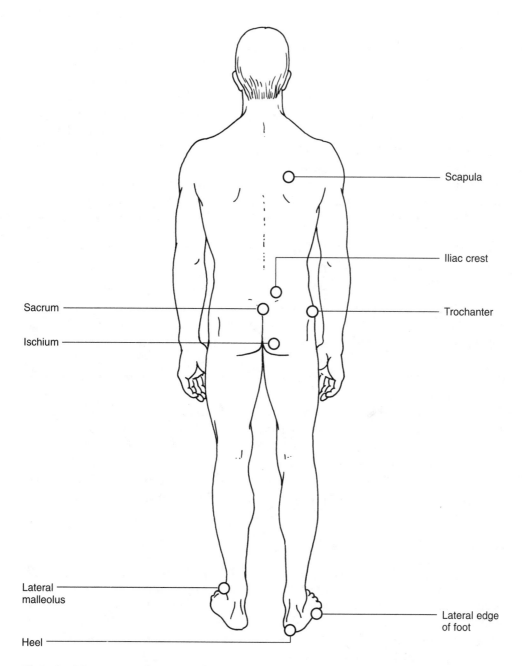

Figure 3.3 Most common locations of pressure ulcers.

atric chair and proper lumbar support to prevent the kyphotic or slumping position. If a footstool is used, care must be taken to avoid positioning the feet high enough for body weight to be shifted from the posterior thighs to the ischial tuberosities.

Pressure gradient

When blood vessels, muscle, subcutaneous fat, and skin are compressed between bone and a lying or sitting surface, pressure is transmitted from the body surface toward the bone. The external surface produces pressure, and the bone produces counterpressure. These opposing forces result in a cone-shaped pressure gradient, as shown in Figure 3.4. All of the tissue between the external surface and the skeletal anatomy is involved. However, the greatest tissue destruction is beneath the skin surface at the bony interface.[1,2,5,9] Because they do not tolerate decreased blood flow, fat and muscle are less resistant to pressure than skin. Therefore, there may be greater destruction in the subcutaneous tissues and muscle than the surface damage indicates.[2,24] This is called the "tip of the iceberg" effect. When assessing the size of a pressure ulcer, one must consider the presence of necrotic undermining or tracts from the pressure gradient.

Pressure ulcer formation

There are two schools of thought regarding where and how pressure ulcers begin. The traditional view is a top-to-bottom approach where ulceration occurs first in the epidermis and later in the deeper tissue layers. Witkowski and Parish,[25] in histologic examinations of pressure ulcers, showed that first tissue damage was in the upper dermis. Among the histologic changes were leukocyte infiltration, edema, hemorrhage, and blood vessel proliferation. The earliest discernible clinical sign of damage in the Witkowski model was blanchable erythema. The second school of thought regarding pressure ulcer formation is a bottom-to-top model where skeletal muscle is injured before damage is evident on the skin surface. This model is supported by the work of Kosiak,[2] Husain,[1] Nola and Vistnes,[5] and Salcido,[9] among others. It is possible that both models of pressure necrosis are correct, and that there are different etiologies for superficial and deep pressure ulcers. Only continued research on the basic science of pressure ulceration will determine the true etiologic model.

Shear

Shearing force is another factor that contributes to the mechanical destruction of tissue.[10] Shear is defined as a mechanical force that is parallel rather than perpendicular to an area. The main shear effect is on deep tissues. Elevating the head of the bed increases shear and pressure in the sacral and coccygeal areas.[10,15] The tissues attached to the bone are pulled in one direction because of body weight, while the surface tissues stick to the sheets and remain stationary. The body skeleton actually slides downward inside the skin, as shown in Figure 3.5. Puckering of the skin may be noticed in the gluteal area. Blood vessels can become either obstructed and torn or stretched. This is most likely to happen when patients are dragged along the surface of the sheets during repositioning or are placed in high-Fowler's position and allowed to slide down. To avoid shearing forces, the head of the bed should be raised

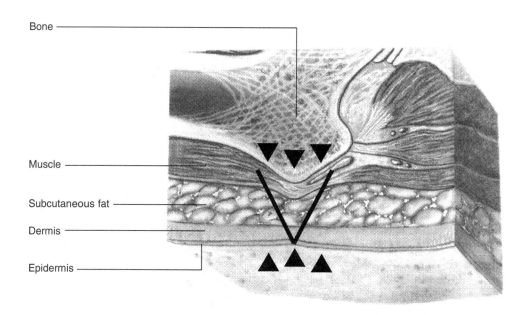

Figure 3.4 Pressure gradient

to no more than a 30-degree angle, except for short periods during eating.[8]

The presence of shearing forces decreases the time that tissue can be subjected to pressure before ischemia or destruction occurs.[6,10] A sufficiently high level of shear may reduce by one half the amount of pressure needed to produce vascular occlusion. Shearing forces are said to account for the high incidence of triangular-shaped sacral ulcers. Shear also may account for clinical observations of large areas of tunneling or deep sinus tracts beneath sacral ulcers.

Friction

Friction is another factor causing mechanical destruction of cutaneous tissue. Friction is created by the force of two surfaces moving across one another, often creating a wound resembling an abrasion. Friction commonly occurs in patients who are unable to lift themselves sufficiently for repositioning. If a patient is pulled across the bed linen, the outer protective layer of skin may be rubbed away.[3,15] This mechanical wearing away of surface tissue increases the potential for deeper tissue damage.[11] Removal of the outer stratum corneum decreases the fibrinolytic activity of the dermis. Increased transcutaneous water loss allows moisture to accumulate on the surface of the body. If the body-support surface interface is moist, there is a sharp rise in the coefficient of friction which, if it becomes great enough, actually causes adherence. If the head of the bed is high, moist skin adheres to the bed linen, the skeleton moves forward due to gravitational force, and then friction and shearing forces act together to contribute to necrosis of tissue in the sacral area.

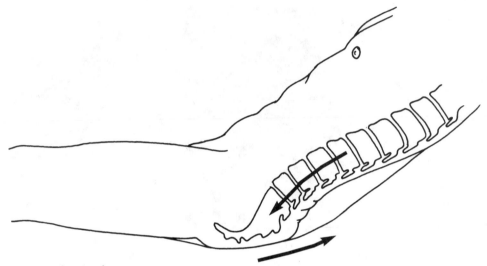

Figure 3.5 Shearing force over sacrum.

Patients who have uncontrollable movements or spastic conditions, patients who wear braces or appliances that rub against the skin, and the elderly are at high risk for tissue damage by friction. Dry lubricants, such as cornstarch, and adherent dressings with slippery backings can aid in decreasing frictional forces against the skin.[7,8]

Excessive moisture

Constant exposure to wetness can waterlog or macerate the skin. Maceration is a contributing factor in the etiology of pressure ulcers primarily because the excessive moisture softens the connective tissue. Once macerated, the epidermis is more easily eroded.[11] Eventually, degenerative changes take place, and the tissue sloughs. Because of the adhesiveness of wet skin surfaces to bed linen, moist skin is five times as likely to become ulcerated as dry skin.[15] This adherency increases the risk of friction as the patient is moved across the surface of the bed linen.[10]

Excessive moisture may be the result of perspiration, wound drainage, soaking the skin during bathing, and fecal or urinary incontinence. Fecal incontinence exposes the skin to bacteria in the stool and contributes the added risk of infection. If the patient is incontinent of both urine and stool, the urea from the urine reacts chemically with the stool and causes further damage.

Infection

The role of infection in pressure ulceration is not fully understood. Robson and associates[12] believe that infection has a role in pressure ulcer causation. Aside from clinical observation, he cites the work of Groth, who conducted animal studies on the combined roles of pressure and infection. Compression alone allowed local increases in bacterial concentration. Bacteria that were injected intravenously localized at the site of compression, resulting in necrosis at pressures lower than those needed to cause necrosis in animals not given a bacterial load. Husain injected streptococci in animals prior to local application of pressure. Histologic studies demonstrated localization of bacteria to the sites of compression. Robson and Krizek[26] quantified the effect of pressure on bacterial count. Incisions created in areas of applied controlled pressure and innoculated with known quantities of organisms per gram of tissue allowed a 100-fold greater bacterial growth than similar wounds created in areas not subjected to pressure. They concluded that compressed skin lowers local resistance to bacterial infection and that compression-induced ischemia inhibits the first line of defense against bacterial invasion.

Researchers at the University of Texas studied the role of denervation in soft tissue infection on pedicle flaps performed on the buttocks of ewes.[13] They conducted these experiments by dividing the animals into three groups: one with the cutaneous nerve intact, one with the nerve severed acutely, and one with the nerve severed 7 days before the flap was done. All flaps received intradermal innoculations of 10^7 Staph aureus. Ninety six hours later, quantitative bacteriology showed a 25-fold increase in bacterial counts seen in the prolonged denervation group. The investigators state that this helps explain why the neurologically impaired are more susceptible to infection and pressure ulceration.

Summary

The unquestionable cause of pressure ulcers is compression of soft tissue sufficient to cause irreversible ischemia. Other significant contributors are shear, friction, moisture, and possibly infection. Tissues vary in their ability to withstand the effects of pressure. Although clinical awareness of impending necrosis occurs only when skin becomes inflamed, it is most likely that deep necrosis has occurred in areas not apparent on visual inspection. Certain individuals are at a higher risk than others to develop pressure ulcers. High-risk individuals, whether in an institution or at home, should be assessed regularly for the development of pressure ulcers. Understanding the etiology of pressure ulcer development is the foundation for planning prevention and treatment.

References

1. Husain, T. "Experimental Study of Some Pressure Effects on Tissues, with Reference to the Bedsore Problem," *Journal of Pathology and Bacteriology* 66: 347-358, 1953.

2. Kosiak, M. "Etiology and Pathology of Ischemic Ulcers," *Archives of Physical Medicine and Rehabilitation* 40(2): 62-69, February 1959.

3. Dinsdale, S.M. "Decubitus Ulcers: Role of Pressure and Friction in Causation," *Archives of Physical Medicine and Rehabilitation* 55: 147-153, 1974.

4. Daniel, R.K., et al. "Etiologic Factors in Pressure Sores: An Experimental Model," *Archives of Physical Medicine and Rehabilitation,* 54: 51-56, 1981.

5. Nola, G.T., and Vistnes, L.M. "Differential Response of Skin and Muscle in the Experimental Production of Pressure Sores," *Plastic and Reconstructive Surgery,* 66: 728-735, 1980.

6. Constantian, M.B. "Etiology: Gross Effects of Pressure," in Constantian, M.B., ed. *Pressure Ulcers: Principles and Techniques of Management.* Boston: Little, Brown & Co., 1980.

7. National Pressure Ulcer Advisory Panel (NPUAP). Pressure Ulcer Prevalence, Cost, and Risk Assessment: Consensus Development Conference Statement. *Decubitus* 2(2): 24-28, May 1989.

8. Bergstrom, N., et al. *Treatment of Pressure Ulcers.* Clinical Practice Guideline No. 15. Rockville, Md.: U.S. Department of Health and Human Services. Public Health Service, Agency for Health Care Policy and Research, AHCPR Publication No. 95-0652. December 1994.

9. Salcido, R., et al. "Histopathology of Decubitus Ulcers as a Result of Sequential Pressure Sessions in a Computer-Controlled Fuzzy Rat Model," *Advances in Wound Care* 7(5): 40, May 1993.

10. Bennett, L., and Lee, B.Y. "Pressure versus Shear in Pressure Sore Causation," in Lee, B.Y., ed. *Chronic Ulcers of the Skin.* New York: McGraw-Hill, 1985.

11. Dinsdale, S.M. "Decubitus Ulcers: Role of Pressure and Friction in Causation," *Archives of Physical Medicine and Rehabilitation* 55: 147, 1974.

12. Phillips, L.G., and Robson, M.C. "Pressure Ulcerations," in Jurkiewicz, M.J., et al., eds. *Plastic Surgery: Principles and Practice.* St Louis: C.V. Mosby Co., 1990.

13. Alison, W.E., et al. "The Effect of Denervation on Soft Tissue Infection Pathology," *Plastic & Reconstructive Surgery* 90(6): 1031-1035, June 1992.

14. Landis, E. "Studies of Capillary Blood Pressure in Human Skin," *Heart* 15: 209, 1930.

15. Roaf, R. "The Causation and Prevention of Bed Sores," in Kenedi, R.M., et al., eds. *Bedsore Biomechanics.* London: University Park Press, 5-9, 1976.

16. Scales, J.T. "Pressure on the Patient," in Kenedi, R.M., et al., eds. *Bedsore Biomechanics.* London: University Park Press, 11-17, 1976.

17. Parish, L.C., et al. *The Decubitus Ulcer.* New York: Masson Publishing, 1983.

18. Reuler, J.B., and Cooney, T.G. "The Pressure Sore: Pathophysiology and Principles of Management," *Annals of Internal Medicine* 94:5-661, 1981.

19. Lindan, O., et al. "Pressure Distributor on the Surface of the Human Body," *Archives of Physical Medicine and Rehabilitation* 46: 378, 1965.

20. Ames, A., et al. "Cerebral Ischemia II: the No Reflow Phenomenon," *American Journal of Pathology* 52:437, 1968.

21. Exton-Smith, A.N., and Sherwin, R.W. "The Prevention of Pressure Sores: Significance of Spontaneous Bodily Movements," *Lancet* 2:1124, 1961.

22. Knight, D.B., and Scott, H. "Contracture and Pressure Necrosis," *Ostomy/Wound Management* 26:60-67, January-February 1990.

23. Zacharkow, D. "Effect of Posture and Distribution of Pressure in the Prevention of Pressure Sores," in Lee, B.Y., ed. *Chronic Ulcers of the Skin.* New York: McGraw-Hill, 1985.

24. Vasconez, L., et al. "Pressure Sores," *Curr Prob Surg* 14:1, 1977.

25. Witkowski, J.A., and Parish, L.C. "Histopathology of the Decubitus Ulcer," *Journal of the American Academy of Dermatology* 6: 1014-1021, 1982.

26. Krizek, T., and Robson, M.C. "Biology of Surgical Infection," *Surgical Clinics of North America* 55(6): 1261-1267, 1975.

CHAPTER 4

Wound Healing

Understanding the nature of wound healing is fundamental to the scientific care of persons who have pressure ulcers. Like so many other areas of study, multiple disciplines have claimed the territory of wounds and wound healing. Communication with and among these professions will facilitate progress toward understanding the problem and developing solutions together.

In an effort to provide a universal language for research, clinical practice, regulatory agencies, and payers, the Wound Healing Society, Richmond, Virginia, has proposed common terminology for defining a wound and the process of wound healing.[1]

A wound is defined as the disruption of the normal anatomical structure and function of a tissue. Acute wounds proceed through an orderly and timely repair process that results in sustained restoration of anatomic and functional integrity. Chronic wounds have failed to proceed through an orderly and timely process to produce anatomic and functional integrity, or proceeded through the repair process without establishing a sustained anatomic and functional result.[1]

The term "orderliness" in this definition refers to the sequence of wound healing events that includes inflammation, angiogenesis, tissue matrix regeneration, contraction, epithelialization, and remodeling. Timeliness is determined by the nature of the pathologic process. Length of time to healing may vary, given the uniqueness of each wound and the status of the patient and the environment.

Lazarus et al define healing as a complex dynamic process that results in the restoration of anatomic continuity and function. An ideally healed wound is one that has returned to normal anatomic structure, function, and appearance. An acceptably healed wound is characterized by restoration of sustained functional and anatomic continuity. A minimally healed wound is characterized by the restoration of anatomic continuity, but without a sustained functional result and therefore subject to recurrence.[1]

Wounds are classified as one of two types with regard to closure: (a) those with minimal tissue loss, such as surgical incisions, and (b) those with substantial tissue loss, such as burns or pressure ulcers. The major differences between the two wound types are the length of time required and the amount of granulation tissue and contraction necessary to close the defect. With no tissue loss, a wound may be sutured, and it will heal by direct union. This is called first or primary intention healing. With tissue loss, a skin or muscle graft may be used to promote healing by delayed primary intention. If the defect cannot be corrected surgically, the wound must heal by indirect union or secondary intention healing. Wounds into the epidermis or dermis can heal by tissue regeneration. Wounds that are through the dermis heal by scar formation because deeper structures, such as subcutaneous tissue, glands, and hair follicles, are not able to regenerate. Contraction is the main mechanism by which a large defect is closed during secondary intention healing. In both wound types, the disrupted anatomy is restored through a process that includes inflammation, proliferation, and differentiation.[2] The process of wound healing begins the moment a wound is made and continues for years. Careful assessment and continuous monitoring of these wound healing processes are essential to wound care.

Phases of wound healing

The body responds to wounding by an ongoing sequential reparative process, with much overlap. This process includes three general phases: inflammation, proliferation, and differentiation.

Inflammatory phase

The inflammatory phase of the healing process is important in activating the tissue repair cascade (see Figure 4.1). A chemical action occurs during this phase that stimulates the healing process. The first response of the body to wounding is local vasoconstriction that lasts about 5-10 minutes. Simultaneously, several cell types are recruited to the wounded area to defend and revitalize traumatized tissue. First, platelets aggregate and deposit granules that affect clotting and stimulate growth factors. The granules promote fibrin deposition to form a thrombus or clot to seal the wound. The surrounding tissues become ischemic and vasodilation occurs. Vascular permeability increases, allowing leakage of neutrophils into the wound space. Enzymes, fluid, and protein enter and are trapped in the extracellular space, where they cause inflammation.

Next, leukocytes, a type of white blood cell, migrate into the interstitial space and begin to digest and transport organic debris from the wound site. Leucocytes start to recede after about 24 hours as monocytes enter the wound. Monocytes are soon converted to macrophages, key cells in wound healing. These cells are responsible for debriding the wound, regulating fibroplasia, and degrading collagen in the wound healing process. In addition, the macrophages release an angiogenic factor, which stimulates formulation of new blood vessels to feed the growing new tissue, and a growth factor, which stimulates fibroblast production and promotes collagen synthesis in the second phase of wound healing.[3] The main function of the inflammatory phase of healing is to initiate the wound healing cascade, remove the debris, and prepare the wound for the regeneration of new tissue.[3,4] Clinically, the inflammatory phase is characterized by local erythema, edema, and tenderness of the affected tissue.

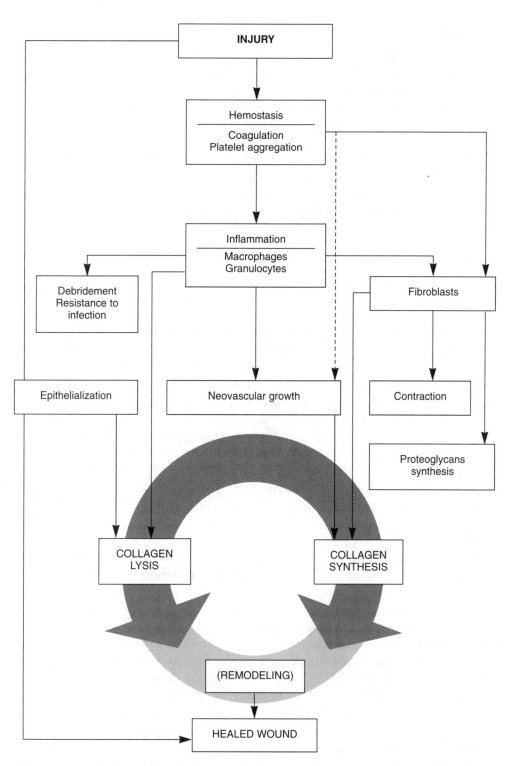

Figure 4.1 Cascade of wound-healing events

Proliferative phase

The proliferative phase of wound healing overlaps the inflammatory phase. It begins 3 to 4 days after wounding and lasts for approximately 15 or 16 days. The main functions during this phase are deposition of connective tissue and collagen cross linking. During this time, epithelial cells migrate across the wound surface. Cellular migration is guided by the wound matrix and anatomical tissue planes.

Fibroblasts, the key cell type in this phase, must multiply and actively synthesize collagen, the principal component of connective tissue. Collagen is responsible for filling the wound and providing strength. If the process of collagen building and breaking down is not kept in balance, there can be an overgrowth of scar tissue or a weak scar that is easily ruptured. Factors that decrease collagen synthesis are listed in Table 4.1.

Granulation

During collagen production, capillaries are forming as bud-like structures from nearby vessels. Stimulated by a relatively hypoxic environment, capillaries penetrate the wound, grow into loops, and provide the nutritional source for the newly generating tissue. These bright red loops of blood vessels impart a granular appearance to the wound surface. For this reason the wound is often described as granulating. Granulation tissue provides a good defense against invasion by surface contaminants, but it produces a difficult terrain for advancing epithelial cells. Occasionally, excessive amounts of granulation tissue, or "proud flesh," will form over a wound. This will prevent epithelial cells from migrating across the surface. The granulation buds can be dehydrated by the use of gauze dressings in order to promote continued wound healing. As the wound matures and the synthesis of collagen decreases, these new vascular channels regress, and the wound undergoes a transformation from capillary-rich, highly cellular tissue to comparatively avascular, cell-free scar composed of dense collagen bundles.[3,4]

Epithelialization

In surface defects, the replacement of dead or damaged tissue by new and healthy cells begins by a fundamental process called epithelialization. When tissue is wounded, the epithelial cells from the wound margins migrate across the wound surface from both sides in order to seal the wound. Cells are driven by an insatiable desire to contact cells of their own type. Epithelial cells are guided in their migration by a network of fibrin strands, which functions as a scaffolding over which the cells creep. Sheets of epithelial cells continue to migrate until they come into contact with other masses of epithelial cells moving across the wound from other directions. This epithelialization is necessary in the repair of all wounds if a watertight seal is to occur. In a primary healing wound, fibrin closes the wound in a few hours and epithelialization begins in 1 to 2 days. Epithelial cells may arise from the hair follicles in a partial-thickness wound if the shaft of the follicle still is intact. In a secondary healing wound, migration of cells is rapid at first, but progress becomes

Table 4.1 Factors That Decrease Collagen Synthesis

Advanced age	Traumatic injuries	Uremia
Malnutrition	Hypoxemia	Diabetes mellitus
Steroids	Radiation injuries	Emotional stress
Infection		

slower so that days or weeks may lapse before epithelialization is complete. If a scab is present over the surface of the wound, the epithelial cells must migrate under the scab. A wound covered by epithelial cells will stop weeping body fluid and electrolytes. As long as the epithelium is intact, the wound will be protected against direct bacterial invasion. However, the slightest trauma will wipe off new epithelial tissue because it is hardly more than a gelatinous film.

Contraction

The size and shape of the scar in a wound that has healed by secondary intention diminishes by a process called wound contraction. Contraction of scar tissue occurs as a wound lessens in size by movement of the surrounding tissue toward the center of the wound. Contraction begins around the fifth day after wounding. It overlaps the proliferation and differentiation phases. Special contractile cells called myofibroblasts appear in contracting wounds. These cells exhibit both collagen synthesis and contractility. Myofibroblasts, thought to be responsible for wound contraction, are not found in sutured wounds but are common in granulating wounds. The fact that skin itself has a tendency to contract is a principle that can be used in determining the line of incision for a surgical wound. Contracting skin occurs in the plane perpendicular to lines of tension in the skin called Langer's lines. Incisions made along Langer's lines place little tension on the skin. Experiments have shown that the scar resulting from wound contraction is influenced by the surrounding skin tension. A reduction in tension produces a less noticeable scar. Contraction is an important part of secondary intention wound healing. The volume of the open wound is reduced by the contracting borders so there is less need for granulation tissue and a smaller surface area for epithelial cells to cover. Contraction ceases when the counteracting force of the surrounding skin begins to exceed the force of the contracting wound.[5] These wounds continue with the dynamic remodeling of collagen for months or even years. Over time, collagen fibril diameter increases, and the fibrils become more compact.

In the proliferative phase, there is collagen synthesis and tissue growth. In the next phase, the tissue begins to take on its permanent form.

Differentiation phase

In the differentiation, or remodeling, phase of wound healing, a wound matures and the collagen in the scar undergoes repeated degradation and resynthesis. Differentiation is the longest phase of wound healing. It usually begins about day 21 but progresses differently for each of the two wound types.

In primary healing wounds, the maximum amount of total collagen is formed by day 42.[4] At this point, equilibrium is established between collagen synthesis and collagen breakdown. The collagen fibers and fibrils become dehydrated and reweave into a tight pattern. The scar becomes less and less bulky and continues to gain tensile strength for 2 years. During this time, the neovascularization of granulation tissue retracts, and the scar will fade from a deep red to a silvery white as the granulation buds retract. The tensile strength of the scar increases during the differentiation phase. Between the 1st and the 14th day, the tissues regain approximately 30%-50% of their original strength. Wounds continue to increase in tensile strength, eventually reaching approximately 80% of normal tissue strength. Wounds never completely regain the tensile strength of prewounded tissue.[6]

The differentiation phase includes growth and development of new tissue and strengthening of the scar. In order to ensure maximum possible healing during the differentiation phase, vitamins are required for cellular activity and amino acids are necessary for tissue regeneration.

Intrinsic factors affecting wound healing

Many conditions—and the effects of these conditions—can compromise wound healing, as shown in Table 4.2. The process of wound healing is influenced by factors within the patient or the wound, such as tissue oxygenation, nutrition, stress, and infection. These factors often can be modified through specific interventions. A number of factors are discussed below.

Tissue oxygenation

Oxygen is necessary for wound healing. It is involved in the destruction of bacteria by neutrophils and macrophages. It is used by amino acids in the process of tissue regeneration. Oxygen tension at the wound site correlates directly with the rate of healing.[7] Healing is impaired by hypoxic conditions that are the result of either inadequate blood flow to the wound or decreased blood oxygen. A patent vasculature is essential to supply the wound with oxygen and nutrients and to remove carbon dioxide and metabolic byproducts. Any condition that reduces blood flow to a wound, such as arterial occlusion, vasoconstriction, or external pressure, has the potential to impede the healing process. If blood volume is low, tissue oxygenation will be low, and wound healing will be impaired.[7]

In addition to an adequate blood supply to the wound, the blood itself must contain sufficient amounts of oxygen. Oxygen is essential for collagen synthesis and fibroblast differentiation. There are four major factors that contribute to wound hypoxia: occluded vessels, hypotension, edema, and anemia. Atherosclerosis is the most common cause of arterial vessel occlusion. Atherosclerosis combined with hypotension can cause low blood flow to the peripheral tissues. When edema is present, there is an increase in the diffusion distance from the capillary to the cell. The pO_2 decreases by as much as 50%.[8,9] With anemia, the availability of the hemoglobin-carrying red blood cell is reduced because of a decrease in blood volume. Even temporary anoxia may result in less stable collagen fiber production.

Table 4.2 Conditions and Effects That Compromise Wound Healing

Condition	Effects
Arteroslerosis	Hypoxia
Cardiac insufficiency	Hypoxia
Collagen vascular disease	Chronic vasculitis
Diabetes mellitus	Thickened capillary membrane
Immunocompromise	Impaired immune response
Malnutrition	Anemia, edema, impaired protein stores
Age	Hypoxia, anemia
Medications	Steroids (alter inflammatory response)
Smoking	Vasoconstriction, hypoxia

Tissue fluid oxygen tensions of 30-40 mm Hg are necessary for wounds to heal.[9] At lower oxygen tensions, metabolic functions associated with the healing process cannot take place. Provided it does not go below critical pressures, the relative hypoxia of ischemic wounds stimulates production of angiogenesis and growth factor by the macrophage. This angiogenesis factor produces the new blood vessels of granulation tissue. It is thought that the mediator of neovascularization and collagen synthesis is lactate. Lactate stimulates angiogenic factor production by the macrophage whether or not oxygen is present. The major source of energy for the metabolism of granulation tissue is an anaerobic process of increased glucose consumption and lactate production.[10] Hypoxia also causes fibroblasts to activate the enzymes for collagen syntheses. Recent studies have shown that wound healing is stimulated by a relatively hypoxic environment.[11] Optimal growth of fibroblasts occurs at low partial pressures of oxygen. Chronic tissue hypoxia is a potent stimulator of capillary proliferation, growing from the wound edge to the more hypoxic center.[12] The process continues until hypoxia subsides. Local hypoxic conditions stimulate the macrophage to release growth factors. Patients at increased risk for nonhealing wounds include those who are oxygen deficient, with tissue oxygen tensions below 30 mm Hg; those who are hypotensive; those who have certain medical conditions, such as diabetes or atherosclerosis; and those who are critically ill with anemia or edema. Topical application of oxygen, even under pressure, has not shown to be of value to wound healing.[7]

Stress

The sympathetic nervous system and adrenal responses to stress include neural, hormonal, and metabolic changes that are thought to have a negative effect on wound healing. The exact mechanism is not clearly understood. However, the mediators of the stress response include catecholamines, norepinephrine, and epinephrine; the increase in these mediators may influence the healing process. Excess norepinephrine levels during the stress response cause vasoconstriction, thereby decreasing the oxygen to the peripheral tissues.[13] During times of stress or activity, additional adrenaline is produced and circulated. Adrenaline increases the production of chalone, a water-soluble inhibitor that is produced by the tissue on which it selectively acts. Chalones depress the regeneration of epidermal tissue. During times of sleep or relaxation, a decreased amount of adrenaline is produced. The chalone is then decreased, and the rate of epidermal cell division and maturation increases. The result is more rapid wound healing. Therefore, a plan that provides sleep and rest for the patient with a pressure ulcer will promote wound healing.[13,14,15]

Advanced age

Aging affects almost all aspects of the healing response.[12] There is a fourfold decrease in wound healing in the elderly, because of decreased epidermal turnover and increased skin fragility. The repair rate in elderly skin declines, as measured by cell proliferation, development of wound tensile strength, collagen deposition, wound contraction, or healing of experimentally induced blisters. This may be the reason for the increased prevalence of pressure ulcers in the skin of older persons.

Geriatric individuals may have difficulty healing because often they are less well nourished and hydrated than their younger counterparts. The combination of medical conditions that occur in the elderly adversely affects healing. Also, older people are more likely than younger people to have impaired respiratory or immune systems, which interfere with oxygen transport and stimulation of the inflammatory phase necessary for wound healing.

An age-related decrease in the number of dermal blood vessels makes the older individual at particularly high risk for ischemic injury. A decrease in dermal and subcutaneous mass further increases the risk for pressure-induced tissue injury.[16]

Malnutrition

Wound healing and the immune response both are contingent upon an adequate supply of various nutrients, including protein, vitamins, and minerals. A deficiency of dietary protein interferes with neovascularization, lymphatic formation, fibroblastic proliferation, collagen synthesis, and wound remodeling. The edema that results from hypoalbuminemia further impairs fibroplasia. In addition, antibody response, immune function, and phagocytosis are impaired in the presence of protein deficiency, increasing the risk of wound infection.[17-20] Immunosuppression negatively affects the inflammatory phase of healing.

Protein

Clinically significant malnutrition is diagnosed if (a) the serum albumin level is less than 3.5 g/dl, (b) the total lymphocyte count is less than 1,500/mm³, or (c) body weight has recently decreased by more than 15%. Concentrations of serum albumin less than 3.0 g/dl are recognized as a screening indicator of nutritional status. Serum albumin levels below 2.5 g/dl are associated with severe protein depletion. Low serum albumin levels represent late manifestation of protein deficiency. Persons with extensive pressure ulcers are often protein deficient. Patients with wounds will require additional calories and protein (30-35 calories per kilogram of body weight and 1.25-1.50 grams of protein per kilogram of body weight per day) to build new tissue for wound healing. Pinchcofsky-Devin and Kaminski[17] studied the nutritional status of 232 nursing home patients and found that, of the 17 who had pressure ulcers, all were severely malnourished. Although a correlation has been found between hypoproteinemia and development of pressure ulcers, a recent retrospective study pooling data from four prospective, randomized controlled clinical trials has concluded that baseline serum albumin ≥2.0 g/dl, a laboratory test frequently used to determine hypoproteinemia, has little prognostic value for pressure ulcer healing.[21]

Protein metabolism is altered in the presence of severe trauma and systemic infection, resulting in increased urinary excretion of nitrogens. In addition, protein intake often is insufficient in persons subject to pressure ulcer development, such as the hospitalized elderly, immobile, or critically ill person.[16] Malnutrition with hypoproteinemia plays a greater role in pressure ulcer development in the elderly population than in the neurologically impaired, where pressure is more significant.[20]

Vitamins

Vitamins, particularly Vitamin C and Vitamin A, are thought to be necessary for wound healing. Vitamin C (ascorbic acid) deficiency is associated with impaired fibroblastic function and decreased collagen synthesis, resulting in delayed healing, capillary fragility, and breakdown of old wounds.[7] An age-associated decrease in ascorbic acid levels may increase the fragility of vessels and connective tissue and lower the threshold for pressure-induced injury.[16] Vitamin C deficiency also is associated with impaired immune function, decreasing the individual's ability to resist infection.[7,18] Because Vitamin C is a water-soluble vitamin and cannot be stored in the body, deficiencies can develop quickly if adequate intake is not maintained.

Deficiencies of Vitamin A have been associated with retarded epithelialization and decreased collagen synthesis. Unlike Vitamin C, Vitamin A is a fat-soluble vitamin and is stored in the liver. Therefore, deficiencies are rare. Patients at highest risk for vitamin A deficiencies are those under severe stress or those with chronic lack of vitamin intake.[22] Other vitamins, such as thiamine and riboflavin, are necessary for collagen organization and the resultant tensile strength of the wound.[7,23]

Minerals

Various minerals, such as iron, copper, manganese, and magnesium, play a role in wound healing, but the nature of their influence is unclear.[24] Zinc deficiencies have been associated with delayed healing and appear to act by reducing the rate of epithelialization and fibroblast proliferation. Deficiencies require replacement, but there is no indication that supplemental zinc is useful if a deficiency does not exist.[4,25] Studies indicate that malnutrition is a risk for pressure ulcer development and an impediment to healing.[26] Attention to nutritional status is crucial in the management of all patients with wounds.

Steroids

Steroid treatment suppresses the inflammatory response in a wound. Inflammation is necessary to trigger the wound-healing cascade, and those patients taking steroids often will undergo a long healing time. Steroids impair capillary budding, inhibit fibroblast proliferation, and decrease protein synthesis and epithelial growth. Steroids given after the inflammatory phase of healing (usually 4 to 5 days after wounding) have a minimal effect on the healing wound. Patients on planned steroid or chemotherapy treatment schedules must consider the effect on wound healing. If possible, the schedule should be altered to avoid these medications during the inflammatory phase of wound healing. Vitamin A is thought to counteract the anti-inflammatory effect of steroids by its effect on lysosomes within inflammatory cells. Systemic therapy with vitamin A has been shown to reverse the steroid influence on inflammation and may be used for patients with wounds who require steroid therapy.[22,27]

Smoking

Smoking has an adverse effect on wound healing. Nicotine interferes with blood flow in two ways: it is a vasoconstrictor, and it increases platelet adhesiveness, causing clot formation. In addition to the nicotine, the smoke of cigarettes is harmful to wound healing. Cigarette smoke influences tissue oxygenation by vasoconstriction and reduces the O_2 available to wounds because carbon monoxide prevents oxygen from binding to the hemoglobin molecule.[3] Smoking is also thought to create endothelial changes in the vessel wall and increased platelet adhesiveness, which may lead to further limitation of blood flow. Cigarette smoke contains toxins in the form of carbon monoxide and hydrogen cyanide, among others. Carbon monoxide has an affinity to bind with the hemoglobin molecule that is 200 times greater than that of oxygen. Breathed oxygen is not available if it cannot be carried by the hemoglobin molecule to the wound tissues. Hydrogen cyanide inhibits enzymes needed for oxygen transport and oxidative metabolism.[28] Patients who are preparing for surgical repair of pressure ulcers or other chronic wounds should be assisted to cease smoking and be informed of the higher risk for skin or muscle graft failure if smoking is continued.[29]

Diabetes

Diabetes influences wound healing by mechanical and metabolic effects.[7] Chronic hyperglycemia may be both the cause and the effect of poor wound healing. Animal studies have shown that high levels of glucose compete with cellular transport of ascorbic acid into cells. Ascorbic acid is necessary for the deposition of collagen. Animal studies also have shown that diabetic rats had significantly reduced tensile strength and connective tissue production compared to nondiabetic controls. Treatment with insulin reversed the effects on wound healing in these animals.[30] Occlusive arterial disease is a common comorbid condition in diabetic patients. This reduction in blood flow to the peripheral tissues can lead to impaired healing. The reduced sensation of diabetic neuropathy frequently leads to development of wounds due to trauma. Diabetes has been shown to alter the function of leukocytes in a way that decreases the effect on bacteria.[31] The inflammatory response is therefore decreased and the healing cascade impaired. The altered leukocyte function may also influence the ability of the diabetic patient to resist infection. Infection is a problem frequently associated with both diabetes and pressure ulceration. Patients with diabetes have more difficulty resisting infection and their wounds heal more slowly than those without diabetes.[32]

Infection

Infectious complications of pressure ulcers include sepsis and osteomyelitis. Debridement, drainage, and removal of the necrotic tissue alone will control most infections. Many organisms may be found on the surface of a chronic open wound. Topical antibiotic treatments are widely used, even without a solid scientific basis. Identified infections should be treated with antibiotics, but the mere presence of organisms in the wound may represent colonization of organisms, not infection. Open wounds do not have to be sterile to heal, and an effort to use topical antibiotics may render the individual insensitive to the antibiotic and produce resistant strains of organisms. A way to determine the presence of true wound infection must be established to guide the treatment decision.

The combination of local tissue response to infection and the accumulation of bacterial metabolic end-products prolongs the inflammatory phase of healing and interferes with neovascularization and collagen synthesis. Devitalized tissue and extravasated blood act as bacterial substrates and increase the risk of infection. Polymorphonuclear leukocytes and monocytes eliminate invading organisms. These white blood cells consume oxygen as they control the bacteria. Hypoxia inhibits the ability of the leukocyte to destroy the bacteria and supports bacterial growth. Sufficient oxygenation is necessary to support the defense against wound infection.[33] Moist necrotic tissue is a medium for bacterial growth and should be removed from the wound. Necrotic tissue also prevents the wound from granulating and forming epithelial tissue.[34] Healing cannot proceed until all necrotic tissue has been removed from the wound.

Wounds with tissue loss, such as pressure ulcers, are contaminated with bacteria because of the loss of the skin's protective covering. This contamination becomes significant and interferes with wound healing when the colony count becomes $>10^5$ organisms per gram of tissue.[33] It is generally recognized in the surgical literature that tissue biopsies with colony counts this high are considered infected. When local defense mechanisms no longer contain the infection, cellulitis, purulence, and fever may be evident. See Table 4.3 for clinical signs of wound infection.

Systemic antibiotics are not beneficial for reducing the bacterial load of the pressure ulcer wound bed because there is reduced vascularity in the local tissues. Use of parenteral antibiotics is indicated only when there is evidence of cellulitis, sepsis, or osteomyelitis. No scientifically designed study has documented that topical antibiotics have reduced the bacteria in the tissue surrounding the wound. The use of topical antibiotics may increase the proliferation of antibiotic-resistant bacteria.[35,36]

Table 4.3 "IFEE Wound" Signs of Infection

I	Induration
F	Fever
E	Erythema
E	Edema

From Alvarez, O., et al. "Moist Environment for Healing: Matching the Dressing to the Wound," *Wounds* 1(1): 40, 1989. Used with permission.

Wound dehydration

Wound healing occurs more rapidly when dehydration is prevented. As shown in Figure 4.2, epidermal cells migrate faster and cover the wound surface sooner in a moist environment than under a scab.[37] Wound fluid has been shown to promote fibroblast proliferation.[38] Dressings designed to promote the retention of moisture at the wound surface are beneficial to the healing process.

Evaluation of healing

Evaluation of healing requires the analysis of wound assessments. The simplest and most obvious method is to examine the wound and compare the observation with previous observations or reports of the wound. The best way to monitor the healing process is to use a systematic, consistent method. Examination should include measurement of the wound's size, including its length, width, and depth. Wound characteristics, such as inflammation, wound contraction, granulation, and epithelialization, are documented in an ongoing and systematic way.[1] Investigators are developing tools to measure wound characteristics and their relation to healing.

Wound healing times are variable. Etiology, patient characteristics, and wound management all affect the healing rate. Chapter 5 provides measurements of wound healing.

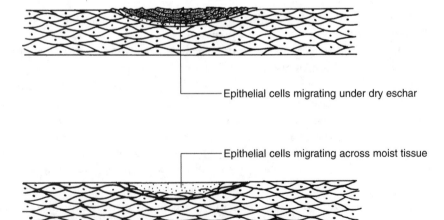

Epithelial cells migrating under dry eschar

Epithelial cells migrating across moist tissue

Figure 4.2 Environmental-epidermal cell migration

Summary

The wound healing sequence follows an expected course if the intrinsic and extrinsic conditions are optimal. Wounds go through inflammatory, proliferative, and differentiation phases. The factors that can interfere with wound healing include malnutrition, infection, stress, and concomitant medical diagnoses. Dressings can provide an immediate environment that either supports or impedes wound healing. All products that go on or into a wound should be nontraumatic. Careful monitoring of the wound healing process without too much interference seems to serve the wound best. Those factors that promote optimum healing, such as protection from trauma or provision of a moist environment, should be supported. Whenever possible, the body should be allowed to heal itself. New techniques for wound care must stand up to scientific scrutiny before their impact upon wound management is realized.

References

1. Lazarus, G.S., et al. "Definitions and Guidelines for Assessment of Wounds and Evaluation of Healing," *Arch Derm* 130(4): 489-493, 1994.

2. Sieggreen, M.Y. "Healing of Physical Wounds," *Nur Clin North Am* 22(2):439-447, 1987.

3. Hotter, A.N. "Physiologic Aspects and Clinical Implications of Wound Healing," *Heart and Lung* 11(6): 522-530, 1982.

4. Goodson, W.H., and Hunt, T.K. "Wound Healing," in Kyle, J., and Hardy, J.D., eds. *Scientific Foundations of Surgery,* 3rd ed. Philadelphia: W.B. Saunders, 1980.

5. Peacock, E.E. "Wound Healing and Wound Care, in Schwartz, S.I., et al., eds. *Principles of Surgery,* 4th ed. New York: McGraw Hill, 1984.

6. Schumann, D. "The Nature of Wound Healing," *AORN J* 35(6): 1068-1077, 1982.

7. Hunt, T.K., and Hussain, Z. "Wound Microenvironment," in Cohen, I.K., et al. *Wound Healing.* Philadelphia: W.B. Saunders, 1992.

8. Timberlake, G.A. "Wound Healing: The Physiology of Scar Formation," *Curr Concepts in Wound Care* 9(2): 4-14, Summer 1986.

9. Rodeheaver, R. "Topical Wound Management," *Ostomy/Wound Management* 20: 58-68, Fall 1988.

10. Hoopes, J.E. "Energy Metabolism in Healing Skin Wounds," *J Surg Res* 10: 459, 1970.

11. Sheffield, P.J. "Tissue Oxygen Measurements with Respect to Soft Tissue Wound Healing with Normobaric and Hyperbaric Oxygen," *Hyperbaric Oxygen Rev* 6:18, 46, 1985.

12. Varghese, M.C., et al. "Local Environment of Chronic Wounds under Synthetic Dressings," *Arch Dermatol* 122:52-57, 1986.

13. Knighton, D.R., et al. "The Use of Topically Applied Platelet Growth Factors in Chronic Nonhealing Wounds," *Wounds* 4:71-78, April 1989.

14. West, J.M. "Wound Healing in the Surgical Patient: Influence of the Perioperative Stress Response on Perfusion," *AACN,* Clinical Issues 1(3): 595-601, November 1990.

15. Carpenito, L.J. *Nursing Diagnosis: Application to Clinical Practice,* 3rd ed. Philadelphia: J.B. Lippincott, 1989.

16. North, A. "The Effect of Sleep on Wound Healing," *Ostomy/Wound Management* 27:57-58, March-April 1990.

17. Goode, P., and Allman, R.M. "The Prevention and Management of Pressure Ulcer," *Med Clin of North Am* 73(6): 1511-1524, 1989.

18. Pinchcofsky-Devin, G., and Kaminski, M.V., Jr. "Correlation of Pressure Sores and Nutritional Status," *Am Geriatr Soc* 34:435-440, 1986.

19. Bobel, L.M. "Nutritional Implications in the Patient with Pressure Sores," *Nur Clin North Am* 22(2): 379-390, 1987.

20. Pinchcofsky-Devin, G. "Why Won't This Wound Heal?" *Ostomy/Wound Management* 24:42-51, Fall 1989.

21. Morley, J.E. "Nutritional Status of the Elderly," *Am J Med* 81: 679-696, 1986.

22. Hill, D.P., et al. "Serum Albumin Is a Poor Prognostic Factor for Pressure Ulcer Healing in Controlled Clinical Trials," *Wounds,* 6(5): 174-178, 1994.

23. Ehrlich, H.P., and Hunt, T.K. "Effects of Cortisone and Vitamin A on Wound Healing," *Ann Surg* 167(3): 324-328, 1968.

24. Alvarez, O.M., and Gilbreath, R.L. "Thiamine Influence on Collagen During the Granulation of Skin Wounds," *Surg Res* 32: 24, 1982.

25. Chvapil, M. "Zinc and Other Factors of the Pharmacology of Wound Healing," in Hunt, T.K., ed. *Wound Healing and Wound Infection: Theory and Surgical Practice.* New York: Appleton-Century Crofts, 1980.

26. Ruberg, R.L. "Role of Nutrition in Wound Healing," *Surg Clin North Am* 64: 705, 1984.

27. Allman, R.M., et al. "Pressure Sores among Hospitalized Patients," *Ann Intern Med* 105(3): 337-42, September 1986.

28. Kottra, C. "Wound Healing in the Immunosuppressed Host," *AORN J* 35(6): 1142-1148, 1982.

29. Silverstein, P., et al. "Cigarette Smoking: Impairment of Digital Blood Flow and Wound Healing in the Hand," *Hand* 9: 97-101, 1992.

30. Silverstein, P. "Smoking and Wound Healing," *Am J of Medicine* 93 (suppl 1A), July 15, 1992, 1A-22S-1A-224s.

31. Goodson, W.H., and Hunt, T.K. "Studies of Wound Healing in Experimental Diabetes Mellitus," *J. Surg Res* 22: 221-227, 1977.

32. Carrico, T.J., et al. "Biology of Wound Healing," *Surg Clin North Am* 64: 721-733, 1984.

33. Ferrell, B.A., et al. "Medical Management of Advanced Pressure Sores," *Geriatr Med Today* 8(1): 81-88, 1989.

34. Stotts, N. "Impaired Wound Healing," in Carrieri, V.K., et al. *Pathophysiological Phenomena in Nursing: Human Responses to Illness.* Philadelphia: W.B. Saunders, 1986.

35. Alterescu, V., and Alterescu, K. "Etiology and Treatment of Pressure Ulcers," *Decubitus* 1(1): 28-35, 1988.

36. Rodeheaver, G. "Topical Wound Management," *Ostomy/Wound Management* : 58-68, Fall 1988.

37. Rodeheaver, G., et al. "Bactericidal Activity and Toxicity of Iodine-Containing Solutions in Wounds," *Arch Surg*, 117: 181-186, February 1982.

38. Winter, G.D., and Scales, J.T. "Effect of Air Drying and Dressings on the Surface of a Wound," *Nature* 197: 91-92, 1963.

CHAPTER 5

Assessment

Assessment is defined as "taking stock of" or evaluating a situation. Assessment is the first step in formulating diagnoses and determining a plan of care. Nursing assessment usually includes a comprehensive approach to the patient as an individual. Assessment of patients with a pressure ulcer problem includes multiple variables and must be done in systematic fashion. Data gathering should include a complete history and physical examination, including psychosocial assessment, evaluation of factors commonly associated with pressure ulcer risk, a thorough examination of the skin, and a precise description of the pressure ulcer.

Assessment of pressure ulcer risk

Soft tissue breaks down more readily in the presence of certain intrinsic patient conditions. Pressure ulcer risk assessment is based on an understanding of those conditions or factors that predispose individuals to pressure ulceration. Patients who are at risk for developing pressure ulcers can be identified by assessing the following variables:
- Number and type of medical diagnoses
- Chronicity of health problems
- Chronological age
- Immobility/ability to move independently
- Mental status/level of consciousness
- Malnutrition/nutritional status
- Incontinence/bladder and bowel control
- Presence of infection and/or fever
- Adequacy of circulation.[1]

Pressure ulcer risk increases as the number of patient problems within each variable increases. Certain high-risk groups are reported to be at great risk for pressure ulceration. Approximately 66% of elderly patients admitted to hospitals for fractured femur[2] and 33% of patients in intensive care units[3] developed pressure ulcers. Patients with chronic underlying pathology, such as diabetes mellitus, Alzheimer's disease, arteriosclerosis, and spinal cord injury often are unable to withstand the forces of pressure and shear because of one or more risk factors. One study reported a 60% pressure ulcer prevalence rate for patients with quadriplegia.[4] Allman et al,[5] in a prospective study of hospitalized bedridden and chairbound persons, found that nonblanchable erythema, lymphopenia, immobility, dry skin, and decreased body weight were independent and significant risk factors for hospitalized patients with limited activity. All health care professionals should be aware of factors that place patients at risk for pressure ulceration so that appropriate prophylactic measures can be instituted.

Immobility/ability to move independently

Independent mobility contributes to both physical and psychological well-being of all individuals. Immobility probably is the greatest threat of all for pressure ulceration. The AHCPR Pressure Ulcer Prediction and Prevention Guideline recommends identification of all bedridden and chairbound patients.[6] Feedar[7] suggests the following areas for evaluation of a patient's mobility and activity: reflexive body adjustment in bed and wheelchair, active bed mobility, active wheelchair repositioning, activity, transfers, ambulation, and distance/endurance. See Table 5.1 for Harper Hospital's physical therapy evaluation of patient strength and mobility.

Patients who are weak and out of condition should be given enough assistance and encouragement to recondition themselves and attain their full potential. Nursing units can hang wall charts indicating individual patient ambulation times and distance. Patients can credit themselves for walking or exercising by placing stars or numbers for every "lap around the hall." Often, health care professionals and family members contribute to positive feedback for patients who are progressing in activity. Activity intolerance needs to be evaluated. Individuals who have been on bedrest for long periods may feel weak and dizzy when ambulated.[8] Chair exercises are useful for groups of debilitated or chairbound patients. Progressive reconditioning may take physical training and psychological coaching. Nurses and physical therapists must try to ensure the highest possible level of mobility for all patients.

Persons who cannot independently reposition themselves must have local pressure over bony prominences alleviated by at least one of the following mechanisms:
• Passive repositioning
• Pillow bridging
• Pressure-relieving sleep and sitting surfaces.[9]

Mental status/consciousness/sensation

Patients who have decreased mental status may not feel discomfort from pressure, may not be alert enough to move spontaneously, may not be motivated to move, may not remember to move, may be too confused to respond to commands to move, or may be physically incapable of changing position. Patients who have decreased mental status often are restrained for their own safety or given sedatives to "calm them down." When patients are restrained or sedated, they have fewer spontaneous movements and are less likely to change position.[1] This results in unrelieved pressure over bony prominences and significantly increases the risk for pressure ulceration of soft tissue. Cautious use of physical restraints and medication may enable more spontaneous movement in persons with altered mental status.

Table 5.1 Evaluating Patient Strength and Mobility

Wayne State University

DMC Harper
Hospital

Name:

DEPARTMENT OF PHYSICAL THERAPY
❑ Initial Evaluation   ❑ Re-Evaluation (Page 1)   MR#:

DATE:	ADMITTED:	REFERRAL RECEIVED:

DATA BASE: AGE: SEX: CODE STATUS: ACTIVITY ORDER:
REASON FOR ADMISSION:

DIAGNOSIS:

PERTINENT PAST MEDICAL/SURGICAL HISTORY:	PERTINENT TESTS/PROCEDURES:

SUBJECTIVE:

FUNCTIONAL STATUS PRIOR TO ADMISSION:

HOME ENVIRONMENT:

AVAILABLE DURABLE MEDICAL EQUIPMENT:

INTERDISCIPLINARY CONTACTS:

OBJECTIVE:

COGNITION/COMMUNICATION/ORIENTATION:

ROM:	STRENGTH:
MUSCLE TONE:	SENSATION:
CARDIOVASCULAR:	PULMONARY:

0167MR111894   White = Medical Record   Yellow = Department Copy   Pink = Department Copy

Continued

Table 5.1 Evaluating Patient Strength and Mobility *(continued)*

Wayne State University **DMC** Harper Hospital	Name:
DEPARTMENT OF PHYSICAL THERAPY ❏ Initial Evaluation ❏ Re-Evaluation (Page 2)	MR#:

BED MOBILITY:	**GAIT:**		
Rolls Rt.	**SURFACE:**	**LEVEL**	**STAIRS**
Rolls Lt.	DISTANCE:_____		
Sit → Supine	ASSISTIVE DEVICE:_____		
Supine → Sit	ASSIST:_____		
Scooting, Supine	DURATION:_____		
Scooting, Sitting	**GAIT DEVIATIONS:**		
Bridging			

TRANSFERS:

Assist: Indep = Independent   SBA = Standby Assist
CG = Contact Guard   MIN = Minimal   MOD = Moderate
MAX = Maximum

COORDINATION:	**SKIN/INCISION/STUMP:**

BALANCE:	STATIC	DYNAMIC	**EXERCISE/TREATMENT GIVEN THIS DATE:**
SHORT SITTING			
STANDING			
ASSISTIVE DEVICE:			

W/C PREPARATION AND MOBILITY:

Continued

Table 5.1 Evaluating Patient Strength and Mobility *(continued)*

Wayne State University

DMC Harper
Hospital

Name:

DEPARTMENT OF PHYSICAL THERAPY
❑ **Initial Evaluation**   ❑ **Re-Evaluation** (Page 3)   MR#:

ASSESSMENT/PROBLEM LIST:

ACTIVITY TOLERANCE:

SAFETY:

PATIENT/FAMILY INDEPENDENT WITH EXERCISE PROGRAM: ❑ YES ❑ NO ❑ N/A AT THIS TIME

GOALS OF TREATMENT:

POTENTIAL: ESTIMATED DURATION:

RECOMMENDATIONS:

DISCHARGE:

EQUIPMENT:

REFERRALS:

PLAN:

TREATMENT:

❑ To be followed by Physical Therapy Assistant

FREQUENCY: INTERVENTION TIME:

_____
Signature/Date   Pager #

0167MR111894   White = Medical Record   Yellow = Department Copy   Pink = Department Copy

Healthy people with intact nervous systems feel persistent local pressure, become uncomfortable, and shift body weight before ischemia occurs.[10] Patients with paraplegia or quadriplegia are unable to sense increased pressure over bony prominences. If they do not, or are unable to move, the unrelieved pressure leads to tissue ulceration. People with sensory deprivation need to be assisted to turn on a regular basis to relieve local pressure over the sacrum and trochanters. Caregivers must be educated to reposition these patients on a regular basis.

Malnutrition/nutritional status

Malnutrition is a widespread problem in America and becoming more so as our society ages. Elderly individuals often decrease dietary intake to the point of becoming malnourished. At the opposite end of the spectrum are those individuals who are overly nourished. Surveys indicate that malnutrition in hospitalized patients may be a common problem.[11] Many ill patients enter the hospital in an already malnourished state, and patients in a well-nourished state who enter the hospital for elective procedures may develop malnutrition during hospitalization. Malnutrition is considered to be one of the primary factors related to pressure ulceration because it contributes to diminished tissue tolerance for pressure.[12,13,14,15] Allman and associates[13] found a significant relationship between a low serum albumin level and pressure ulcers. They suggested that the odds of having a pressure ulcer increase threefold with every decrease of 1 gram in the serum albumin level. The normal albumin concentration of the serum is 3.5-5.0 g/dl. Serum albumin deficit levels are rated as severe (<2.5 g/dl), moderate (<2.5-3.0 g/dl), and mild (<3.0-3.5 g/dl). Research has demonstrated a fourfold increase in morbidity and a sixfold increase in mortality in patients with serum albumin concentrations <2.5 g/dl.[16]

The Nutrition Screening Initiative of Healthy People 2000 recommends use of nutrition screening tools to provide an important frame of reference for individuals and health care providers.[17] Nutritional assessment should include dental health, oral and gastrointestinal history, chewing and swallowing ability, quality and frequency of foods eaten, history of involuntary weight loss or gain, serum albumin levels, nutritionally pertinent medications, and any psychosocial factors affecting nutritional intake. Other important factors include a person's ability to acquire and pay for food, food preferences, cultural and lifestyle influences on food selection, ability to cook, facilities for cooking, and environment for eating. Persons determined to be at risk for malnutrition should have nutritional screening assessments performed at least every 3 months.[18] (See the Harper Hospital nutritional assessment tool in Chapter 6 for clinical and laboratory assessment parameters).

Incontinence

Incontinence increases the risk for pressure ulceration by creation of excessively moist tissue and by chemical irritation.[19] If the skin is kept constantly wet from either fecal or urinary incontinence, the tissue becomes overly soft and wet. The outer layer of wet skin is easily rubbed away as a person is given skin care or moved across the bed linen. One acute care study showed the odds of having a pressure ulcer were 22 times greater in patients who were fecally incontinent compared to patients who were not incontinent.[20] Another study found increased odds of pressure ulcers among fecally incontinent elderly residents of nursing homes.[21] According to Allman[13] and Shannon,[22] fecal incontinence is more significant in pressure ulceration than urinary incontinence. It was surmised that this was because of bacteria and toxins in the stool.[13] In patients with both urinary and fecal incontinence, the pH in the perineal area is increased when fecal enzymes convert urea into ammonia. This rise in pH increases the activity of fecal proteases and lipases, which in turn makes the skin more permeable to other irritants, such as bile salts.[19] The skin is then compromised by these caustic substances. One study of geropsychiatric inpatients suggests that the interaction of urine and stool may contribute to perineal dermatitis in elderly incontinent patients.[23] Also, it is possible that vigorous skin cleansing and use of multiple incontinent products contribute to further skin breakdown.

The etiology of incontinence needs to be determined. It should not be assumed that incontinence is a normal part of aging. Incontinence assessment includes evaluation of reversible causes, including urinary tract infections, medications, confusion, fecal impaction, polyuria related to glycosuria or hypercalcemia, and restricted mobility with inability to get to a toilet.[24] It may be that the incontinent patient is confused about the location of a strange bathroom, too embarrassed to ask for a bedpan, or lacking in the functional skills to perform self-toileting. Table 5.2 represents a comprehensive functional assessment tool for patients with urinary incontinence.[25] Tracking the amount and frequency of urination and stooling is important in determining an appropriate incontinence management plan. All incontinent individuals should have a bowel and/or bladder program initiated.

Psychological factors

Studies have demonstrated that pressure ulcer formation in paraplegics and quadriplegics is associated with self-concept.[26] Also, there is evidence that mean depression scores are high among spinal cord-injured patients at risk for pressure ulcers.[27] Young patients with spinal cord injuries often become angry at their situation. If these patients become depressed and uninterested in self-care, they may have repeated tissue breakdown due to apathy and neglect. Depression has been known to lead to alcoholism and chemical abuse among spinal cord-injured individuals with pressure ulcers.[28] Occasionally, the pressure sore is seen as a means to gain additional attention from family and health professionals. Health care professionals must be vigilant with regard to the emotional status of patients who are at risk for pressure ulceration. If depression is a factor, the patient should be referred for psychological counseling.

Chronic emotional stress has been cited as a factor that contributes to pressure sore susceptibility. When a person is emotionally stressed, the adrenal glands increase production of glucocorticoids. Collagen production is then inhibited, and this makes the soft tissue more susceptible to pressure ulceration.[26] Patients should be

Table 5.2 Assessing Urinary Incontinence

Name _____ Room number _____

Age _____ Sex _____ Race _____ Date of admission _____

History of the incontinence

1. Approximate date of onset of incontinence _____

2. How frequent are the incontinent episodes in 24 hours? _____

3. How often does the patient urinate (continent and incontinent) in 24 hours? _____

4. Does the patient urinate regularly?   Yes _____ No _____

5. Does the patient urinate at night?   Yes _____ No _____

6. Is the patient incontinent at night?   Yes _____ No _____

7. Is the patient incontinent during the day?   Yes _____ No _____

8. What is the usual amount of urine passed?

    Small _____ Moderate _____ Large _____ Varies_____

9. Is the patient's fluid intake regular?   Yes _____ No _____

10. What is the patient's fluid intake in 24 hours?

    Small _____ Moderate _____ Large _____ Varies_____

Cognitive abilities

11. Does the patient ask to go to the toilet?   Yes _____ No _____

12. Does the patient ever go to the toilet for self?   Yes _____ No _____

13. Does the patient know where the bathroom is?   Yes _____ No _____

14. If placed on a toilet, does the patient urinate?   Yes _____ No _____

15. Does the patient seem aware of being wet?   Yes _____ No _____

16. Is the patient restless before an incontinent episode?   Yes _____ No _____

17. Is the patient more confused before an incontinent episode?   Yes _____ No _____

18. Is the patient concerned after an incontinent episode? Yes No

19. Does the patient ask to go to the toilet?   Yes _____ No _____

Mobility

20. Can the patient get in and out of a chair alone?   Yes _____ No _____

21. Can the patient walk to the bathroom alone?   Yes _____ No _____

22. Can the patient walk with the assistance of one person?   Yes _____ No _____

23. Must the patient be lifted onto the toilet?   Yes _____ No _____

24. Can the patient maintain balance without holding on?   Yes _____ No _____

25. Is the patient free to move about at will?   Yes _____ No _____

26. Does the patient walk very slowly?   Yes _____ No _____

Activities of daily living

27. Is the patient able to manipulate clothing?   Yes _____ No _____

28. Is the patient able to button and zipper clothing?   Yes _____ No _____

29. Does the patient perform hygiene activities for self?   Yes _____ No _____

30. Does the patient use a diaper that can be removed?

     None used _____ Easily removed _____ Difficult to remove _____

Used with permission. Jirovec, M., Brink, C., Wells, T. (1988). Functional Assessment of a Patient with Urinary Incontinence. *Nursing Clinics of North America* 23(1): 224-225.

encouraged to discuss situations that are causing them stress. Often this information needs to be elicited by careful questioning from qualified health care professionals.

Pressure ulcer risk assessment scales

Nurses often are able to foresee the consequences of risk and disability and to prevent a problem before it happens. Based on experience, one may be able to readily identify patients who are at risk for pressure ulceration. It may be more difficult to explain exactly why each patient is at risk. There are several risk assessment scales available to help identify a patient's degree of pressure ulcer risk. Nurse researchers created these risk assessment tools to objectively rate factors that contribute to the development of pressure ulcers. Most pressure ulcer risk assessment scales are based on the original work of Doreen Norton,[29] who studied the pressure ulcer problem in Great Britain. Gosnell[30] and Braden[31] developed risk assessment scales based on the findings and limitations of existing tools. Variations of pressure ulcer risk assessment tools are available from manufacturers of pressure relief and wound care products. Most pressure ulcer risk assessment scales identify immobility, inactivity, incontinence, malnutrition, and decreased mental status or decreased sensation as major factors that predispose patients to pressure ulceration. When the various risk factors are scored and summed, the resulting number indicates the degree of pressure ulcer risk for that individual.[3] The specificity and intensity of nursing interventions are then determined by the pressure ulcer risk assessment score. Many health care agencies are mandating pressure ulcer risk assessment on every patient admitted to their facility.

Norton Scale

The Norton Scale[29] consists of five parameters: physical condition, mental state, activity, mobility, and incontinence. Each of the five parameters is rated on an ordinal scale of 1-4, with total scores ranging from 5 to 20. With the Norton Scale, the lower the score, the higher the risk for pressure ulceration. The Norton "cutoff" score originally was placed at 14. In view of modern medications, preventive equipment, and continued feedback on use of the Norton Scale, Doreen Norton now places the onset of risk at a Norton score of 16 or below.[32] The Norton Scale has been criticized for not including nutrition. In fact, nutrition was included in the original data collection form subsumed under the general condition category.[32] One benefit of the Norton Scale is its simplicity and ease of use. Rater agreement was seen as achievable with few elements to assess. (For a more detailed look at the Norton Scale, see the Appendices.)

Gosnell Scale

The Gosnell Scale[33] was based on further research and refinement of the Norton Scale. The general condition category was changed to nutrition, and the incontinence category was renamed continence. General skin appearance, detailed medication, diet and fluid balance, and intervention categories were added to the instrument but not rated in ordinal fashion. Gosnell developed a rater's guide containing descriptors to clarify and make more precise the meaning of each numbered risk factor. A reverse ordering of the five rated risk factors resulted in scoring that reflects greater pressure ulcer risk with a higher score. A Gosnell score of 5 is the lowest and 20 is the highest possible score. Work is still in progress to determine the critical cutoff score, although it was determined to be 11 or greater in one acute care study.[34] (For a more detailed look at the Gosnell Scale, see the Appendices.)

Braden Scale

The Braden Scale[35] conceptualizes both the etiologic factors contributing to prolonged pressure and the factors contributing to diminished tissue tolerance for pressure. It was developed in response to difficulties encountered by staff in long-term care facilities when rating nutrition and continence on other risk scales.[36] The Braden Scale is composed of six subscales: sensory perception, moisture, activity, mobility, nutrition, and friction/shear. Each factor is described and rated on an ordinal scale of 1-4, with the exception of friction/shear, which is rated on a 3-point scale. The maximum possible score is 23. Like the Norton Scale, the Braden Scale uses lower scores to reflect higher risks for pressure ulceration. The cutoff score to denote risk for pressure ulceration is ≤16.[36] The Braden scale continues to be tested extensively. (For a more detailed look at the Braden Scale, see the Appendices.)

Testing of pressure ulcer risk assessment scales

It is important for pressure sore risk assessment scales to accurately predict which patients will develop pressure ulcers. There is fear that some scales may overpredict pressure ulcers, and that scarce resources will be wasted in preventive measures for patients who really are not at risk. The three most popular risk assessment scales have had varying degrees of testing for interrater reliability and predictive validity. There is good interrater reliability for the Braden Scale when used by registered nurses.[3] The interrater agreement was disappointing when the Braden Scale was used by LPNs and unlicensed personnel. Reliability data are not available for the Norton Scale. One study conducted in extended care showed good reliability of the Gosnell Scale when used by registered nurses.[37,38]

Common measures of predictive validity are sensitivity and specificity. Sensitivity reflects the percentage of people developing pressure ulcers who were determined to be at risk by a formal pressure ulcer risk scale. Specificity reflects the percentage of people not developing pressure ulcers who were determined to be not at risk by a formal pressure ulcer risk assessment scale.[3] The reported sensitivity and specificity of the three most popular tools varies greatly.[18] Possibly this is because of different study settings, populations, and outcome measures. Because these tools have been tested in specific health care settings, they may not be generalizable to all others. Each agency should select a risk assessment tool to pilot test and use at their institution. The assessment tool must be validated for the specific type of patient population. Cutoff scores to determine at-risk status may be altered based on findings for populations in a particular setting.[3]

Based on current reliability and validity testing, the AHCPR Guideline for Pressure Ulcer Prediction and Prevention recommends use of either the Norton or Braden Pressure Sore Risk Assessment Scales.[6] Xakellis, Frantz, Arteaga et al[39] used both the Norton and Braden Scales to measure pressure ulcer risk of 504 residents of a state-supported long-term care facility. Patient classification agreement between the Norton and Braden Scales was 0.73. Agreement between staff nurse preventive interventions and determination of at-risk status was 0.41 for the Braden Scale and 0.43 for the Norton Scale. It is important to determine this relationship, because the purpose of assessing pressure ulcer risk is to carry out preventive interventions. These interventions will not be without cost, and the magnitude of cost will be directly related to the number of people defined as at risk.[39]

The absolute frequency of reassessment for pressure ulcer risk has not been established scientifically. Because the majority of pressure ulcers develop within the first 2 weeks after admission to a nursing home, it is logical to identify at-risk patients early.[14] The literature suggests weekly reassessment for patients determined to be at risk for pressure ulceration.[6] However, common sense indicates that whenever patient conditions change or patients become chairbound or bedridden, they should be reassessed for pressure ulcer risk.

Skin inspection

Pressure against the tissue causes pallor to the skin, indicating interrupted blood flow to a localized area of tissue. This skin pallor reflects tissue ischemia that, when prolonged, can result in extensive tissue damage. Often the first external sign of ischemia due to pressure is reactive hyperemia. When skin becomes ischemic under pressure for over 1 minute, it becomes reddened, or hyperemic, after the pressure is removed. Because this rush of blood results from a period of blocked blood flow, it is called reactive hyperemia. This protective mechanism dilates the vessels and increases the amount of blood available to nourish and oxygenate the tissue. Increased blood flow to the tissue also assists in removing accumulated waste products. Reactive hyperemia first presents itself as a bright flush, which generally lasts from one-half to three-fourths of the duration of an ischemic period. If pressure exceeds tissue tolerance, the mechanism of reactive hyperemia becomes insufficient to meet the demands of the compromised circulation.[40]

Blanchable erythema, the earliest sign of ischemia, appears as a pink to red area of skin. In light-skinned individuals, compressing the reddened area with a finger causes the color to blanch or turn white. When the finger is removed, redness reappears immediately. When the pressure that caused blanchable erythema is removed, the tissue should resume its normal color within 24 hours. There are no long-term effects on the tissue from blanchable erythema. Blood flow recovery time after relief from pressure can be considered as a measure of pressure ulcer susceptibility. In dark-skinned individuals, erythema is more difficult to discern. Bennett[41] developed a shading strip to facilitate assessment of subtle color changes in darkly pigmented skin.

Individuals who are debilitated or at extremely high risk for pressure ulcers may exhibit nonblanchable tissue changes in less than 2 hours.[40] Nonblanchable erythema is more serious than blanchable erythema. The color intensity of nonblanchable erythema is greater than in blanchable erythema. The color of nonblanchable erythema does not fade when compressed by the finger. Nonblanchable erythema is reversible if it is recognized early and treated. Nonblanchable erythema may be the first outward sign of tissue destruction. As the tissues are deprived of oxygen beyond the critical period, cell death occurs.[40]

As the epidermal tissue continues to be destroyed, vesicles appear. A shiny, erythematous base with indistinct borders may be noted. The skin surrounding the shiny base has nonblanchable erythema. Intervention is required to prevent progression of this lesion to a chronic pressure ulcer.

Assessment of the person with a pressure ulcer

Assessing the individual with a pressure ulcer includes assessment of the patient's physical and psychosocial health, mental status, learning ability, stress, depression, social support, medication, smoking habit, alcohol or drug use, goals, values, lifestyle, sexuality, culture and ethnicity, pressure ulcer risk factors, nutritional assessment, and any pressure ulcer-related pain or complications.[18] After a complete health history and physical examination, the ulcer itself must be thoroughly assessed. Any pain associated with the pressure ulcer or the pressure ulcer treatment regimen also should be assessed, using a visual analog scale.[42] If necessary, topical, oral, or parenteral pain medication should be administered prior to pressure ulcer examination or treatment.

Ulcer assessment

Pressure ulcers range from blanchable erythema of intact skin to deep destruction and loss of tissue that occurs in Stage IV ulcers. A chronic pressure ulcer has a well-defined border with surrounding nonblanchable erythema. There may be induration of tissue extending far beyond the open wound. Often, extent of the ulcer cannot be determined by inspection, as there may be extensive undermining along fascial planes. Ulcers present over the sacrum may be connected by a tunnel to ulcers over the trochanter of the femur or the ischial tuberosities. There may be extensive necrotic tissue present in the ulcer cavity.[40]

Assessment of the pressure ulcer should include a history (including etiology, duration, and prior treatment), anatomic location, stage, size (including length, width, and depth measured in centimeters), sinus tracts, undermining, tunneling, exudate or drainage, necrotic tissue (slough and eschar), presence or absence of granulation tissue, and epithelialization or new skin growth.[18] In addition, the borders of the ulcer can provide clues to healing potential. Intact skin surrounding the ulcer should be assessed for redness, warmth, induration or hardness, swelling, and any obvious signs of clinical infection. Table 5.3 depicts a sample pressure ulcer documentation form.

Table 5.3 Pressure Ulcer Assessment Guide

Patient name _____

Date _____ Time _____

ULCER (1)	ULCER (2) _____	Indicate Ulcer Sites
Site _____	Site _____	
Stage _____	Stage _____	
Size (cm)_____	Size (cm) _____	
Length _____	Length _____	
Width_____	Width _____	
Depth _____	Depth _____	

(If Yes, describe in space provided below)

	No	Yes		No	Yes
Sinus tract	____	____	Sinus tract	____	____
Tunneling	____	____	Tunneling	____	____
Necrotic tissue	____	____	Necrotic tissue	____	____
Slough	____	____	Slough	____	____
Eschar	____	____	Eschar	____	____
Exudate	____	____	Exudate	____	____
Serous	____	____	Serous	____	____
Serosanguineous	____	____	Serosanguineous	____	____
Purulent	____	____	Purulent	____	____
Granulation	____	____	Granulation	____	____
Epithelialization	____	____	Epithelialization	____	____
Pain	____	____	Pain	____	____
SURROUNDING SKIN					
Erythema	____	____	Erythema	____	____
Maceration	____	____	Maceration	____	____
Induration	____	____	Induration	____	____

Anterior

Description of ulcer(s)_____

_____

_____

_____

_____

Posterior

CLASSIFICATION OF PRESSURE ULCERS

Stage I: Nonblanchable erythema of intact skin, the heralding lesion of skin ulceration. In individuals with darker skin, discoloration of the skin, warmth, edema, induration, or hardness may also be indicators.

Stage II: Partial-thickness skin loss involving epidermis and/or dermis.

Stage III: Full-thickness skin loss involving damage to or necrosis of subcutaneous tissue that may extend down to, but not through, underlying fascia. The ulcer presents clinically as a deep crater with or without undermining adjacent tissue.

Stage IV: Full-thickness skin loss with extensive destruction, tissue necrosis, or damage to muscle, bone, or supporting structures (for example, tendon or joint capsule).

Source: U.S.Department of Health and Human Services. Public Health Service. Agency for Health Care Policy and Research (AHCPR). *Clinical Practice Guideline. Number 15: Treatment of Pressure Ulcers* Rockville, MD., December 1994. AHCPR Publication No. 95-0652.

Ayello[43] uses the word *assessment* as a mnemonic to teach neophytes the parameters for pressure ulcer assessment and documentation. The letters in *assessment* serve as the first letters of data elements included in comprehensive pressure ulcer evaluation, as shown here:

A = Anatomical location, age of ulcer
S = Size, stage
S = Sepsis
E = Exudate type and amount, erythema
S = Surrounding skin color, swelling, saturation of dressing
S = Sinus tracts, undermining
M = Maceration
E = Edges, epithelialization
N = Nose (odor), necrotic tissue type and amount, neovascularization
T = Tenderness to touch, tension (induration), tautness, tissue bed (granulation tissue)

Measuring pressure ulcer size

Pressure ulcer size can be measured with simple or sophisticated methods. Bohannon[44] assessed the practicality and accuracy of graph paper counting, weighing, and planimeter techniques to determine wound area from perimeter tracings. The simplest way to determine wound size in the clinical setting is to take linear measurements of length and width in centimeters or millimeters. Some clinicians prefer to trace the wound perimeter and then transfer a copy to the medical record. To determine gross wound depth, it is preferable to insert a gloved finger into the ulcer at the deepest part and then measure the length of finger able to be inserted. Iatrogenic injuries can be caused by placing cotton tipped applicators and tongue blades into deep wounds without adequate knowledge of anatomical structures. Figure 5.1 shows a commercially available wound measuring device with concentric circles. Paper measuring tapes also are available from many companies.

Another useful measurement of size is wound volume. Researchers often use dental alginate to create molds of the wound.[45] Clinically, wound volume can be measured by placing a film dressing over the wound cavity, adhering it to the intact skin and instilling saline through the film via syringe until fluid reaches the film level. When the saline is aspirated through the film, the amount of fluid is measured in cubic centimeters and recorded.

Serial color photographs also are helpful in measuring progress during pressure ulcer treatment. Some commercially available Polaroid cameras have film with metric squares superimposed on the film, so the wound size can be determined by counting the squares. In order to gain a consistent perspective, it is important for the photographer to hold the camera the same distance from the wound bed each time a picture is taken. Sophisticated camera equipment will give longer lasting photographs of truer color; however, expensive photographic equipment may not be readily available in many clinical settings.

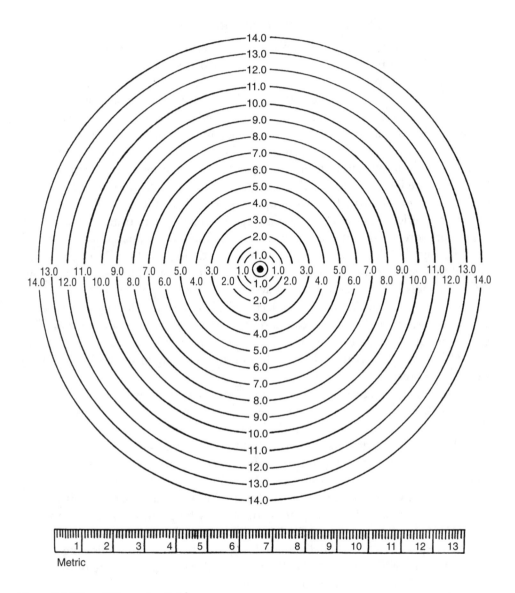

Figure 5.1 Wound Measuring Guide

Pressure ulcer classification systems/staging

On initial inspection, the depth of a pressure ulcer also is indicated by staging. Stage is indicated by noting the deepest layer of exposed tissue. An ulcer should not be restaged unless deeper layers of tissue become exposed, such as after debridement.[46,47] The literature discusses many classification systems for staging or grading pressure ulcers. In 1975, Darrell Shea, an orthopedic surgeon at the University of Miami, published a landmark paper describing a method of classifying and managing pressure sores.[48] He believed that a pathology-based pressure sore classification system would simplify communication for all disciplines, provide an effective means of pressure sore identification in clinical practice and research, and serve as a broad guide for determining whether or not operative treatment was needed.

Shea's numeric classification or grading system suggested an orderly evolution of the pressure sore. Each pressure sore grade was defined by the anatomic limit of soft tissue damage that could be observed after the pathology had declared itself. Shea believed that all layers of soft tissue were involved in a Grade I pressure sore. However, in his pressure sore classification system, the clinical presentation of Grade I pressure damage is limited to the epidermis. This epidermal damage ranges from soft tissue swelling, induration, heat, and erythema of unbroken skin to moist, superficial, irregular ulceration. Grades II, III, and IV pressure sores also gave anatomic limits of involved soft tissue based on Shea's understanding of the pathophysiology of soft tissue breakdown.

Over the intervening years, Shea's original work was modified. A Consensus Development Conference sponsored by the National Pressure Ulcer Advisory Panel (NPUAP) was held in Washington, D.C., in March 1989. Physicians, nurses, biomedical engineers, researchers, and other health professionals who attended the conference reached consensus on pressure ulcer risk factors, prevalence, and cost, as well as a pressure ulcer classification system.[49] The NPUAP classification schema was recommended as a universal staging system for use by all professional disciplines. This staging system has since been adopted by the Agency for Health Care Policy and Research (AHCPR) Pressure Ulcer Guideline Panels and is published in both sets of AHCPR Clinical Practice Guidelines for Pressure Ulcers.[6,18] The following definitions represent the NPUAP and AHCPR Pressure Ulcer Stages. (See the full-color illustrations of all pressure ulcer stages later in this chapter.)

Stage I. Nonblanchable erythema of intact skin: the heralding lesion of skin ulceration. In individuals with darker skin, discoloration of the skin, warmth, edema, induration, or hardness also may be indicators.

Stage II. Partial-thickness skin loss involving the epidermis, dermis, or both. The ulcer is superficial and presents clinically as an abrasion, blister, or shallow crater.

Stage III. Full-thickness skin loss involving damage to or necrosis of subcutaneous tissue, which may extend down to but not through underlying fascia. The ulcer presents clinically as a deep crater with or without undermining of adjacent tissue.

Stage IV. Full-thickness skin loss with extensive destruction, tissue necrosis, or damage to muscle, bone, or supporting structures (such as tendon or joint capsule). Undermining and sinus tracts also may be associated with Stage IV pressure ulcers.

In 1995, the National Pressure Ulcer Advisory Panel held a fourth national consensus conference to debate controversial issues surrounding assessment, measurement, and outcomes of pressure ulcer healing.[47] At that time, agreement was reached on several uses and misuses of the current pressure ulcer staging system. Participants agreed that pressure ulcers do not necessarily progress from one stage to another in an orderly fashion and that various stages of pressure ulcers may, in fact, have differing etiologies. They also agreed that pressure ulcer treatment should not be based on stage alone and that ulcers do not heal by reverse staging from Stage IV to Stage I.[47] Pressure ulcer stage is designated by structural layers of exposed tissue. As Stage IV pressure ulcers granulate to progressively more shallow depth, they do not replace lost structural layers of muscle, subcutaneous fat, and dermis before they re-epithelialize.

Although helpful for pressure ulcer classification, staging is only a small part of assessing a patient with a pressure ulcer. When assessing pressure ulcers, it is equally important to examine other ulcer characteristics, including intact skin surrounding the ulcer. The presence of inflammation, induration, or ischemia may give clues to the prognosis of the ulcer. Additionally, a pressure ulcer stage without consideration for the entire person has little predictive value in determining healing and no value at all when the ulcer is isolated from the patient.[50]

Closed pressure ulcers

A special situation exists in the closed pressure ulcer, which differs from an open lesion but still is caused by the same pathophysiological process. The term "closed pressure ulcer" was selected by Shea[48] to characterize an innocent-appearing and frequently overlooked ulcer that conceals a deep and potentially fatal lesion. A closed pressure ulcer may be the result of shearing mechanisms that cause ischemic necrosis in subcutaneous fat without skin ulceration. This results in a walled-off cavity filled with necrotic debris. These lesions are deceivingly extensive. Inflammation creates intense internal pressure. Eventually, the skin ruptures, creating a small, benign-appearing surface defect, which drains a large, contaminated base. Closed pressure ulcers commonly develop in the pelvic area in healthy spinal cord-injured persons who are confined to wheelchairs. Systemic manifestations of infection are not common.[48]

Recognition of chronic closed pressure ulcers is essential. Closed pressure ulcers cannot be classified into a numerical stage or grade because the amount of tissue destruction is not apparent until the defect is surgically opened. The only acceptable treatment is wide surgical excision of the ulcer and closure with a muscle rotation flap.[48]

Assessing complications associated with pressure ulcers

Complications of pressure ulcers can delay healing and may become life-threatening.[51] The major medical complications of pressure ulcers are sepsis and osteomyelitis. Clinically, there is confusion over the difference between colonization and infection. There also is controversy over appropriate methods of diagnosing infectious processes.

Colonization

The polymicrobial nature of pressure ulcers has been emphasized in the literature. All pressure ulcers are colonized with bacteria to a greater or lesser extent. In most cases, debridement and adequate cleansing will prevent the ulcer from becoming infected.[18] In an otherwise healthy individual, a wound can tolerate contamination or colonization of up to 100,000 (10^5) organisms per gram of tissue. If there are greater than 10^5 bacteria/gram of tissue, colonization may lead to wound infection.[52] A 2-week trial of topical antibiotics, such as silver sulfadiazine, should be considered for nonhealing pressure ulcers that have been unresponsive to 2-4 weeks of optimal patient care.[18,53]

Determining infection

Ulcer infection is determined by the classic signs of rubor, calor, dolor, and tumor. Table 5.4 defines the clinical signs of inflamed or infected wounds.[54] The cardinal sign of an infected ulcer is advancing cellulitis, which indicates the offending organism has invaded tissue surrounding the ulcer and is no longer localized.[18]

Sepsis

In a susceptible host, sepsis or bacteremia may occur with any pressure ulcer stage. Sepsis often is caused by anaerobes and gram-negative bacteria. Organisms commonly associated with pressure ulcers are *Staphylococcus aureus,* gram-negative rods, or *Bacteroides fragilis.*[18] Appropriate treatment of sepsis is the administration of systemic antibiotics to cover these organisms empirically. A blood culture is done to identify the causative organisms. If causative organisms can be identified, antibiotic regimens can be ordered specifically for those organisms.[55]

Osteomyelitis

Osteomyelitis is an infection involving the bone. It may occur in a Stage IV pressure ulcer when there is bony involvement. Allman[56] suggests that approximately 25% of nonhealing ulcers have underlying osteomyelitis. Osteomyelitis is a serious infection that delays healing, causes extensive tissue damage, and has a high mortality rate. A bone biopsy and culture are necessary to make the diagnosis.[51] Numerous strategies for noninvasive diagnosis of osteomyelitis are reported in the literature. Bone scans, which have a high false-positive rate, are of questionable value. If the patient's white blood cell count, erythrocyte sedimentation rate, and plain X-ray are all positive, the positive predictive value for osteomyelitis is 69%.[18,51] Treatment for osteomyelitis is long-term systemic antibiotics.[52]

▬Table 5.4 Defining Inflamed or Infected Wounds ▬▬▬▬▬▬

Erythema (rubor, redness)
An inflamed wound will often present with a well-defined border of erythema as the body is responding to trauma; a poorly defined border of erythema may indicate infection. The intensity of the erythema also needs to be examined. A very intense erythema, with well-defined borders, may be a sign of infection. Also, red streaking up or down a particular area usually indicates infection.

Fever (heat, calor)
A systemic fever and complaints of malaise may indicate infection, whereas a local temperature increase may indicate only inflammation.

Foul odor
A very foul smell does not necessarily indicate infection. The odor may be a result of necrotic, nonviable tissue solubilizing during autolytic or enzymatic debridement. A characteristically sweet smell, however, may indicate a Pseudomonas infection, whereas a Proteus infection may smell like ammonia.

Edema
Extravascular edema may be generalized throughout an area or it may be localized in the periwound tissue. Edema may be a sign of chronic heart failure or venous insufficiency if generalized in an extremity and of normal temperature and therefore may not be a sign of either inflammation or infection resulting from the wound. However, if the edematous area is warm and localized, it may be a sign of infection.

Drainage
Drainage should be objectified by the amount of color, viscosity, smell, and nature and duration of its existence. Drainage should be distinguished from tissue sloughing. It should be noted if drainage accumulates quickly or persists after both wound and periwound cleansing. Proper assessment of drainage is important, because it may indicate the presence of infection, or it may be the body's brief, normal inflammatory response to trauma. Drainage may also occur due to the presence of dead tissue or a foreign substance. The amount of drainage should be classified as minimal, moderate, or maximum. More objective measurements may be implemented if clinically necessary. One should expect that moderate to maximal amounts of drainage will collect under a dressing immediately after wounding, and one should expect that this drainage will normally decrease over 3 to 5 days as the wound moves out of the inflammatory or exudative phase into the proliferative phase. Likewise, there is usually minimal drainage present in a subacute noninfected wound.

Color of exudate
The color of the wound drainage should be evaluated. Normally, exudate trapped under a synthetic dressing in an acute wound will have a range in color from red to brown due to the presence of blood, fibrin, and other hemostatic processes. As the wound progresses, the drainage will become either clearer and watery as it progresses toward healing or more yellow and viscous if an infection develops. Infections may also cause the drainage to appear yellow-green or green-blue. Color of drainage should not be confused with necrotic tissue sloughing off secondary to debridement.

Pain (dolor)
Reports of pain are very subjective and may or may not indicate infection. Pain in an arterial insufficient leg, for example, may be due to the insufficiency alone, not infection. Pain that is severe in a wound of a healthy, young patient who suffered a laceration into the subcutaneous fat, for example, may not be normal if the symptoms continue after an unusual amount of time (a day or two) and therefore may indicate infection.

Used with permission. *Topics in Geriatric Rehabilitation* 9(4):37, June 1994.

Culturing

Cultures of the pressure ulcer are necessary to determine infecting organisms. The literature reports several clinically applicable methods of obtaining samples for culture:
- Surface swab
- Needle aspiration after normal saline injection into the wound
- Curettage of the ulcer base after cleansing the surface of the ulcer
- Deep tissue biopsy.[57]

Wound swab cultures are of dubious value and merely detect the presence of colonizing bacteria. Specimens obtained by needle aspiration after saline instillation appear to underestimate the actual number of individual organisms isolated from the deep tissue. The results obtained by curettage of the base of the ulcer show the best correlation with deep tissue culture. Deep tissue biopsy with culture is the most accurate method of determining infecting organisms. If possible, quantitative bacterial cultures of soft tissue and bone should be done when an ulcer does not respond to a course of topical antibiotic therapy. If the bacterial level in the biopsied tissue is greater than 10^5, healing will be impaired.[57,58]

Assessment of pressure ulcer healing or deterioration

Over the years, clinicians have offered numerous definitions of "wounding" and "wound healing," but these definitions lacked clarity about what constituted a "healed" wound. Recently, the Wound Healing Society, in an attempt to create common language, published useful definitions of a minimally healed wound (restoration of anatomic continuity but without sustained function), an acceptably healed wound (restoration of sustained function and anatomic continuity), and an ideally healed wound (normal anatomic function, structure, and appearance).[59] Assessment of wound status and improvement or deterioration includes multiple attributes of the wound and quantification of wound parameters.[47]

Tracing wounds on clear plastic film provides a viable option for recording wound surface area, although inferring the rate of healing after taking successive measurements can be problematic. Gilman,[60] attempting to quantify the rate of healing, suggests that wound margins advance at a constant linear rate. If the area and perimeter of large and small wounds are measured at intervals and used to calculate absolute reduction in area, it would erroneously show that large wounds heal faster than small wounds. If these same measurements are used to calculate the percentage of reduction in wound area, it would erroneously show that small wounds heal faster than large wounds. To accurately measure the average progress toward wound closure, Gilman devised the following formula to calculate the rate of wound healing:

$$\bar{d} = \Delta A / \bar{p}$$

where $\bar{d}$ represents the average distance of advance of the wound margin, ΔA represents the change in area of the wound, and $\bar{p}$ is the average perimeter of the wound. Table 5.5 illustrates these concepts in large and small wounds.

Table 5.5 Assessing and Analyzing Wound Healing

Which of the wounds shown below is healing faster? Three analyses of the relative healing rate give three different answers.

Wound tracings at the beginning (solid) and at the end (dotted) of study period.

#1. Large ulcer

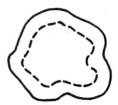

Initial area = 42.73   Final area = 21.81
Initial perimeter = 24.52   Final perimeter = 19.20

#2. Small ulcer

Initial area = 8.90   Final area = 1.37
Initial perimeter = 10.95   Final perimeter = 4.75

Analysis A
Comparison using reduction in absolute area
    Wound #1 reduction in area = 20.9 cm^2
    Wound #2 reduction in area = 7.5 cm^2
    Ratio #1/#2 = 2.8
This analysis concludes that wound #1 is healing about 3 times faster than wound #2.

Analysis B
Comparison using % reduction in area
    Wound #1 reduction in area = 49%
    Wound #2 reduction in area = 85%
    Ratio #2/#1 = 1.7
This analysis concludes that wound #2 is healing about 2 times faster than wound #1.

Analysis C
Comparison using d = $\Delta A/\bar{p}$
    Wound #1 $\bar{d}$ = .96 cm
    Wound #2 $\bar{d}$ = .96 cm
This analysis shows that the two wounds are healing at about the same rate.

To quantify multiple indices, Bates-Jensen developed a Pressure Sore Status Tool (PSST) with 15 parameters for assessing a pressure ulcer.[61,62,63] The PSST is a paper-and-pencil instrument used to identify location, shape, necrotic tissue amount, exudate type, exudate amount, surrounding skin color, peripheral tissue edema, peripheral tissue induration, granulation tissue, and epithelialization. Two items—location and shape—are not scored. The remaining items are scored on a 5-point likert scale. The individual items are summed, and the total score indicates overall wound status. Total scores range from 13 to 65. The tool allows for temporal tracking of individual characteristics as well as the total wound. Multiple scores show regeneration or degeneration of the ulcer. Reliability and validity studies of the PSST are ongoing. The tool has been automated and incorporates graphic capabilities and computerized tracking ability for monitoring progress or deterioration of pressure ulcers. (For a detailed look at the Bates-Jensen Pressure Sore Status Tool, see the Appendices.)

Cooper developed a 17-item Wound Characteristics Instrument (WCI) to assess open soft tissue post-surgical wounds healing by secondary intention.[64] She states that crucial indices reflecting the status of pressure ulcers have yet to be identified. According to Cooper, physical pressure ulcer assessment measures include size, visual appraisal of tissue and exudate, surrounding skin, ability of the patient to be involved in care, sensory state, edema, bacterial population, bacterial status, nutritional status, position of ulcer on body, duration of ulcer, and patient mobility.[65] The purpose of assessing the pressure ulcer must be identified because researchers and clinicians may need different measures. Cooper points to difficulties in measuring some of the requisite pressure ulcer indices.

Recently, the Sessing Scale was published as a simple, easy-to-use observational instrument that measures granulation tissue, infection, drainage, necrosis, and eschar on a 7-point scale to assess pressure ulcer healing.[66] The scale is scored by calculating the change in numerical values over successive wound assessments. Positive scores indicate ulcer improvement, and negative scores indicate worsening ulcers. The Sessing Scale has validity and reliability for assessment of the progression of pressure ulcers in clinical and research settings. Further reliability testing of the Sessing Scale is in progress.

Based on predictors of time to healing, VanRijswijk[67] estimates that the frequency of pressure ulcer reassessment should be at least weekly by a qualified health care professional. If other caregivers are caring for the patient, they should be taught to monitor the ulcer for signs of improvement or deterioration each time the dressing is changed.

Summary

Because assessment determines all other care given to patients with pressure ulcers, it must be comprehensive and orderly. The importance of risk assessment should not be underestimated. Patients must be assessed for pressure ulcer risk on admission to any health care agency and reassessed periodically as their condition changes.

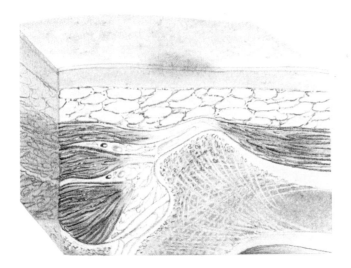

Stage I pressure ulcer: nonblanchable erythema of intact skin; the heralding lesion of skin ulceration.

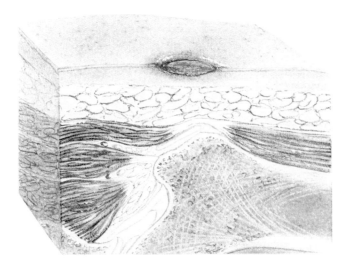

Stage II pressure ulcer: partial-thickness skin loss involving epidermis and/or dermis. The ulcer is superficial and presents clinically as an abrasion, blister, or shallow crater.

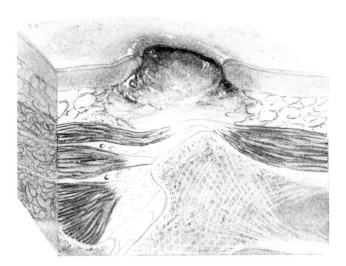

Stage III pressure ulcer: full-thickness skin loss involving damage or necrosis of subcutaneous tissue which may extend down to, but not through, underlying fascia. The ulcer presents clinically as a deep crater with or without undermining of adjacent tissue.

Stage IV pressure ulcer:
full-thickness skin loss with extensive destruction, tissue necrosis or damage to muscle, bone, or supporting structures (e.g., tendon, joint capsule, etc.)

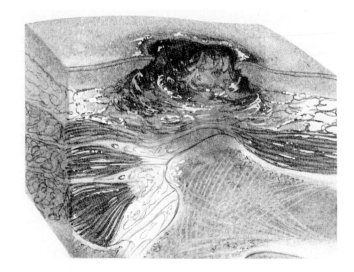

Closed pressure ulcer:
a large bursa-like cavity lined by chronic fibrosis extending to deep fascia or bone. There is drainage through a small sinus tract.

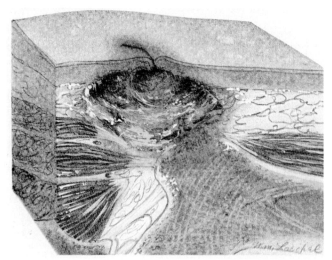

Pressure ulcer treatment may terminate, but risk assessment and prevention never do.

Staging systems are communication tools that provide information about the type of exposed tissue in the pressure ulcer. Staging is only a method for describing tissue and not a method for prescribing treatment or measuring pressure ulcer healing. Stage is a static measurement that is taken when the bottom of the ulcer becomes fully exposed. A four-stage pressure ulcer classification system does not address the problem of a closed pressure ulcer. Swab cultures of the wound surface should not be used to assess for infecting organisms. Currently, researchers are developing tools to more fully describe pressure ulcer characteristics and to measure pressure ulcer improvement or deterioration. The results of this work will improve communication among health care clinicians, educators, researchers, policy makers, regulating bodies, and third-party payors.

References

1. Shannon, M.L. "Pressure Sores," in Norris, C.M., ed. *Concept Clarification in Nursing.* Rockville, Md.: Aspen, 1982.

2. Versluysen, M. "How Elderly Patients with Femoral Fractures Develop Pressure Sores in Hospitals," *British Medical Journal of Clinical Research and Education* 292(6531): 1311-13, May 17, 1986.

3. Bergstrom, N., et al. "A Clinical Trial of the Braden Scale for Predicting Pressure Sore Risk," *Nursing Clinics of North America* 22(2): 417-28, 1987.

4. Richardson, R.R., and Meyer, P.R. "Prevalence and Incidence of Pressure Sores in Acute Spinal Cord Injuries," *Paraplegia* 19(4): 235-47, 1981.

5. Allman, R.M., et al. "Pressure Ulcer Risk Factors Among Hospitalized Patients with Activity Limitation," *JAMA* 273(11): 865-870, 1995.

6. Panel for the Prediction and Prevention of Pressure Ulcers in Adults. "Pressure Ulcer in Adults: Prediction and Prevention." Clinical Practice Guideline, No. 3. AHCPR Publication No. 92-0047. Rockville, Md.: U.S. Department of Health and Human Services, Agency for Health Care Policy and Research, May 1992.

7. Feedar, J.A. "Physical Therapy Modalities in Wound Healing," *Topics in Geriatric Rehabilitation* 9(4): 16, 1994.

8. Magnan, M.A. "Activity Intolerance," in Carpenito, L.J. *Nursing Diagnosis: Application to Clinical Practice,* 5th ed. Philadelphia: J.B. Lippincott, 1995.

9. Maklebust, J. "Pressure Ulcers: Etiology and Prevention," *Nursing Clinics of North America* 22(2): 359-377, 1987.

10. Krouskop, T.A. "A Synthesis of Factors That Contribute to Pressure Sore Formation," *Med Hypothesis* 11(2): 255-267, 1983.

11. Smith, T., et al. "Hospital Malnutrition," *Lancet* 1: 689-693, 1977.

12. Natow, A. "Nutrition in Prevention and Treatment of Pressure Sores," *Topics in Clinical Nursing,* 39-44, 1983.

13. Allman, R.M., et al. "Pressure Sores Among Hospitalized Patients," *Annals of Internal Medicine* 105(3): 337-42, 1986.

14. Bergstrom, N., and Braden, B.A. "A Prospective Study of Pressure Sore Risk Among Institutionalized Elderly," *Journal of the American Geriatric Society* 40(8): 747-758, 1992.

15. Breslow, R.A., et al. "The Importance of Dietary Protein in Healing Pressure Ulcers," *Journal of the American Geriatric Society* 41(4): 357-362, April 1993.

16. Pinchofsky-Devin, G.D., and Kaminski, M. "Correlation of Pressure Sores and Nutritional Status," *Journal of the American Geriatric Society* 34(6): 435-40, 1986.

17. Nutritional Screening Manual for Professionals Caring for Older Americans (1991). Nutrition Screening Initiative, 2626 Pennsylvania Ave. NW, Suite 301 Washington D.C., 20037.

18. Bergstrom, N., et al. "Treatment of Pressure Ulcers," Clinical Practice Guideline, No. 15. AHCPR Publication No. 95-0652. Rockville, Md.: U.S. Department of Health and Human Services, Public Health Service, Agency for Health Care Policy and Research. December 1994.

19. Kemp, M.G. "Protecting the Skin from Moisture," *Journal of Gerontological Nursing* 20(9): 8-14, 1994.

20. Maklebust, J., and Magnan, M. "Risk Factors Associated with Having a Pressure Ulcer: A Secondary Data Analysis," *Advances in Wound Care* 7(6): 25-42, 1994.

21. Brandeis, G.H., et al. "A Longitudinal Study of Risk Factors Associated with Formation of Pressure Ulcers in Nursing Homes," *Journal of the American Geriatric Society* 42(4): 388-93, 1994.

22. Shannon, M.L., and Skoga, P. "Pressure Ulcer Prevalence in Two General Hospitals," *Decubitus* 2(4): 38-40, 1989.

23. Lyder, C., et al. "Structured Skin Care Regimen to Prevent Perineal Dermatitis in the Elderly," *Journal of ET Nursing* 19: 12-16, 1992.

24. National Pressure Ulcer Advisory Panel. "Statement on Pressure Ulcer Prevention." NPUAP, 1992.

25. Jirovec, M.M., et al. "Nursing Assessments in the Inpatient Geriatric Population," *Nursing Clin of North America* 23(1): 219-225, 1988.

26. Anderson, T.P., and Andberg, M.M. "Psychosocial Factors Associated with Pressure Sores," *Arch Phys Med Rehabil* 60(8): 341-346, 1979.

27. Fuhrer, M.J., et al. "Depressive Symptomology in Persons with Spinal Cord Injury Who Reside in the Community," *Archives of Physical Medicine and Rehabilitation* 74(3): 255-60, March 1993.

28. Vidal, J., and Sarrias, M. "An Analysis of the Diverse Factors Concerned with the Development of Pressure Sores in Spinal Cord Patients," *Paraplegia* 29(4): 261-267, May 1991.

29. Norton, D., et al. *An Investigation of Geriatric Nursing Problems in Hospitals.* London: Churchill Livingstone, 1975 (original work published in 1962).

30. Gosnell, D.J. "An Assessment Tool to Identify Pressure Sores," *Nursing Research* 22: 55, 1973.

31. Braden, B.J., and Bergstrom, N. "A Conceptual Schema for the Study of the Etiology of Pressure Sores," *Rehabilitation Nursing* 12(1): 8-12, 1987.

32. Norton, D. "Calculating the Risk: Reflections on the Norton Scale," *Decubitus* 2(3): 24-31, 1989.

33. Gosnell, D.J. "Client Risk for Pressure Sores," Chapter 9 in Waltz, C.F., and Strickland, O.L., eds. *Measurement of Nursing Outcomes,* vol. 1: *Measuring Client Outcomes.* New York: Springer Publishing Co., 1988.

34. Maklebust, J., et al. "Pressure Ulcer Incidence in High-Risk Patients Managed on a Special Three-Layered Air Cushion," *Decubitus* 1(4): 30-40, 1988.

35. Bergstrom, N., et al. "The Braden Scale for Predicting Pressure Sore Risk," *Nursing Research* 36(4): 205-10, 1987.

36. Braden, B.J., and Bergstrom, N. "Clinical Utility of the Braden Scale for Predicting Pressure Sore Risk," *Decubitus* 2(3): 44-51, 1989.

37. Gosnell, D.J. "Assessment and Evaluation of Pressure Sores," *Nursing Clinics of North America* 22(2): 399-416, 1987.

38. Gosnell, D.J. "Pressure Sore Risk Assessment: A Critique. Part 1: the Gosnell Scale," *Decubitus* 2(3): 24-31, 1989.

39. Xakellis, G.C., et al. "A Comparison of Patient Risk for Pressure Ulcer Development with Nursing Use of Preventive Interventions," *Journal of the American Geriatrics Society* 40(12): 1250-1254, 1992.

40. Parish, L.C., et al. *The Decubitus Ulcer.* New York: Masson Publishing USA, 1980.

41. Bennett, M.A. "A Shading Strip to Facilitate Assessment of Darkly Pigmented Skin." Personal communication, 1995.

42. Vanni, L. "A Visual Analog Scale for Assessing Pain," Harper Hospital, 1994.

43. Ayello, E. "Teaching the Assessment of Patients with Pressure Ulcers," *Decubitus* 5(4): 53-54, 1992.

44. Bohannon, R.W., and Pfaller, B.A. "Documentation of Wound Surface Area from Tracings of Wound Perimeter," *Physical Therapy* 83(10): 1622-24, 1983.

45. Resch, C.S., et al. "Pressure Sore Volume Measurement," *Journal of the American Geriatric Society* 36: 444-446, 1988.

46. Maklebust, J. "Pressure Ulcer Staging Systems: Intent, Limitations, Expectations," *Advances in Wound Care* 8(4): 1995.

47. National Pressure Ulcer Advisory Panel. "Pressure Ulcers, Assessment Measurement, and Outcomes: Controversy to Consensus Proceedings of the Fourth National Conference," *Advances in Wound Care* 8(4): entire issue, July 1995.

48. Shea, J.D. "Pressure Sores: Classification and Management," *Clin Orthop Related Res* 12: 89-100, 1975.

49. National Pressure Ulcer Advisory Panel. "Pressure Ulcers: Incidence, Economics, Risk Assessment: Consensus Development Conference Statement." West Dundee, Ill.: S-N Publications, 1989.

50. Jeter, K.F. "1990: The Decade for New Definitions," *Gaymar pressure ulcer forum* 4(4): 1-3, 1989.

51. Lewis, V.L., et al. "The Diagnosis of Osteomyelitis in Patients with Pressure Sores," *Plastic and Reconstructive Surgery,* 81(2): 229-32, December 1988.

52. Rousseau, P. "Pressure Ulcers in an Aging Society," *Wounds* 1(2): 135-141, 1989.

53. Kucan, J.O., et al. "Comparison of Silver Sulfadiazine, Povidone Iodine, and Physiologic Saline in the Treatment of Chronic Pressure Ulcers," *Journal of the American Geriatric Society* 29(5): 232-35, May 1981.

54. Feedar, J.A. "Wound Evaluation and Treatment Planning," *Topics in Geriatric Rehabilitation* 9(4): 35-42, 1994.

55. Bryan, C.S., et al. "Bacteremia Associated with Decubitus Ulcers," *Archives of Internal Medicine* 143(11): 2093-95, November 1983.

56. Allman, R.M. "Epidemiology of Pressure Sores in Different Populations," *Decubitus* 2(2): 30-33, 1989.

57. Sapico, F.L., et al. "Quantitative Microbiology of Pressure Sores in Different Stages of Healing," *Diagnosis and Microbiology of Infectious Diseases* 5(1): 31-38, May 1986.

58. Krizek, T.J., and Robson, M.C. "Biology of Surgical Infection," *Surg Clinics of North America* 55(6): 1261-67, December 1975.

59. Lazarus, G.S., et al. "Definitions and Guidelines for Assessment of Wounds and Evaluation of Healing," *Archives of Dermatology* 130: 489-493, April 1994.

60. Gilman, T.H. "Parameter for Measurement of Wound Closure," *Wounds* 2(3): 95-101, May-June, 1990.

61. Bates-Jensen, B.M., et al. "Validity and Reliability of the Pressure Sore Status Tool," *Decubitus* 5(6): 20-28, 1992.

62. Bates-Jensen, B.M. "The Pressure Sore Status Tool," *Topics in Geriatric Rehabilitation* 9(4): 17-34, 1994.

63. Bates-Jensen, B.M. "Indices for Pressure Ulcer Assessment: The Pressure Sore Status Tool," *Advances in Wound Care* 8(4): 1995.

64. Cooper, D.M. "Human Wound Assessment: Status Report and Implications for Clinicians," *AACN Clinical Issues in Critical Care Nursing* 1(3): 533-563.

65. Cooper, D.M. "Pressure Ulcer Assessment: Requisite Indices," *Advances in Wound Care* 8(4): 1995.

66. Ferrell, B.A., et al. "The Sessing Scale for Assessment of Pressure Ulcer Healing," *Journal of the American Geriatric Society* 43(1): 37-40, 1995.

67. VanRijswjk, L. "Pressure Ulcers: Frequency of Reassessment," *Advances in Wound Care* 8(4): 1995.

CHAPTER 6

Pressure Ulcer Prevention

In the 1990s, pressure ulcers continue to be a major cause of patient morbidity and mortality. The pressure ulcer problem offers nursing and other health care disciplines both an opportunity and a responsibility to help reduce its incidence. The team approach is recommended by clinical experts in the field.[1-5] Nurses should step forward and initiate skin care teams with members from all interested disciplines. Nurses also can help raise the level of pressure ulcer awareness and pressure ulcer prevention within their nursing units and health care settings.

The primary purpose of pressure ulcer prevention programs is to reduce the occurrence of pressure ulcers. Preventing pressure ulcers may not be easy, but there are many interventions that one can use to assist in preserving patients' skin and underlying tissue. The first step is knowing which patients are at risk for skin breakdown. It is important to identify each patient's internal risk factors so that care plans for prevention can be individually tailored. Knowing which factors are implicated helps one select specific prophylactic nursing interventions to reduce pressure ulcer risk. Whenever a patient's condition changes, risk should be re-evaluated so that prevention measures can be updated.[2-4] Research demonstrates that nursing care devoted to the prevention of pressure ulcers in terms of time and frequency is significantly related to effective outcomes.[6]

For any plan to be effective, it must include patient and family education about pressure ulcer prevention.[7] Teaching may be the most important intervention. Prior to selecting prevention strategies, mutual nurse-patient-family decisions must be made about:
- Goals of care
- Educational needs
- Nutritional management
- Correct body positions
- Turning and repositioning schedules
- Support surfaces
- Skin care
- Monitoring changes in risk status

Goals of care

Goals of care need to be established before determining a plan for pressure ulcer prevention.[2,7,8] If a terminally ill individual desires only comfort measures and if pressure ulcer prevention procedures are painful and burdensome, the patient's wishes should be documented and supported.[8] However, many terminally ill patients prefer to have pressure ulcer prevention measures instituted.[9] Some hospice organizations have established nursing standards of care for hospice patients that include both pressure ulcer prevention and treatment. One of these standards prescribes nursing actions to achieve the goals mutually derived by the patient and the nurse.[10]

Educational needs

Learning needs should be established with the individual or the caregiver.[7] For information on adult learning principles and patient and family education, see Chapter 11.

Nutritional management

Nutrition is important for maintaining tissue integrity. There is a strong relationship between nutritional status and pressure ulceration, and yet nutrition is an area that often is overlooked by nurses and doctors.[11] Patients and caregivers need to be taught the significance of good nutrition and the relationship between nutritional status and pressure ulcers. Overall goals of care and patient and family preferences should guide decisions for nutritional management.[2,5]

Dietary intake

Whenever possible, individuals should have a well-balanced diet that includes foods from all four basic food groups. Studies suggest that protein needs of healthy adults are met by the Nutritional Screening Initiative.[12] This consists of 0.8 grams of protein per kilogram of body weight. The average-size healthy adult can meet this by eating one or two 3-ounce servings of protein in the form of meat, meal, cheese, or eggs each day.

Sufficient nutrients to meet individual metabolic needs must be available.[11,13] One of the guiding principles of good nutitional support is maintenance of positive nitrogen balance. An adequate diet will provide enough calories for energy needs and additional protein for restoring muscle mass and wound healing. This is anabolism and positive nitrogen balance.

Adequate dietary intake to prevent malnutrition greatly reduces the risk for new pressure ulcer formation. For patients on oral intake, it is important that nursing personnel monitor both the quantity and quality of food eaten. If intake is questionable, dietary consultation is indicated for complete nutritional evaluation. A daily calorie count can help the dietitian evaluate the patient's actual intake. A patient who is not receiving adequate calories will break down glycogen and fat reserves and also will start metabolizing the body's proteins for energy. When this occurs, the body is in a state of catabolism and negative nitrogen balance.[13] In malnourished individuals, nurses and dietitians should cater to patients' food likes and dislikes and any special dietary needs. Assistance with meals, monitoring of patients' swallowing ability, and assessment of dietary tolerance must be ongoing by both bedside caregivers and dietary personnel.[2,3,4,5]

Laboratory tests

No single biochemical or physical measure indicates a person's nutritional health. Laboratory tests, when combined with physical measures, can have nutritional implications. Depressed serum protein, serum albumin, and transferrin levels are indicators of poor nutritional status. In general, the longer a starvation period, the greater the drop in standard plasma levels of these substances. Significant hypoproteinemia will result in interstitial edema. The resulting edema interposes fluid between the cells and subsequently reduces tissue oxygenation. This edema may play a role in the genesis of pressure ulceration in elderly, malnourished individuals.[13]

Albumin is a body protein, and its concentration in the serum is used as a gross indicator of nutritional state. Serum albumin, with its relatively long half-life of about 20 days, decreases slowly during malnutrition. Normal serum albumin levels range from 3.5-5.0 g/dl. Serum albumin deficits are rated as mild, moderate, or severe (see Table 6.1).[11] A subnormal serum albumin level represents late manifestation of protein deficiency.

Pressure ulcers have been found to be associated with severely malnourished patients.[11,14,15] In one study, the stage of pressure ulcer was correlated with the degree of hypoalbuminemia.[11] Hypoalbuminemia refers to serum albumin concentrations <3.5 g/dl. Serum albumin levels of patients at risk for pressure ulcers should be monitored by nurses. Patients with significant hypoproteinemia need alternative methods of feeding.

Body weight

Many patients are unable to eat because of their illness or NPO status. At-risk individuals should be weighed weekly. Change from previous weight to present weight, together with onset of illness, provides a valuable index of nutritional assessment. A history of unintentional weight loss and/or weight for height of less than 85% of standard has been related to functional consequences of malnutrition.[13] (See Table 6.2 for recommended weight/height on the Nutrition Information Form developed at Harper Hospital in the Detroit Medical Center.)

Body weight can be measured on an upright scale for ambulatory patients. Bedscales should be used for measuring weight of bedfast patients. A physician, nurse, or dietitian should be notified of a 10-pound or greater weight loss during any 6-month period. In patients at risk for malnutrition, an involuntary change of 5% of body weight is predictive of a drop in serum albumin.[5]

Table 6.1 Serum Albumin Deficit Levels

Mild	3.0 - 3.5 g/dl
Moderate	2.5 - 3.0 g/dl
Severe	<2.5 g/dl

Table 6.2 Assessment Recommendations for Determining Proper Weight, Caloric Levels, and Degree of Nutritional Depletion

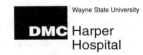 Wayne State University
DMC Harper Hospital

FOOD AND NUTRITION SERVICES
Nutritional Assessment

Recommended Weight for Height:
Female: 100 lbs per 5 ft + 5 lbs per inch > 5 ft
Male: 106 lbs per 5 ft + 6 lbs per inch > 5 ft

> Estimated daily calorie levels are determined by multiplying the BEE and the appropriate Stress and/or Activity Factor.

**Basal Energy Expenditure
Female: 655 + (9.6 x wt in kg) + (1.8 x ht in cm) - (4.7 x age in years)
Male: 66 + (13.7 x wt in kg) + (5.0 x ht in cm) - (6.8 x age in years)

**Stress Factor:

	Stress Factor	gms Protein per kg IBW
Surgery:	1.1 - 1.3	1.5 - 2.0
Infection:	1.3 - 1.5	1.5 - 2.5
Maintenance:	1.3	0.8 - 1.2
Repletion:	1.5	1.2 - 2.0
Pulmonary:	1.0 - 1.6	1.0 - 2.0
Cancer:	1.3 - 1.5	0.8 - 2.0
AIDS:	1.3 - 1.5	1.0 - 2.0
Liver Failure:	1.5 - 1.75	0.5 - 1.5
Cardiac Failure:	1.0 - 1.2	1.2 - 1.5
Renal Failure:	1.3 - 1.8	0.5 - 1.0
		HD: 1.0 - 1.2
		PD: 1.2 - 1.5
Cystic Fibrosis	1.5 - 2.0	1.5 - 2.0

Activity Factor:
Bed rest: 1.0
Active without stress: 1.3
Cardiac Failure: 1.2 - 1.3

Fluid Requirements:
<50 years old: 1500 cc for first 20 kg
20 cc per kg for remaining kg ABW
>50 years old: 1500 cc for first 20 kg
15 cc per kg for remaining kg ABW

Degree of Nutritional Depletion/Risk/Needs:

	Mild	Moderate	Severe
Age:	18 - 64 yrs	<18 yrs or > 64 yrs	<18 yrs or >64 yrs
Weight:	<5% loss/6 mo.	5% - 10% loss/1 mo.-6 mo.	>5% loss/1 mo.
			>10% loss/6 mo.
	<5% - 10% of IBW with no hx. of unplanned wt. loss in past yr. 85-90% UBW	10% - 20% above or 20 - 30% below IBW 75 - 84% UBW	>20% IBW <70% IBW <74% UBW
Feeding Regimen:	Decresed Oral Intake	Poor Intake/NPO x 5 days Parenteral/Enteral	Poor Intake/NPO x 5 days Parenteral/Enteral
Albumin:	2.8 - 3.5	2.1 - 2.7	<2.1
TLC:	1500 - 1800	900 - 1500	<900
Transferrin:	150 - 200	100 - 150	<100
Diagnosis:	Minor Surgery/ Minor Infection	High Risk Diagnosis/ Problems*	High Risk Diagnosis/ Problems*

*High Risk Diagnosis/Problems May Include:

Major Surgery	Cancer	Decubitus Ulcer	Persistent Nausea,
Major Trauma	AIDS	Inflammatory Bowel	Vomiting, Diarrhea
Gastrointestinal Fistula	Respiratory Failure	Renal Failure/Dialysis	
Abdominal Surgery/ Resection	Malabsorption	Substance Abuse	

** ASPEN Certified Nutrition Support Dietician Review Manual, 1989, 1993
ADA Manual of Clinical Dietetics, 1988
ADA Dietitians in Nutrition Support Conference, 1990

Nutritional goals

The nutritional goal is to ensure a diet containing adequate nutrients to maintain tissue integrity. Oral and cutaneous signs of vitamin and mineral deficiencies should be monitored.[5,13] Some clinical experts recommend supplementing or supporting the intake of protein, calories, Vitamin C, and zinc. Also, a daily high-potency vitamin and mineral supplement is recommended if the person has suspected vitamin deficiency. If an individual has inadequate dietary intake, an involuntary weight loss of 5% of body weight, or a serum albumin level lower than 3.5 g/dl, a dietitian should be consulted for more thorough nutritional screening. (See Table 6.3 for individual patient nutritional screening.)

If thorough nutritional assessment confirms malnutrition, assisted oral feedings, dietary supplements, or tube feedings may be recommended to achieve positive nitrogen balance. This will require approximately 30-35 calories per kilogram of body weight per day and 1.25 to 1.5 grams of protein per kilogram of body weight per day. As much as 2 grams of protein per kilogam of body weight per day may be needed to place a malnourished individual into positive nitrogen balance.[5] (See Table 6.4 for the caloric content of various nutritional supplements and Table 6.5 for recommended tube feeding rates and concentrations.)

Persons at risk for malnutrition need to have a nutritional screening assessment repeated at least every 3 months.[5] Repeat measurements of serial protein markers, such as serum albumin, should be used to evaluate efforts of nutritional support.[13]

Managing pressure

Pressure management begins with an understanding of proper body positioning, the importance of turning and repositioning, and the advantages of suitable support surfaces for sleeping (overlays, mattresses, specialty beds) and sitting.

Pressure and body position

It is generally accepted that unrelieved pressure of sufficient intensity and duration to cause tissue necrosis leads to pressure ulceration.[2,5] Compression of soft tissue is thought to alter perfusion of the capillaries. Using a laser doppler to study the response to constant, low-level, compressive pressure, investigators found a great deal of skin blood flow variability over the trochanters of elderly persons at risk for pressure ulcers.[16] Another study used thermography to examine the effects of reactive hyperemia in skin overlying the greater trochanter of the femur. This experiment showed that subjects had significantly increased skin blood flow over the trochanteric region after lying for 1-2 hours on a hospital mattress. There was good correlation between magnitudes of pressure and vascular response within each individual subject. The longer the pressure application, the longer it took for the temperature to return to baseline levels after relief of pressure.[17] The authors suggest that temperature of a traumatized area of skin does not return to baseline until long after skin color returns to normal. They also propose that visual determination of erythema

Table 6.3 Assessing Patient Nutrition

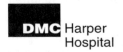 Harper Hospital

FOOD AND NUTRITION SERVICES
Nutritional Assessment

S:

O: Age_____ Sex _____ Ht _____ Weight: ABW _____ UBW _____ Adjusted Wt _____

Admit _____ IBW _____

Diagnosis: _____   PMH: _____

_____   _____

Lab Values: Nutritinally Pertinent Medication:

Albumin_____   Cholesterol _____   (   ) Insulin   (   ) Coumadin

BUN _____   Creatinine _____   (   ) Steroids   (   ) Oral Hypoglycemics

Glucose_____   Other_____   (   ) MAO   (   ) Vitamins/Minerals

(   ) None   (   ) Other_____

Current Diet: _____   Feeding Problems: (   ) Chewing

Food Allergies: Y   N   (   ) Swallowing

Special Diet at Home: Y   N   (   ) Other

Previously Instructed: Y   N   (   ) None

Diet Instruction Given: _____

GI: _____ Nausea _____ Emesis _____ Diarrhea _____ Constipation _____ N/A

Current Nutrition Support:

(   ) TPN Calories _____ NP Cal: _____ Pro: _____ gm CHO: _____ gm

(   ) TF Fat: _____ gm _____ cc Free Water _____% RDA Vit/Min

A: Wt is _____ % IBW/UBW

    Estimated Needs: _____ Cal_____ gm Protein   Fluid: _____ cc

    BEE: _____ Stress Factor: _____ Progm/kg IBW: _____

Nutrition Status: (   ) High Risk   (   ) Moderate Risk

(   ) Low Risk   (   ) Not Currently Compromised

Comments:

P. Recommendation/Plan:

(   ) Continue present regimen

(   ) Change diet or nutritional therapy

(   ) Oral supplements: _____

(   ) Calorie count x _____days

(   ) Will remain available for further consultation as needed.

Goal Nutrition Support: Product Name: _____ Rate:_____

Cal: _____   NP Cal:_____ Pro: _____ gm   CHO:_____ gm

Fat: _____gm _____cc Free Water _____% RDA Vit/Min

Date: _____ R.D. Beeper#_____

Table 6.4 Caloric Content of Nutritional Supplements

HARPER HOSPITAL ENTERAL FORMULARY

3990 John R
Detroit, Michigan 48201

PRODUCT	ENSURE® Liquid Nutrition	PROMOTE™ High Protein Liquid Nutrition	OSMOLITE® Isotonic Liquid Nutrition	ENSURE PLUS® High Calorie Liquid Nutrition	PULMOCARE® Specialized Nutrition for Pulmonary Patients	VITAL® HN Nutritionally Complete Partially Hydrolyzed Diet	CARNATION INSTANT BREAKFAST
Calories Liter/Can/Pkg	1060/254	1000/237	1060/254	1500/355	1500/355	1000/300	1120/280
Protein (g) Liter/Can/Pkg	37.2/8.8	62.4/14.8	37.2/8.8	55/13	62.6/14.8	41.7/12.5	58/15
Fat (g) Liter/Can/Pkg	37.2/8.8	26/6.2	38.5/9.1	53.3/12.6	92.1/21.8	10.8/3.2	35/8
CHO (g) Liter/Can/Pkg	145/34.3	130/30.8	145/34.3	200/47.3	106/25	185/55.4	136/35
Protein Source	Sodium & Calcium Caseinates, Soy Protein Isolate	Sodium & Calcium Caseinates. Soy Protein Isolate	Sodium & Calcium Caseinates. Soy Protein Isolate	Sodium & Calcium Caseinates. Soy Protein Isolate	Sodium & Calcium Caseinates	Partially Hydrolyzed Whey, Meat, and Soy. Free Amino Acids	Nonfat Dry Milk, Calcium Caseinate, Sweet Dairy Whey
Fat Source	Corn Oil	High-Oleic Safflower Oil (50%) *Canola Oil (30%) MCT Oil (20%)	MCT Oil (50%) Corn Oil (40%) Soy Oil (10%)	Corn Oil	Corn Oil	Safflower Oil (55%) MCT Oil (45%)	Milk Fat
Carbohydrate Source	Corn Syrup, Sucrose	Hydrolyzed Cornstarch, Sucrose	Hydrolyzed Cornstarch	Corn Syrup, Sucrose	Hydrolyzed Cornstarch, Sucrose	Hydrolyzed Cornstarch, Sucrose	Lactose, Sucrose Corn Syrup Solids
Na (mEq/L)	36.8	40.4	27.6	49.6	57	20.3	11.3/8 oz.
K (mEq/L)	40	50.6	25.9	54	48.6	34.1	18.7/8 oz.
Osmolality	470	350	300	690	490	500	720
NP Cal Liter	911	751	911	1280	1250	833	888
Amt to meet RDA (ml)	1887	1250	1887	1420	947	1500	1060
Cost Per 8 oz. Serving	.55	.99	.90	.95	1.22	4.03	.48
Comments	Lactose Free. All Purpose, Low Residue. Can be used on Clear Liquid Diets. Good Taste.	High Protein. Lactose Free. Low Residue. *Source of Omega 6 F.A.	Isotonic. Low Residue. Bland Taste. Lactose Free.	Lactose Free. High Calorie. Low Residue. Normal Pro. Good Taste.	55% Fat 28% CHO Good for Pumonary Patients Reduce CO2	Chemically Defined. Peptides and Free Amino Acids. Use for Malabsorption.	Contains Lactose Oral. Above Analysis when Mixed with Whole Milk.
Tube/Oral	Tube/Oral	Tube/Oral	Tube/Oil	Tube/Oral	Tube/Oral	Tube/Oral	Oral

(continued)

Table 6.4 Caloric Content of Nutritional Supplements *(continued)*

HARPER HOSPITAL ENTERAL FORMULARY

3990 John R
Detroit, Michigan 48201

PRODUCT	JEVITY® Isotonic Liquid Nutrition with Fiber	VIVONEX T.E.N. Elemental	AMIN AID	HEPATC AID II	POLYCOSE® Glucose Polymers (Liquid)	PROMOD® Protein Supplement
Calories Liter/Can/Pkg	1060/250	1000/300	1956/665/pkg	1180/400/Pkg	2000/380	/560
Protein (g) Liter/Can/Pkg	44.4/10.5	38.2/11.4	19.4/6.6/Pkg	44/15/Pkg	-/	-75/100 gm
Fat (g) Liter/Can/Pkg	36.8/8.7	2.7/0.8	46.2/15.7/Pkg	36/12.3/Pkg	-	-/12/100 gm
CHO (g) Liter/Can/Pkg	151.7/35.9	205.5/61.6	366/124/pkg	168/57.3/Pkg	500/94/100 gm	/13.4/100 gm
Protein Source	Sodium & Calcium Caseinates	Free Amino Acids	Essential Amino Acids plus Histidine	Essential & Non-Essential Amino Acids	-0-	Whey
Fat Source	MCT Oil(50%) Corn Oil (40%) Soy Oil (10%)	Safflower Oil	Partially Hydrogenated Soybean Oil	Partially Hydrogenated Soybean Oil	-0-	None added
Carbohydrate Source	Hydrolyzed Cornstarch, Soy Polysaccharide	Maltodextrin Modified Starch	Maltodextrin, Sucrose	Maltodextrin, Sucrose	Glucose Polymers	None Added
Na (mEq/L)	40.4	20	<15	<14	30/L <5 (100 gm)	11 (100 gm)
K (mEq/L)	40.0	20	0	0	0	33 (100 gm)
Osmolality	300	630	700	560		
NP Cal Liter	882	847	1882	1004		
Amt to meet RDA (ml)	1321	2000	-	-		
Cost Per 8 oz. Serving	1.00	4.28	7.81	14.41	0.30 per oz	0.19 per 5 gm Pro
Comments	Contains Fiber, Lactose Free, Gluten Free. Isotonic. 50% MCT. Use to normalize bowel function.	Elemental 100% Free Amino Acids. Use for Malabsorption. Very Low Fat.	Renal Failure. High Cal. Low Pro. Essential, Amino Acids. Negligible Electrolytes. No Vitamins.	Liver Failure. High BCAA. Lessens Risk of Protein Induced Encephalopathy. No Vitamins.	CHO Supplement, Powder	Protein Supplement 10 gm in 240 cc fluid 5 gm pro in 1 scoop 6.6 gm weight
Tube/Oral	Tube	Tube	Tube	Tube/Oral	Tube/Oral	Tube/Oral

Table 6.4 Caloric Content of Nutritional Supplements *(continued)*

HARPER HOSPITAL ENTERAL FORMULARY

3990 John R
Detroit, Michigan 48201

PRODUCT	ENSURE® PUDDING	MCT OIL	GLUCERNA® Specialized Nutrition with Fiber for Patients with Abnormal Glucose Tolerance	CITRISOURCE	NEPRO™ Specialized Liquid Nutrition (Renal Dialyis)	SUPLENA™ Specialized Liquid Nutrition (Renal Pre-Dialysis)
Calories Liter/Can/Pkg	/250/5 oz can	7667/	1000/237	-/180/serv	2000/475	2000/475
Protein (g) Liter/Can/Pkg	6.8/5 oz can/	-	41.8/9.9	/8.8/serv	69.9/16.6	30/7.1
Fat (g) Liter/Can/Pkg	/9.7/5 oz can	-	55.7/13.2	/0/serv	95.6/22.7	95.6/22.7
CHO (g) Liter/Can/Pkg	/34/5 oz can	-	93.7/22.2	/36/serv	215.2/51.1	255.2/60.6
Protein Source	Nonfat Milk	-0-	Sodium & Calcium Caseinates	Whey Protein Concentrate	Calcium Magnesium, Sodium Caseinates	Sodium & Calcium Caseinates
Fat Source	Partially Hydrogenated Soybean Oil	Coconut Oil	High-Oleic Safflower Oil (85%) Unhydrogenated Soy Oil (15%)	-0-	High-Oleic Safflower Oil (90%) Soy Oil (10%)	High-Oleic Safflower Oil (90%) Soy Oil (10%)
Carbohydrate Source	Lactose, Sucrose, Modified Food Starch	-0-	Hydrolyzed Cornstarch, Soy Polysaccharide, Fructose	Hydrolyzed Cornstarch, Sucrose	Hydrolyzed Cornstarch, Sucrose	Hydrolyzed Cornstarch, Sucrose
Na (mEq/L)	10.4/5 oz can	-	40	1.5/serv	36.1	34
K (mEq/L)	8.4/5 oz can	-	40	0.2/serv	27.0	28.5
Osmolality			375	700	635	600
NP Cal Liter			833		1720	1880
Amt to meet RDA (ml)	-	-	1422	-	946*	946*
Cost Per 8 oz. Serving	0.67	0.75 per oz	1.54	0.98	2.06	1.51
Comments	Pudding Supplement. Contains Milk. Gluten Free.	Does not contain EFA	Low Cho for abnormal Glucose Tolerance. Contains Fiber. Lactose Free.	Fat Free for Clear Liquid Diets Lactose Free Oral Supplement	Hi Cal Mod Pro Low Lytes for dialysis patients. *except Mg, P, Vit A, Vit D	For predialysis renal patients. High Cal. Low Pro. Low Lytes *except Mg, P, Vit A, Vit D
Tube/Oral	Oral	Tube/Oral	Tube/Oral	Oral	Tube/Oral	Tube/Oral

Table 6.4 Recommended Guidelines for Starting Tube Feedings

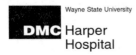
Wayne State University

DMC Harper
Hospital

RECOMMENDED GUIDELINES FOR STARTING TUBE FEEDINGS

- Iso-osmolar formulations may be started at full strength. Use pump with fiber-containing products.
- Hyperosmolar products should be started at 1/2 strength and advance to full strength as tolerated.
- Continuous —start at 25-50 ml/hour and increase by 10-25 ml increments every 24 hours until fluid and caloric goals are achieved.
  —flush tube every 4-6 hours.
- Bolus —start at 100 ml every 4 hours and increase as above every 4-6 hours.
  —check residuals prior to each feeding.
  —flush tube after each feeding.
- Do not increase rate and strength at same time.
- If feeding not tolerated, reduce rate and strength and gradually increase.
- Elevate head 45 degrees or Semi Fowler position.

1. Diet Manuals are located in each nursing station and in the hospital library.
2. Diet Manuals state the interpretation of the order and also indicate usual nutritional adequacy of the diet.
3. Clear Liquid Diets are high in sodium, provide minimum calories or nutrients, unless supplemented.
4. Full Liquid Diets are high in lactose. They can be modified if needed.
5. A Regular, No Added Salt Diet order will be interpreted as 4 Gram Na.
6. Cardiac Diet will be interpreted as a Low Cholesterol, 4 Gram Na.
7. Fat Controlled Diet for Cardiology should be written as a Low Cholesterol, Low Saturated Fat Diet.
8. Low Fat Diet order will be interpreted as a Low Fat Diet for GI patients, containing 40 to 50 grams of fat, both saturated and polyunsaturated.
9. Low Protein Diet orders will be interpreted as 40 gm. Pro.
10. Nutrition assessments are completed on a pink nutrition assessment form and placed in the progress notes.
11. Diet orders entered directly into Technicon will usually be implemented sooner. (Delays due to transcription are avoided).
12. Changes in diet orders need to be entered into HOWIE promptly and previous diet orders need to be deleted for changes to be processed correctly.
13. Trays cannot be served unless there is a written order on the diet sheet.
14. Nonselective admission trays are usually served for the first two to three meals. The number of admission trays a patient receives depends on his time of admission and when a written diet order is received by the dietary office.
15. Diet technicians pick-up patients' menus and assist patients with selections, if patient is available. Menus need to be completed by 10:00 a.m. Menus are distributed the evening before.
16. Registered dietitians are available to provide nutrition education for patients and family, inservice programs, nutritional assessments, etc. Requests should be entered through HOWIE, as a consult. Mis-O-Grams should not be used for this purpose.
17. Please feel free to contact the dietitians for your assigned area to have your questions answered or to assist with patient feeding problems. Dietitians do carry beepers. Beeper numbers are available at the nursing station.
18. Food and beverages sent to the floors are for patient use.

does not indicate the full extent of damage and may be an inadequate assessment of hyperemia. The intrinsic features of each person's vascular response to normal mechanical forces experienced in the sidelying position appear to be a sensitive measure of the individual's susceptibility to pressure ulceration.[17]

Findings from a study of the effects of different turn intervals on skin of healthy older adults showed the greatest increase in skin surface temperature at the end of 2-hour turn intervals when compared with shorter turn intervals of 1 and 1½ hours.[18] The authors were attempting to substantiate the traditional 2-hour turning regimen taught in schools of nursing.

If patients are at risk because of immobility, they must be repositioned frequently enough to prevent persistent reddened or hyperemic areas of skin. The temperature of previous hyperemic areas may provide additional cues to skin recovery from pressure. Repetitive pressure against the skin and underlying tissue, without adequate recovery time, contributes greatly to pressure-induced ischemia and necrosis. Both duration and intensity of pressure need to be reduced in individuals at risk for pressure ulcers.

Body positioning to manage pressure

Body positioning techniques can be an important way to decrease pressure on vulnerable soft tissue over bony prominences.

Correct body positions while in bed

Individuals should be positioned so that they are not lying on a reddened area of the body. All donut-shaped products or ring cushions that totally surround an ischemic area should be avoided. Such products tend to reduce the blood flow to an even wider area of tissue.[19] If the reddened area is on an extremity, pressure to the area can be reduced by suspending the extremity with a pillow.[5] Pillows also can be placed between the legs so that apposing knees and ankles do not exert pressure on one another (see Figure 6.1). When resting in the sidelying position, persons should never be placed directly on the greater trochanter of the femur.[2,5] Caregivers should be taught to place patients in a 30-degree laterally inclined position (see Figure 6.1) so as to simultaneously avoid pressure over the sacrum and trochanter.[20] Pillows or foam positioning wedges can be used to maintain this 30-degree sidelying position until the patient is repositioned. One investigator found that hyperemic response to pressure over the trochanter was reduced in the sidelying position when the legs were flexed compared to the same sidelying position with the legs extended.[17] Practitioners at one Veterans Hospital have determined that eliminating the 90-degree sidelying position is the responsibility of every person caring for an individual who is at risk for pressure ulcers.[21]

Research findings have demonstrated that pressure over heels was difficult to reduce below capillary closing pressure, even on specialty support surfaces.[22] Consequently, heels should be suspended totally to avoid pressure on the small surface area of the rounded bony prominence[2,5] (see Figure 6.1). This can be accomplished by

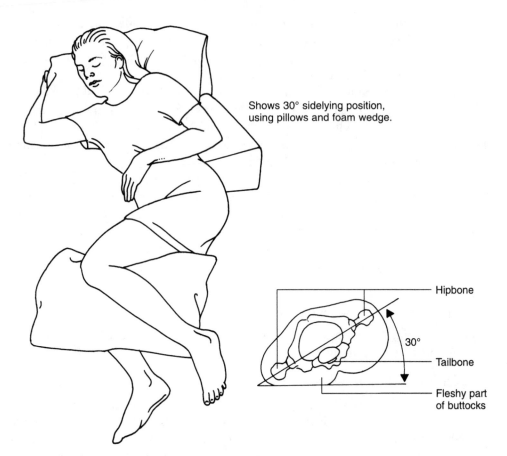

Shows 30° sidelying position, using pillows and foam wedge.

Hipbone

30°

Tailbone

Fleshy part of buttocks

30-degree laterally inclined position with proper pillow positioning

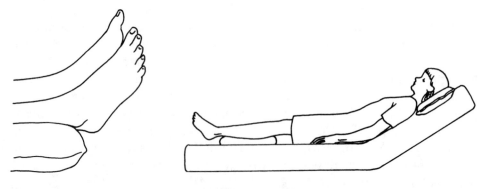

Proper heel placement

Head of bed elevation limited to 30° or less

Figure 6.1 Proper Positioning in Bed

supporting the back of the calves with pillows or foam devices, although care should be taken to avoid knee contraction. Clinicians have found innovative ways to elevate heels off the mattress by using inflatable water wings or swim floats and by using partially filled I.V. bags under the Achilles tendon and heels.

The angle of the supporting bed surface affects the patient's risk for mechanical damage to the skin. The head of the bed should be raised as little as possible (no more than 30 degrees) so that it does not cause the patient to slide down in bed (see Figure 6.1). Sliding while in a semi-reclining position can cause frictional and shear forces that disrupt blood flow to soft tissue in the sacral region.[2,5] Individuals who must have the head of the bed elevated during meals or tube feedings usually can have the head lowered about 1 hour after eating. People who must have the head elevated for other medical reasons must have skin in the sacral region monitored frequently for pressure areas. If there is a question about proper positioning, a physical therapist can offer valuable suggestions.

Turning and repositioning to decrease pressure duration

Through its sensory system, the body normally detects persistent local pressure before ischemia occurs. A person with an intact nervous system compensates for local pressure by shifting weight frequently while sitting, standing, or even during sleep.[23] Healthy people change position as frequently as every 15 minutes. Patients who have mental status changes or spinal cord injuries may not feel pressure and, consequently, do not move to avoid discomfort. These patients need to be reminded to turn or need to be repositioned at least every 2 hours by nursing personnel. Some patients need turning more frequently than every 2 hours; repositioning depends on the ability of soft tissue to tolerate the effects of pressure.

To avoid effects of friction and shear forces, patients should be lifted, rather than dragged, across the bed surface. For additional protection from abrasive frictional forces, film or hydrocolloid dressings can be placed on the skin over susceptible pressure points of the body.[2,3] A practical way to decrease friction over the elbows and heels is to have the patient wear socks and long sleeves.

To help avoid the hazards of immobility, patients should be rehabilitated to their maximum level of functioning.[2] Physical therapists should be consulted to teach bed mobility to bedbound patients. Patients should move or be repositioned frequently enough to allow any reddened areas of skin to recover from the effects of pressure. Usually, turning is done at least every 2 hours, but it may be more frequent, depending on the tissue's tolerance to pressure. A turn clock may be a helpful reminder of correct body positions and turning times[24] (see Figure 6.2). Both persons at risk for pressure ulcers and their caregivers can be taught to supplement full body turning schedules with smaller shifts in body weight.[25]

There are devices that can help some bed patients assist with repositioning. Siderails are helpful in increasing bed mobility of many bedbound individuals. Persons can either turn independently while holding on to siderails or hold them to assist caregivers with turning. An overbed frame with attached trapeze assists some pa-

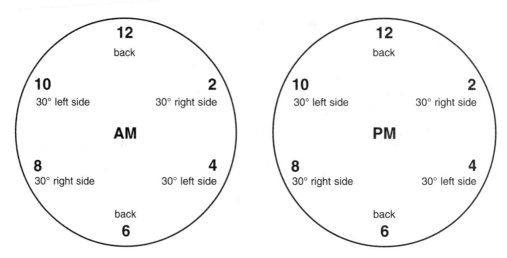

Figure 6.2 Using a turn clock for a turning schedule

tients to shift body weight independently. They can use upper body strength to lift their buttocks off the bed and avoid abrasive friction burns to the skin.

Body positioning while sitting

People who are at risk for pressure ulcers are at greater risk while sitting than when they are lying down. Because of gravitational force, there is greater body weight over a smaller surface area when one is sitting. When the body is flat in bed, there is more surface over which to disperse pressure.[2,4,5]

When people are sitting, it is important to emphasize good body posture and alignment. Sitting directly on a reddened area should be avoided. The top of a person's thighs should be kept horizontal so that the weight is evenly distributed along the back of the thighs. If the knees are higher than the hips, body weight is shifted to the ischial tuberosities, placing them at risk for pressure ulceration. To reduce this risk, ankles, elbows, forearms, and wrists should be adequately supported in a neutral position. Knees should be separated so that they do not rub together.[2,5] For individuals who need a wheelchair, attention to certain criteria will assure a chair that matches user needs. Figure 6.3 illustrates important measurements that influence posture and propulsion efficiency and also shows the correct placement of the leg to ensure that weight is equally distributed over the length of the thigh. Too great a seat angle, with knees higher than buttocks, can increase ischial/sacral pressure, causing tissue damage.

Body posture and orientation can dramatically affect the pressure or shear forces generated between a seated individual and the seating surface. Changes in posture can effectively reduce the maximum pressures present in a neutral sitting position.[26] If possible, patients who are sitting in a chair need to reposition themselves every 15 minutes. Paraplegic patients often are taught to do wheelchair pushups to relieve pressure. If individuals have the upper body strength, they can do pushups inter-

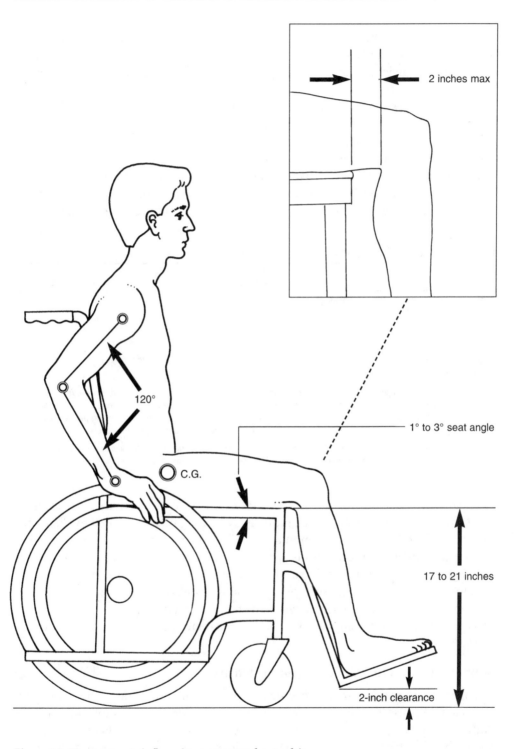

Figure 6.3 Measurements influencing posture and propulsion

mittently whenever they are seated. If done every 15 minutes, chair pushups allow blood flow to the buttocks and sacrum to be reestablished. Not all seated spinal cord-injured individuals can do pushups to relieve pressure. A recent study showed that having the person lean forward toward the thighs reduced the pressure over the ischial tuberosities to 34 mm Hg from 189 mm Hg in a normal position. Pressure on the tissue around the ischium dropped from 114 mm Hg to 33 mm Hg.[27] Clinicians need to use judgment about the safety of individual patients leaning forward. After 1 hour of chair sitting, patients who are unable to lift themselves or shift their own weight should be assisted back to bed, where they are less vulnerable to the forces of pressure.[2] See Table 6.6 for recommended maximum acceptable interface pressures over susceptible bony locations on spinal cord-injured individuals.

Table 6.6 Recommended Maximum Pressures

Level of risk	Ischial tuberosities	Trochanters	Sacrum	Coccyx
High—no sensation; history of sores at site of measurement	40	60	<20	<20
Moderate—no sensation; no history of tissue breakdown	60	80	40	40
Low—partial or full sensation; no history of tissue breakdown	80	80	40	40

Note—These maximum recommended pressures assume a normal clinical status, pushups performed every 15 minutes, and no other factors that would increase the risk of breakdown. Prolonged sitting (>10 hrs) and infrequent pressure relief are weighted by reducing each of the maximum allowable pressures by 10 mm Hg per factor. If risk is already high, then sitting time and/or pressure relief frequency must be brought to normal levels.

Source: Department of Veterans Affairs. "Choosing a Wheelchair System," *Journal of Rehabilitation Research and Development,* Veterans Health Services and Research Administration, March 1990.

If patients are at risk for pressure ulceration because of inactivity, one needs to assist them to become more active gradually by helping them from bed to chair, and then from the chair to assisted ambulation. While the patient is chairsitting, repositioning still remains critical. Because pressure on ischial tuberosities is of the greatest magnitude while sitting, it is crucial that special chair cushions be used to redistribute pressure to the larger surface of the buttocks. Patients who are inactive may need incentive to move; assistive devices, such as overhead frames, trapezes, walkers, and canes; or merely nursing personnel to help maneuver I.V. poles and other equipment.[28,29]

Support surfaces to reduce pressure intensity

Whether at-risk patients are in a bed or a chair, pressure points of the body must be protected. Historically, pillows have been used for bridging vulnerable areas of the body to eliminate pressure (see Figure 6.4). A vast array of special beds, mattresses, and cushions currently is available to help reduce the intensity of pressure. Pressure-reducing surfaces include foam, gel, water, and air mattresses; alternating pressure pads; low air-loss, high air-loss, and oscillating beds; and turning frames.

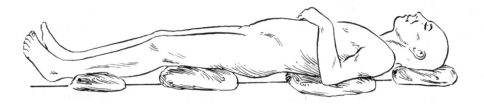

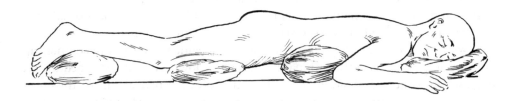

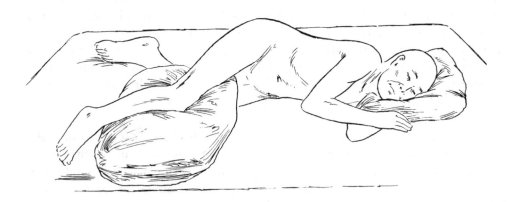

Figure 6.4 Pillow bridging

Horizontal support surfaces

Horizontal support surfaces include mattress overlays, mattresses, and specialty beds.

Mattress overlays

Foam, air, and gel products generally are used for pressure ulcer prevention. Two-inch foam mattress overlays are comfort items only and not suitable for patients at risk for pressure ulceration.[5] Good foam overlay products for a person of average weight are at least 3-4 inches thick, have a density of 1.3 pounds per cubic foot, and have 25% indentation load deformation (ILD) of 30 pounds.[30,31] These values measure both softness and stiffness of foam and determine efficacy and durability. Solid foam mattress overlays are superior to convoluted foam mattress overlays. Good quality foam does not fatigue or wear out as readily as inexpensive foam. It must allow adequate deformation and still offer a supportive surface.

In a study of 51 hospitalized patients placed on either foam overlays or alternating pressure pads[32] and a randomized control trial comparing alternating pressure pads with silacore mattress overlays,[33] there was no evidence to show that either support surface was superior in eliminating skin breakdown. An ICU provided the setting for comparative evaluation of an alternating pressure pad, an air mattress overlay, and a water mattress overlay. Sacral and heel pressures were found to be excessive on the alternating pressure pad, and the authors cautioned against its use.[34]

Maklebust, Mondoux, and Sieggreen studied the pressure relief characteristics of various support surfaces used for prevention and treatment of pressure ulcers. A special three-layered air cushion had the lowest pressures over the trochanters of healthy subjects.[22] In another study,[35] the same investigators measured differences in interface pressures among subjects on three different surfaces. An air mattress overlay and an air fluidized bed did not have significantly different interface pressures, although both surfaces were superior to the standard hospital mattress with regard to pressure reduction over the sacrum and trochanter. None of the surfaces performed adequately to reduce heel pressures below capillary closing pressure. Clinical nurse specialists at a university hospital conducted a study of high-risk patients on a special three-layered air cushion. Patients on the air cushion developed far fewer pressure ulcers than patients with the same risk factors reported in the literature.[36]

Some clinicians advocate the use of dynamic rather than static pressure relief mattresses. A study to compare the skin microvascular response of healthy persons on a dynamic mattress overlay and a static pressure-reducing mattress found no significant differences in trochanteric skin blood perfusion. Subjects showed increased skin temperature and blood flow on both surfaces.[37]

With any pressure-reducing mattress overlay, it is important to make certain that the overlay does not become fully compressed under the weight of the body. If the overlay compresses enough for the person to rest on the underlying mattress, he is

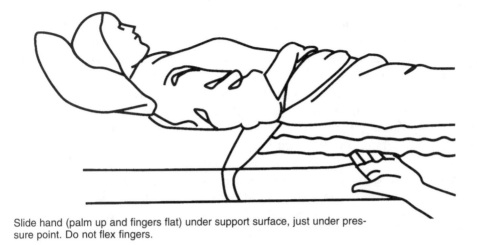

Slide hand (palm up and fingers flat) under support surface, just under pressure point. Do not flex fingers.

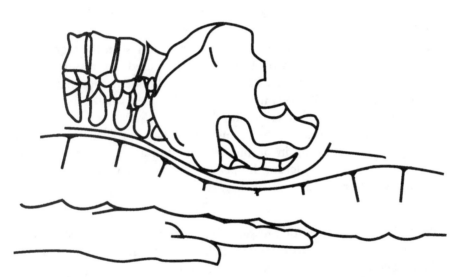

With good support, the patient's bony prominence cannot be felt with a flat hand when the patient is in a "worst-case" position (i.e., head of bed is elevated 30°, patient is side-lying on greater trochanter, etc.). Copyright, 1989. Used with permission of Gaymar Industries, Inc.

Figure 6.5 Handcheck to assess pressure relief

said to "bottom out." Doing a "handcheck" to make certain that the person does not "bottom out" is a way to determine the adequacy of pressure reduction. To correctly perform a "handcheck," the nurse inserts a hand between the mattress overlay and the underlying mattress. The hand must be flat, fingers outstretched, and palm facing upward (see Figure 6.5).[5] If the person's body can be felt through the mattress overlay, it does not offer adequate pressure reduction, and a product with more depth is needed.

Mattresses

Many hospitals have begun replacing their standard staph-check mattresses with pressure-reducing foam-core mattresses to try to eliminate mattress overlays. Their goal is to reduce pressure ulcer incidence and save health care dollars by eliminating costly overlays and specialty beds. One prospective controlled study of 44 high-risk patients evaluated the use of foam replacement mattresses against standard hospital mattresses. Patients on both mattresses developed pressure ulcers; however, there was a statistically significant difference in the number of patients who developed pressure ulcers on the standard hospital mattress compared to the foam replacement mattress.[38] Recently, a study was conducted to evaluate the long-term performance of these foam replacement mattresses.[39] Interface pressures were measured on selected sites of the mattresses at regular 3-month intervals over an extended period of use. Results showed that interface pressures increased at each site on the mattress during the course of study. During the second part of the study, the stiffness of foam was measured at selected points on the mattresses. Patient reports of discomfort in the sacral area and sinking into the mattress prompted the study. Stiffness profiles of 25 new foam mattresses were compared to 25 randomly selected foam mattresses that had been used for at least 2 years. Stiffness in the sacral-coccygeal and heel sections was reduced by 40% in all of the used mattresses. Patient reports of discomfort were consistent with softening of the foam core mattresses. The study concluded that institutions using foam replacement mattresses should monitor them closely for signs of deterioration.[39]

If an individual who is at risk for pressure ulceration has a problem with excessive moisture against the skin from incontinence, wound drainage, or perspiration, a support surface that flows air across the person's skin is recommended. Many portable low air-loss mattresses are available.

Specialty beds

Few specialty beds are necessary for pressure ulcer prevention.[2] However, a study comparing an air suspension bed to a standard ICU bed and mattress found that patients on the air bed had significantly fewer pressure ulcers than the patients who were on a regular mattress. In a randomized controlled trial of 100 at-risk patients, 8 developed pressure ulcers on the air bed, whereas 39 developed pressure ulcers on the regular ICU bed.[40] There are very few randomized controlled studies comparing one type of support surface to another. Too often, dissimilar types of surfaces are compared. What is needed are comparative investigations of low air-loss and air-fluidized surfaces or low air-loss overlays compared to low air-loss beds.

Seating support surfaces

Special chair cushions are designed to reduce pressure on the ischial tuberosities while sitting. One study found no statistical differences in the ability of seven wheelchair cushions to reduce reactive hyperemia over the ischium. The investigators recommended intermittent total weight-bearing pressure relief even with the use of expensive wheelchair cushions.[41]

People who are wheelchair dependent need durable cushions that can withstand everyday use. For wheelchair users who weigh between 50 and 300 pounds, the recommended specifications for foam wheelchair cushions are a thickness of 3-4 inches, a 25% indentation load deformation (ILD) between 40 and 70 pounds, and a density between 1.8 and 2.8 pounds per cubic foot.30 Some wheelchair seating clinics specialize in making custom-fitted chair cushions.[42,43] These special clinics may have computerized mechanisms both to assess patient characteristics and to design seating surfaces. These cushions are a costly but justifiable expense, given the alternative of pressure ulceration or enforced bedrest.

For spinal cord-injured patients, wheelchair cushion selection is based on pressure evaluation, lifestyle, postural stability, continence of bladder and bowel, and cost.[31] Individuals who use wheelchairs should be encouraged to seek replacement cushions when older cushions fatigue and lose the capacity to adequately reduce pressure. A "handcheck" can be performed to determine the pressure-reducing adequacy of the chair cushion.

Choosing support surfaces for pressure ulcer prevention

There is no scientific evidence that one support surface consistently works better than all others. The best way to match a support surface to a particular individual's needs is to learn the special characteristics of each type of surface (see Table 6.7).[5] To become knowledgeable, learn the generic categories of beds, mattresses, and cushions, and then determine which commercial products fall into each category of support surface. Advantages and disadvantages of various types of surfaces are given in Table 6.8.

The choice of pressure-reducing equipment for pressure ulcer prevention can be based on the following criteria: clinical effectiveness, financial cost of the equipment,

Table 6.7 Selected characteristics for special support surfaces

Performance characteristics	Support devices					
	Air-fluidized	Low-air-loss	Alternating air	Static floatation (air or water)	Foam	Standard mattress
support area	Yes	Yes	Yes	Yes	Yes	No
Low moisture retention	Yes	Yes	No	No	No	No
Reduced heat accumulation	Yes	Yes	No	No	No	No
Shear reduction	Yes	?	Yes	Yes	No	No
Pressure reduction	Yes	Yes	Yes	Yes	Yes	No
Dynamic	Yes	Yes	Yes	No	No	No
Cost per day	High	High	Moderate	Low	Low	Low

Source: *Treatment of Pressure Ulcers.* Agency for Health Care Policy and Research (AHCPR) Clinical Practice Guideline No. 15. Publication No. 95-0652. Rockville, Md.: U.S. Dept. of Health and Human Services, Public Health Service. December 1994.

Table 6.8 Pressure Reduction Devices: Advantages and Disadvantages

Description	Advantages	Disadvantages
Overlays		
Indications: Critically ill patient with a Norton score of 14 or less, or who will be on bedrest for more than 24 hours		
Foam Varying density, convoluted foam; Highfloat (Pre-foam), Geo-Matt (Span-America); $50-$60	Varying densities provide pressure reduction in high-pressure areas; most patients find foam mattresses comfortable	May be flammable; patients are difficult to reposition due to envelopement; foam may cause increased perspiration; adds height to the bed, which may make it more difficult to get the patient out of bed
Static air mattress Plastic air mattress that is inflated with a blower; Sof Care (Gaymar), Koala Kair (Baxter); $40-$60	May be more effective than foam with heavier patients	Inflation level must be checked regularly; may cause increased perspiration due to plastic surface; adds height to the bed, which may make it more difficult to get the patient out of bed
Alternating pressure air mattress A pump inflates mattress cells in an alternating fashion; Bio Flote (Bio Clinic), Grant PCA Systems (Grant); $35-$55	Usually there is no charge for the motor if the mattress is purchased	Alternating air pressure requires a motor and an electrical source; plastic surface may increase perspiration
Low-air-loss beds		
Indications: Immobile patients who are difficult to turn plus one of the following: decreased serum albumin, anasarca, paralysis and/or sedation, expected prolonged ICU stay, existing skin breakdown, or pain associated with the bed surface, such as cancer or Guillain-Barré patients		
Bed surface consists of inflated air cushions, each section is adjusted for optimal pressure relief for patient's body size; Mediscus (Mediscus Group), KinAir (Kinetic Concepts); $35-$90 per day	Provides pressure relief in any position; most models have built-in scales; surface fabrics are made of low-friction material	Must use incontinence pads recommended by manufacturer; air cushions may make it difficult to transfer patients in and out of bed; patients must still be turned frequently for pulmonary toilet
Air-fluidized beds		
Indications: Immobility associated with posterior surgical grafts, flaps, or burns		
Air is blown through glass beads to "float" the patient; Clinitron (Mediscus Group), FluidAir (Kinetic Concepts); $60-$120 per day	Relieves pressure and reduces shear, friction, and moisture	Extremely heavy and difficult to move; foam wedge is required to elevate the head of the bed, which negates the relief of pressure, shear, friction, and moisture on the upper back and head; difficult to transfer patient; increased air flow may increase evaporative fluid loss, leading to dehydration

Table 6.8 Pressure Reduction Devices: Advantages and Disadvantages *(Continued)*

Description	Advantages	Disadvantages
Pulsating beds Air cushions that alternately inflate and deflate, providing continuous pulsating action; Therapulse (Kinetic Concepts), Rescue (Support Systems International); $50-$145 per day	Not yet well defined	Pulsation may improve peripheral venous return

Oscillating, low-air-loss beds

Indications: Severe immobility, such as hemodynamically unstable patients who do not tolerate turning and/or documented pulmonary pathophysiology requiring frequent position changes for secretion mobilization

Bed surface consists of air cushions that are programmed to alternately inflate and deflate sections so the patient is rotated from side to side; in some models, the bed frame rotates; Biodyne (Kinetic Concepts), Pulmonair (Mediscus Group); $50-199 per day	Pressure relief and low-friction surface are provided with gentle repositioning; most models have built-in scales	Patients must be positioned correctly for effective turning; conscious patients may not tolerate the movement of the bed; patients must have stable spines
Oscillating support surfaces Entire bed frame and surface rotate in an arc; Keane Mobility system (Mediscus Group), Rotorest (Kinetic Concepts); $50-145 per day	Pressure reduction may be provided; frequent turning of patients with unstable spines is possible	Conscious patients may not tolerate the bed movement; bed rotation increases the risk of shearing forces on the tissue; contact with support surfaces during rotation may lead to pressure ulcer development; may be difficult to maintain lines and other invasive devices with bed frame rotation

Note: Due to the cost of specialty beds, the need for the bed should be evaluated daily; when mobility is improved and other indications for the specialty bed no longer exist, the patient should be moved to a regular bed, with an overlay device if needed.

Reprinted with permission of *AACN Clinical Issues in Critical Care Nursing*, Vol 1, No 3, 1990.

ease of use by caregivers, patient comfort, services offered by the equipment supplier, and patient and staff educational materials supplied by the manufacturer.[44] The VA Hospital system investigated the use of expensive support surfaces at their facilities nationwide. A decision-making algorithm was developed to determine if pressure reduction was being sought for pressure ulcer prevention, pressure ulcer treatment, or patient comfort[45] (see Figure 6.6). The AHCPR Guideline for the Prediction and Prevention of Pressure Ulcers provided the basis for decision nodes in the algorithm. In the VA Health Care System, first-line or low-technology devices were emphasized to contain expenditures.

Krouskop and Garber suggest that tissue interface pressure measurements be used to make relative judgments about effectiveness of pressure-reducing support sur-

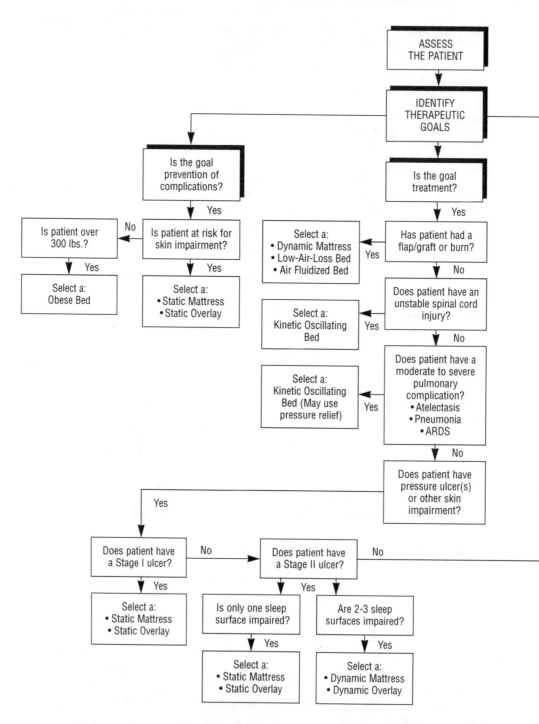

Note: If only one sleep surface is impaired, it is assumed the patient will not be turned on the affected site. A device with pressure relief is indicated if two to three sleep surfaces are impaired.

Figure 6.6 Specialty support surfaces

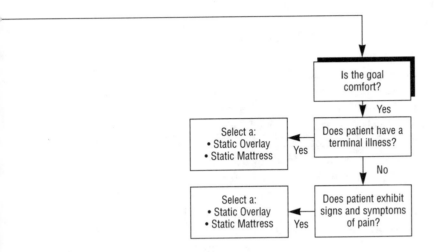

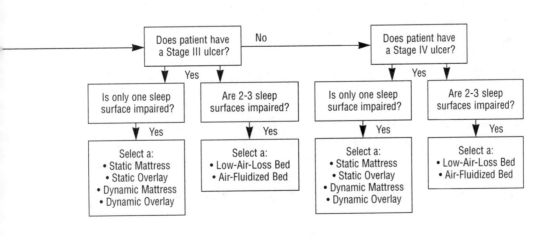

Used with permission. Thomason, S., Hawley, G., Wurzel, J. (1993). *Decubitus,* November, page 37.

faces.[31] Krouskop further suggests that patient environment may be used to determine the potential suitability of a support surface. He used interface pressure measurements as a basis for evaluating use of foam mattress overlays in various health care settings. He provided examples from several different clinical locations. In intensive care units, where a foam overlay would be used for less than 7 days and the patient would not lie on the side for more than 10 minutes and would be repositioned hourly, the upper limits for acceptable interface pressures are given as 45 mm Hg over the sacro-coccygeal area and scapula, 50 mm Hg at the heels, and 70 mm Hg at the trochanters. In acute care settings, where foam mattress overlays are not used for more than 21 days and the patient is repositioned every 2 hours, the maximum interface pressures are 40 mm Hg over the sacro-coccygeal area and scapula and 50 mm Hg over the heels and trochanters. In chronic care settings, such as homes or nursing homes where turning can be expected only every 6 to 8 hours, maximum acceptable interface pressures are 35 mm Hg at the sacro-coccygeal area and scapula and 45 mm Hg at the heels and trochanters.[31]

The cost of mattresses, beds, and chair cushions varies considerably, and the most expensive ones are not always the most effective. Hedrich-Thompson et al found that moderately priced products were preferable for reducing pressure to the sacrum and trochanter. No product, regardless of cost, was acceptable for reducing heel pressures.[46]

Some support surfaces are made for single-patient use, and others are rental items used by many people. Charges can range from a $24.00 one-time fee for a foam overlay, to a daily rental fee of $125.00 for a highly technical therapy bed. Often, with emphasis on decreased resource consumption, cost may inappropriately assume a greater role than clinical effectiveness. It is important for caregivers at the bedside to be vigilant about effectiveness of items used for patients.[47]

Any requests for special support surfaces need to be justified. It is important to give rationales for certain support surface characteristics needed by an individual. See Table 6.9 for Harper Hospital's patient criteria for use of specialty surfaces. Table 6.10 helps clinicians differentiate between low air-loss and high air-loss products. In some settings, a particular product may not be available because of reimbursement restrictions. Other times only certain products are carried by a particular health care agency. Even if a preferred type of support surface is unavailable, documentation should reflect the person's needs.

While use of pressure-reducing surfaces on the bed or chair may allow caregivers to lengthen repositioning intervals, they also may give a false sense of security.[28] It must be remembered that special equipment, while helpful as part of the overall management plan, is not a substitute for attentive nursing care.[31] Patients require individual turning schedules regardless of any pressure-reducing devices in use. The schedule depends on nursing assessment of the patient's tissue tolerance to pressure.[28,30]

Table 6.9 Patient Criteria for High and Low Air-Loss Therapy

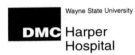

Wayne State University

DMC Harper
Hospital

1. Patients who have plastic surgery operations:

   a. Air-loss therapy is necessary for 2-3 weeks for patients who have whole but-tock/gluteal rotation flaps to the sacrum—then wean to air mattress overlay prior to discharge.

   b. Air-loss therapy is unnecessary for patients who have local/Limberg rotation flaps to the sacrum.

2. Patients with severe or multiple pressure ulcers may be eligible for air-loss therapy after the following criteria have been met:

   a. other less costly pressure relief devices have been tried first (e.g., air mattress overlay) except in cases of new plastics operations that require air-loss therapy

   b. the patient was on an air mattress overlay during a previous admission and developed a pressure ulcer or an existing ulcer deteriorated

   c. there is a nutrition plan in place

   d. there is an incontinence management plan in place

   e. there is a debridement plan in place

   f. there is a topical wound management plan in place

3. Patients with bone metastasis/pathological fractures are eligible for air-loss therapy when severe pain is unrelieved by pain medication and prohibits position changes.

4. Patients who have radical vulvectomy operations with imposed immobility require high air-loss therapy for approximately 10 days postoperatively because of the necessity to do wound irrigations without repositioning the person.

5. Patients who have massive edema leading to generalized weeping and/or slough-ing skin may require high air-loss therapy because of its drying effect.

Harper Hospital

3990 John R Detroit, Michigan 48201 313.745.8040

Table 6.10 Guidelines for Differentiating Use of High and Low Air-Loss Therapy

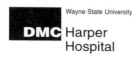

Wayne State University

DMC Harper
Hospital

High air-loss therapy (air-fluidized bed) may be more efficacious than low air-loss therapy in the following circumstances:

1. <u>Uncontrolled incontinence</u> because the increased drying effect of air-fluidized beds reduces maceration of tissue.

2. <u>Repeated extensive dressing changes</u> because air-fluidized beds increase the ease of positioning.

3. <u>Positioning restrictions</u>—Patients who have severe trochanteric ulcers and hip contractures are more easily positioned on air-fluidized beds.

Low air-loss therapy may be more efficacious than high air-loss therapy in the following circumstances:

1. <u>Flotation disorientation</u>—With low air-loss therapy, elderly patients may have less disorientation than with high air-loss therapy.

2. <u>Continuous moist dressings</u>—If saline soaks are ordered, low air-loss therapy may be preferred because high air loss can dry the dressings too rapidly.

3. <u>Risk of aspiration</u>—Patients who require tube feedings are at less risk for aspiration with low air-loss therapy because the head of the bed can be elevated without decreasing pressure relief capability. Air-fluidized beds require the use of foam back wedges to elevate the head—this may decrease the pressure-relieving capability of the air-fluidized bed.

4. <u>Out of bed activity</u>—Patients who need to be out of bed are more easily moved/ambulated from low air-loss surfaces. The low air-loss surfaces deflate in the seat area. The air-fluidized bed has a permanent railing over which patients must be lifted.

˙Note: If all other factors are equal, be aware that the Harper Hospital Department of Epidemiology requires that patients on air-fluidized beds be in private rooms. Patients on low air-loss surfaces may be placed in semi-private rooms.

Harper Hospital
3990 John R Detroit, Michigan 48201 313.745.8040

Skin care

Once a plan is developed to compensate for malnutrition and immobility, one needs to concentrate on individualizing daily skin care. Inspecting patients' skin for pressure areas should be done on a routine basis, depending on assessed risk and ability to tolerate pressure. If reddened areas of skin are found over bony prominences, they should not be massaged. Massage is no longer recommended because recent studies show that it may reduce blood flow and cause tissue damage.[48,49,50]

Older adults have special needs for skin care. Aged people have diminished skin elasticity and a slower rate of epidermal proliferation. These changes in aging skin alter its functional effectiveness as a barrier. Also, with aging, the epidermal-dermal junction flattens, making the epidermis less anchored to the dermis. Gentle handling of the elderly can reduce the likelihood of skin tears caused by epidermis sliding across dermis.[28]

There is a significant association between advanced age and severity of skin dryness, which can result in reduced pliability and cracking of the epidermis. It has been reported that 59% to 80% of the elderly population suffer from dry skin.[51] Investigators have found an association between dry, flaking skin and development of pressure ulcers.[52]

A major environmental contribution to dry skin is lack of moisture in the air. Relatively low humidity is found in overheated hospitals, long-term care facilities, and the homes of many elderly people. Efforts should be taken to add moisture to room air through humidification. Central or room humidifiers can significantly reduce the detrimental effect of low humidity on the stratum corneum.[53]

Cleansing the skin

The skin needs to be cleansed only when soiled. There are many ways to maintain adequate hygiene without a daily shower or tub bath. When possible, individuals need to be given a preference for frequency and type of bathing.[54] For most individuals at risk for pressure ulcers, full body bathing need take place only on an intermittent basis. Often this means "face and fanny care" on a routine basis and more frequent cleansing of the axilla and perineal area as soiling from perspiration, urine, feces, or wound drainage takes place. This is especially important for people with dry, aged, or at-risk skin, in whom more frequent bathing may remove the natural barrier and increase skin dryness. The skin's protective acid mantle should be maintained with nonalkaline cleansing agents. The temperature of bath water should be slightly warm, and the cleansing agent may be a mild soap, such as Dove. In a study of 18 brand-name soaps, irritancy levels were found to be exceedingly low for Dove synthetic detergent bar compared to all others tested. The value of superfatted soaps, thought to be milder because of protective oils, was not supported in this study.[55] In cases of very dry skin, it may be more prudent to use only warm water and avoid cleansing agents altogether.

Minimal force always should be used during skin cleansing.[2,4,5] Gentle washing with a soft cloth and patting the skin dry with a soft towel rather than rubbing works best. Excessive friction and vigorous rubbing against the skin are contraindicated.[2,4,5]

Moisturizing the skin

It is important to keep the skin well lubricated without oversaturating the epidermis. Milk of magnesia and Maalox should not be used because they are drying agents that alter the pH of the skin. Dry skin is caused by loss of moisture from the stratum corneum, which, in turn, decreases skin pliability. Controlling the signs and symptoms of dry skin can be done by applying topical agents.[53] These come in a variety of preparations, such as lotions, creams, and ointments. A pharmacy consult can provide information about types of products that are commercially available.[29] Table 6.11 shows a skin care flowchart developed by the Pressure Ulcer Committee at Harper Hospital. The purpose of the flowchart was to empower the staff nurses by indicating which products were carried by the hospital and which decisions had to be made in order to choose an appropriate item. The flowchart was automated so that nurses could independently order products from the pharmacy or central supply via computer.

Lotions

Of all the moisturizers, lotions have the highest water content, evaporate the most quickly and, therefore, need to be reapplied the most frequently. Lotions are composed of powder crystals dissolved in water and held in suspension by surfactants. They may be more aesthetically pleasing than creams or ointments because they are easy to apply, have a cooling effect, are nonocclusive, and do not leave a greasy film on the skin. Some dermatologists recommend using lotions in a low-humidity environment, believing that the high water content will add more moisture to the skin. Examples of widely available lotions are Aloe Vera Lotion, Eucerin Lotion, Vaseline Intensive Care Lotion, and Alpha Keri Lotion.[53]

Creams

Creams are preparations of oil in water, so they are more occlusive than lotions. They need to be applied about four times daily for maximum effectiveness. Examples of over-the-counter skin creams are Alpha Keri Cream, Lubriderm Cream, Cold Cream USP, and Vaseline Dermatology Formula.[53]

Ointments

Ointments are mixtures of water in oil and, hence, are the most occlusive. The oil component of ointments can be lanolin or petrolatum. Examples of lanolin-based ointments include Nivea, Eucerin, and Keri; petroleum-based ointments include Hydrophyllic Petrolatum USP and Vaseline. Studies have shown that petrolatum is more effective on dry skin than lanolin. Ointments provide a longer lasting effect on skin moisture than either lotions or creams.[53]

Protecting the skin from irritants

Skin that is waterlogged from constant wetness is more easily eroded by friction, more permeable to irritants, and more readily colonized by microorganisms than skin that is not overly wet. Patients who are incontinent of urine are exposed to increased dampness or moisture over time, and this places them at increased risk for skin breakdown.[56] Both urinary and fecal incontinence create problems from excessive moisture and chemical irritation. Because of pathogens in the stool, fecal incontinence may be more damaging to the skin than urinary incontinence.[14,15,57] Most likely, there is an interaction of the urea in urine with chemical enzymes in the stool. A complex chemical interaction between urine and stool may contribute to diaper dermatitis of elderly incontinent patients.[56]

Determine etiology of incontinence

First, it is necessary to determine the etiology of incontinence. One must not assume that incontinence is a normal part of aging. Patients may be incontinent for any number of reasons. Fecal impaction or tube feedings may precipitate diarrheal stools. Urinary incontinence can be traced to several sources. Medication may be the culprit, or the patient may have a urinary tract infection, may be unable to reach the bathroom in time, or may be confused or too embarrassed to ask for the bedpan.[4,28,58]

Once the cause of incontinence is determined, a care plan must be developed to manage the problem. A Foley catheter is not recommended solely for incontinence. If the cause of incontinence is reversible, patients should be given frequent voiding opportunities with positive reinforcement for requesting toileting assistance or staying dry. A prompted timed voiding approach often can decrease incontinence episodes in elderly patients.[58]

Incontinence collectors

If incontinence continues, there are several external urinary and fecal collection devices available on the market. Condom catheters connected to dependent drainage are used to manage urine output by many incontinent men. There are commercially available, but less successful, external urinary collection devices for women. Fecal incontinence collectors are made of pectin skin barriers with attached drainable pouches, much like colostomy pouching systems. A regular schedule for changing these collectors is useful. It is much easier to change an intact fecal collector than a leaking appliance on a patient with diarrhea. For nurses who are unfamiliar with these incontinence collectors, perhaps an Enterostomal Therapy nurse or wound care specialist can demonstrate their application.[28,29] Rectal tubes are not good alternatives for managing fecal incontinence because they may be associated with physiological complications, such as vasovagal responses and ischemia of anal tissue.[1]

Table 6.11 Skin Care Flow Chart

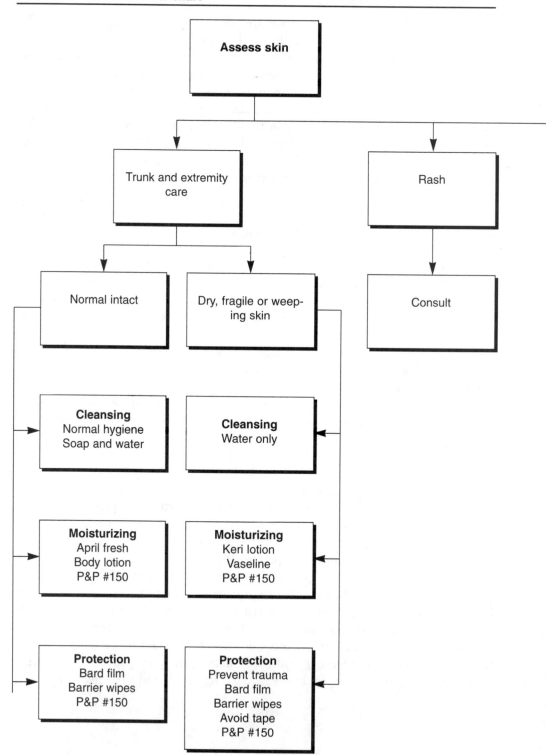

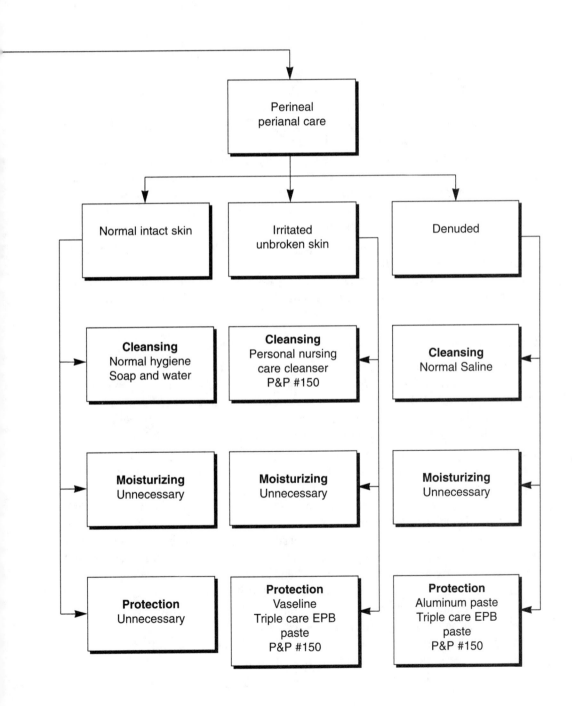

Incontinence underpads

If patients are not candidates for external collection devices, it is important to provide hygiene immediately after soiling. Absorptive underpads must be used to wick moisture away and provide a quick-drying surface to the skin.[2,3,56,59] Studies showed significantly less skin wetness, closer to normal skin pH, and lower degrees of contact dermatitis in infants wearing disposable absorbent gel diapers than those wearing disposable cellulose core diapers or laundered cloth diapers.[60] Nevertheless, many health care facilities, while attempting to control expenditures, will not stock disposable underpads if their cost outweighs the cost of washable, reusable underpads.[61] Nursing personnel must remain vigilant about the effectiveness of various types of underpads used by health care facilities.

Plastic and paper linen savers should never be placed next to the patient because they hold moisture, which irritates the skin surface.[56,62] Nursing personnel sometimes place linen on top of incontinence underpads to avoid completely changing the bed when a patient voids. This practice nullifies the purpose of the underpad, which is to protect the skin, not the bed. Sometimes, incontinence underpads are secured around patients like diapers. Again, this technique disallows the purpose of the underpad. The patient would be better served by lying on top of the pad and letting the uncovered areas of skin air dry. When the patient is repositioned, another skin surface can be air drying.[56]

Diapers and incontinence underpads do not eliminate the need for vigilance on the part of caregivers. An established schedule should determine the time for automatically checking patients who are likely to be incontinent.

Topical skin barriers

Liquid copolymer film barriers can offer protection for unbroken at-risk skin.[63] These liquid barriers come in multiuse spray cannisters or single-foil packets of copolymer-saturated wipes. If the skin is irritated or denuded, the alcohol content of some liquid barriers may sting the patient. The purpose of the liquid barrier is to create a plasic-like film on the skin to protect it from moisture, so it is important to use a barrier that is not water soluble. After application of the liquid barrier, fan the area and separate apposing parts until the skin is completely dry and nontacky. The barrier does not have to be completely removed with cleansing.

Areas of intact skin around open wounds need to be protected from drainage and maceration. Petroleum jelly can be used on the skin if moisture is from water or saline. If the moisture or drainage contains irritants, a paste may be necessary to protect the skin. A paste is composed of ointment with powder added for thickness and durability. Zinc oxide is a common ingredient of commercially available protective barrier pastes. Paste is an excellent skin barrier that is purposely difficult to remove in order to remain effective. Its tenacity makes it more impermeable to irritants. Paste can best be removed with mineral oil.[56]

Avoid using a topical barrier that leaves oil on the skin if an adhesive product, such as a hydrocolloid, will be used. Hydrocolloid wafers are useful as physical barriers to protect skin from moisture or drainage. Moist dressings can be placed directly on top of hydrocolloid wafers. The skin under the wafer will be protected as long as the wafer remains intact.

Monitoring change in risk status

Table 6.12 summarizes the risk factors and illustrates prophylactic nursing interventions to reduce pressure ulcer risk.[2] The interventions can be used as a basis for a generic standard protocol for pressure ulcer prevention. Changes in patient risk status require a revision of the plan of care.

Table 6.12 Preventing Pressure Ulcers: Risk Factors and Interventions

Risk Factors	Nursing Interventions
Immobility	Provide pressure relief surface Establish turning schedule Reduce shear and friction Consult physical therapist
Inactivity	Provide assistive devices to increase activity
Incontinence	Cleanse and dry skin after elimination Assess etiology of incontinence Apply protective skin barriers
Decreased mental status	Assess patient/family ability to provide care Educate caregiver regarding pressure ulcer prevention
Malnutrition	Provide adequate nutritional and fluid intake Consult dietitian for nutritional evaluation
Impaired skin integrity	Avoid pressure, friction, shear, excessive wetness Moisturize skin Do not massage red areas Do not use donuts Do not use heat lamps

Documentation

After the pressure ulcer prevention plan is developed, consider all the factors that may influence patient outcomes, write realistic and measurable goals, and then solicit support from other health care professionals. Try to communicate the importance of consistent care to peers, for if a plan is to be fairly evaluated, all caregivers must implement care in the same manner. If, despite everyone's best efforts, the patient develops a pressure ulcer, the prevention plan must be intensified. The pressure area cannot heal while the area remains ischemic. If adequate pressure relief is not provided and the risk factors, such as malnutrition, are not reduced, pressure ulcer prevention efforts will be futile.[28,29]

References

1. Levine, J.M., et al. "Pressure Sores: A Plan for Primary Care Prevention," *Geriatrics* 44(4): 75-6, 83-7, 90, 1989.
2. Panel for the Prediction and Prevention of Pressure Ulcers in Adults. "*Pressure Ulcers in Adults: Prediction and Prevention.*" Clinical Practice Guideline, No. 3. AHCPR Publication No. 92-0047. Rockville, Md.: U.S. Department of Health and Human Services, Agency for Health Care Policy and Research, May 1992.

3. Bergman-Evans, B., et al. "Clinical Practice Guidelines: Prediction and Prevention," *Journal of Gerontological Nursing,* 20(9): 19-26, 52, 1994.

4. National Pressure Ulcer Advisory Panel. *Monograph on Pressure Ulcer Prevention.* Buffalo: NPUAP, 1992.

5. Bergstrom, N., et al. "*Treatment of Pressure Ulcers.*" Clinical Practice Guideline, No. 15. AHCPR Publication No. 95-0652. Rockville, Md.: U.S. Department of Health and Human Services, Agency for Health Care Policy and Research, December 1994.

6. Clarke, M., and Kadhom, H.M. "The Prevention of Pressure Sores in Hospital and Community Patients," *Journal of Advanced Nursing* 13(3): 365-73, 1988.

7. Maklebust, J., and Magnan, M.A. "Approaches to Patient and Family Education for Pressure Ulcer Management," *Decubitus* 5(4): 18-20, 24, 26, 1992.

8. Lishinsky, E.S. "A Philosophy of Care: Pressure Sores in Hospice Patients," *Today's OR Nurse* 10(4): 20-23, 1988.

9. Colburn, L. "Pressure Ulcer Prevention for the Hospice Patient," *American Journal of Hospice Care* 22-26, 1987.

10. Hoffman, R., et al. "Standards of Care for Hospice Patients with Pressure Ulcers," *Decubitus* 4(4): 19-24, 1991.

11. Pinchcofsky-Devin, G., and Kaminski, M.V. "Correlation of Pressure Sores and Nutritional Status," *J Am Geriatr Soc* 34: 435, 1986.

12. "Nutritional Screening Manual for Professionals Caring for Older Americans: Nutrition Screening Initiative." Washington, D.C.: Greer, Margolis, Mitchell, Grunwald & Associates, 1991.

13. Kaminski, M.V., et al. "Nutritional Management of Decubitus Ulcers in the Elderly, *Decubitus* 2(4): 20-30, 1989.

14. Allman, R.M., et al. "Pressure Sores Among Hospitalized Patients," *Ann Intern Med* 105(3): 337, 1986.

15. Allman, R.M., et al. "Pressure Ulcer Risk Factors Among Hospitalized Patients with Activity Limitation," *JAMA* 273(11): 865-870, 1995.

16. Frantz, R., et al. "The Effects of Prolonged Pressure on Skin Blood Flow in Elderly Patients at Risk for Pressure Ulcers," *Decubitus* 6(6): 16-20, 1993.

17. Barnett, R.I., and Ablarde, J.A. "Skin Vascular Reaction to Standard Patient Positioning on a Hospital Mattress," *Advances in Wound Care* 7(1): 58-65, 1994.

18. Knox, D.O., et al. "Effects of Different Turn Intervals on Skin of Healthy Older Adults," *Advances in Wound Care* 7(1): 48-56, 1994.

19. Crew, R.A. "Problems of Rubber Ring Nursing Cushions and a Clinical Survey of Alternative Cushions for Ill Patients," *Care Science Practice* 5(2): 9-11, 1987.

20. Seiler, W., et al. "Influence of the Thirty Degree Laterally Inclined Position on Skin Oxygen Tension on Areas of Maximum Pressure: Implications for Pressure Sore Prevention," *Gerontology* 32(3): 158-166, 1986.

21. Morton, R.L., and Witmer, D.O. "Just Say No to Pressure Ulcers: Eliminate the Side-Lying Position," *VA Practitioner* 1: 69-72, January 1993.

22. Maklebust, J., et al. "Pressure Relief Characteristics of Various Support Surfaces Used in the Prevention and Treatment of Pressure Ulcers," *Journal of Enterostomal Therapy* 14(3): 85, 1986.

23. Exton-Smith, A.N., and Sherwin, R.W. "The Prevention of Pressure Sores: The Significance of Spontaneous Bodily Movements," *Lancet* 2: 1124, 1961.

24. Lowthian, P.T. "Practical Nursing: Turning Clock System to Prevent Pressure Sores," *Nursing Mirror* 148(21): 30-31, 1979.

25. Smith, A.M., and Malone, J.A. "Preventing Pressure Ulcers in Institutionalized Elders: Assessing the Effects of Small, Unscheduled Shifts in Body Position," *Decubitus* 3(4): 20-24, 1990.

26. Hobson, D. "Comparative Effects of Posture on Pressure and Shear at Body-Seat Interface," *Journal of Rehabilitation Research,* 29(4): 21-31, 1992.

27. Henderson, J., et al. "Efficacy of Three Measures to Relieve Pressure in Seated Patients with Spinal Cord Injury," *Archives of Physical Medicine and Rehabilitation* 75(5): 535-539, 1994.

28. Maklebust, J. "Pressure Ulcers: Etiology and Prevention," *Nursing Clinics of North America* 22(2): 359-377, 1987.

29. Maklebust, J. "Pressure Ulcer Update," *RN* 12: 56-62, December 1991.

30. Kemp, M.G., and Krouskop, T.A. "Pressure Ulcers: Reducing Incidence and Severity by Managing Pressure," *Journal of Gerontological Nursing* 20(9): 27-34, 1994.

31. Krouskop, T.A., and Garber, S.L. "The Role of Technology in the Prevention of Pressure Sores," *Ostomy/Wound Management* 16: 44-45, 48-49, 52-54, 1987.

32. Whitney, J.D., et al. "Do Mattresses Make a Difference?" *Journal of Gerontological Nursing* 10(9): 20-25, 1984.

33. Daechsel, D., and Conine, T.A. "Special Mattresses: Effectiveness in Preventing Decubitus Ulcers in Chronic Neurological Patients," *Archives of Physical Medicine and Rehabilitation* 66(4): 246-248, 1985.

34. Sideranko, S., et al. "Effects of Position and Mattress Overlay on Sacral and Heel Pressures in a Clinical Population," *Research in Nursing and Health* 15: 245-251, 1992.

35. Maklebust, J., et al. "Pressure Relief Capabilities: The Sof-Care Bed Cushion and the Clinitron Bed," *Ostomy/Wound Management* 21(corrected supplement): 32-41, Winter 1988.

36. Maklebust, J., et al. "Pressure Ulcer Incidence in High-Risk Patients Managed on a Special Three-Layered Air Cushion," *Decubitus* 1(4): 30-40, 1988.

37. Mayrovitz, H.N., et al. "Effects of Rhythmically Alternating and Static Pressure Support Surfaces on Skin Microvascular Perfusion," *Wounds* 5(1): 47-55, 1993.

38. Hofman, A., et al. "Pressure Sores and Pressure-Decreasing Mattresses: Controlled Clinical Trial," *The Lancet* 343: 568-571, March 1994.

39. Krouskop, T.A., et al. "Evaluating Long-Term Performance of a Foam-Core Hospital Replacement Mattress," *JWOCN* 21(6): 241-46, 1994.

40. Inman, K.J., et al. "Clinical Utility and Cost-Effectiveness of an Air Suspension Bed in the Prevention of Pressure Ulcers," *JAMA* 269(9): 1139-1143, 1993.

41. DeLateur, B.J., et al. "Wheelchair Cushions Designed to Prevent Pressure Sores: An Evaluation," *Archives of Physical Medicine and Rehabilitation* 57(3): 129-35, 1976.

42. Garber, S.L., et al. "A System for Clinically Evaluating Wheelchair Pressure-Relief Cushions," *American Journal of Occupational Therapy* 32(9): 565-570, 1978.

43. Ferguson-Pell, M., et al. "A Knowledge-Based Program for Pressure Sore Prevention," *Annals of NY Academy of Science* 463: 284-86, 1986.

44. Doughty, D., et al. "Your Patient: Which Therapy?" *Journal of Enterostomal Therapy* 17: 154-159, 1990.

45. Thomason, S., et al. "Special Support Surfaces: A Cost- Containment Perspective," *Decubitus* 6(6): 32-40, 1993.

46. Hedrick-Thompson, J., et al. "Pressure Eduction Products: Making Appropriate Choices," *Journal of ET Nursing* 20(6): 239-244, 1993.

47. Kemp, M.G., et al. "The Role of Support Surfaces and Patient Attributes in Preventing Pressure Ulcers in Elderly Patients," *Research in Nursing and Health* 16: 89-96, 1993.

48. Ek, A.C., et al. "The Local Skin Blood Flow in Areas at Risk for Pressure Sores Treated with Massage," *Scandinavian Journal of Rehabilitation Medicine* 17(1): 81-86, 1985.

49. Olsen, B. "Effects of Massage for Prevention of Pressure Ulcers," *Decubitus* 2(4): 32-37, 1989.

50. Dyson, R. "Bedsores: The Injuries Hospital Staff Inflict on Patients," *Nursing Mirror* 146(24): 30-32, 1978.

51. Frantz, R.A., and Kinney, C.N. "Variables Associated with Dry Skin," *Nursing Research* 35(2): 98-100, 1986.

52. Guralnik, J.M., et al. "Occurrence and Predictors of Pressure Sores in the National Health and Nutrition Examination Survey Follow-up," *Journal of the American Geriatric Society* 36(9): 807-812, 1988.

53. Frantz, R.A., and Gardner, S. "Clinical Concerns: Management of Dry Skin," *Journal of Gerontological Nursing* 20(9): 15-18, 45, 1994.

54. Rader, J. "To Bathe or Not to Bathe: That is the Question," *Journal of Gerontological Nursing* 20(9): 53-54, 1994.

55. Frosch, P.J., and Kligman, A.M. "The Soap Chamber Test: A New Method for Assessing the Irritancy of Soaps," *Journal of American Academy of Dermatology* 1: 35-41, 1979.

56. Kemp, M.G. "Protecting the Skin from Moisture and Associated Irritants," *Journal of Gerontological Nursing* 20(9): 8-14, 1994.

57. Maklebust, J., and Magnan, M.A. "Risk Factors Associated with Having a Pressure Ulcer: A Secondary Analysis," *Advances in Wound Care*, 1994.

58. Jeter, K., et al. *Nursing for Continence*. Philadelphia: W.B. Saunders, 1990.

59. Lowthian, P.T. "Underpads in the Prevention of Decubiti," in Kennedi, R.M., et al., eds. *Bedsore Biomechanics*. London: MacMillan Press, 1976.

60. Campbell, R.L., et al. "Clinical Studies with Disposable Diapers Containing Absorbent Gelling Materials: Evaluation of Effects on Infant Skin Condition," *Journal of American Academy of Dermatology* 17(6): 978-87, 1987.

61. Grant, R. "Washable Pads or Disposable Diapers?" *Geriatric Nursing* 2(4): 248-251, 1982.

62. Maklebust, J. "Impact of AHCPR Pressure Ulcer Guidelines on Nursing Practice," *Decubitus* 4(2): 46-50, 1991.

63. Shipes, E., and Stanley, I. "A Study of a Liquid Copolymer Skin Barrier for Preventing and Alleviating Perineal Irritations in Incontinent Patients," *Journal of Urological Nursing* 2(3): 32-34, 1983.

CHAPTER 7

Pressure Ulcer Treatment

The wound healing process is greatly influenced by the extracellular environment of the wound. Nurses often have the opportunity to favorably manipulate certain environmental factors that can influence this process. Significant extrinsic factors that affect wound treatment include protecting the wound and providing a physiological environment. This is done through pressure relief (including body positioning, repositioning, and use of support surfaces), provision of adequate nutrients, and good local wound care (including wound debridement, adequate cleansing, and selection of appropriate wound dressing materials). Whenever possible, pressure ulcer risk factors should be minimized. (See Chapter 5 for detailed information on assessing pressure ulcers and their risk factors and Chapter 6 for further information on body positions, repositioning, support surfaces, and nutrition.)

Support surfaces

If pressure is not removed or reduced, all other attempts at healing the pressure ulcer will be futile. Pressure-relieving devices work by redistributing pressure at bony prominences over the larger surface area of the entire body. The theoretical principle is Pascal's law, which states that the weight of a body floating on a fluid system is evenly distributed over the entire surface. In this manner, pressure points are eliminated. A second underlying mechanism is deformation. If a support surface is unyielding and unable to deform, the external pressure instead compresses and deforms body tissue. A support surface must be capable of deforming enough to permit prominent areas to sink into the support. Additionally, it must be capable of transmitting the pressure forces from one area to another. A surface must mold to the body to maximize contact and then, via Pascal's law, redistribute the patient's weight as evenly as possible. The redistribution of weight raises the pressure over less prominent areas of the body. This increase in pressure is usually insignificant when compared with the original pressure and is not of concern as long as the pressure remains below capillary-closing pressure.[1,2]

The number of patient support or sleep surfaces marketed as pressure-relieving devices has escalated during recent years. There are specialized mattresses and beds to support the entire body in order to more evenly distribute the pressure. Slabs of polyurethane, foam pads, or mattresses are made in numerous densities, thicknesses, and convolution patterns. Mattress overlays are made of gel, sheepskin, and water- or air-filled vinyl cushions. Sophisticated electronic buoyant support systems have been designed to float, turn, and independently move the patient in and out of bed. (See Table 6.7 for characteristics of various support surfaces and Figure 6.6 for an algorithm to help select an appropriate type.)

It is especially important to reduce pressure on bony prominences when patients spend long periods of time on the operating table. In the operating room, patients tend to be hypothermic and hypoperfused. Often, they are placed in non-neutral positions. There are multiple reports of operating room-acquired pressure ulcers.[3-7] Objective measures are needed to evaluate operating room pads for their effectiveness in reducing pressure over bony prominences. Until there is an adequate body of knowledge generated from controlled outcome studies with the use of various operating room table pads, support surface-tissue interface pressures are an accepted method of determining their pressure-reducing capability. In order to minimize confusion and misrepresentation, biomedical engineers recommend that a standard format be developed for reporting research data on tissue interface pressure measurements.[8,9] If products are selected on the basis of low interface pressures, other factors also must be considered. See Table 6.8 for factors to consider when selecting support surfaces.

Nutrition

Clinicians agree that patients with pressure ulcers should receive aggressive nutritional support. Tissue repair requires both energy and adequate amounts of vitamins and minerals. The role of nutrition in healing pressure ulcers and preventing their recurrence is well accepted clinically, but the research data are incomplete and contradictory.[10]

A sound principle of wound care is to provide the substrates essential for healing. Proteins are needed for repair and regeneration. Amino acids are necessary for angiogenesis, fibroblast activity, collagen synthesis, and scar formation. Adequate carbohydrate and fat intake is needed to prevent amino acids from being used for energy expenditure. One study found that malnourished patients with Stage IV pressure ulcers who consumed 40 kcal/kg of body weight healed their pressure ulcers without gaining a significant amount of weight.[11] The authors concluded that the patient's energy intake was preferentially used for healing the ulcers. Vitamins and minerals should be increased, but specific requirements for wound healing are not known.[12,13] (See Chapter 6 for more information about nutrition and supplements.)

Laboratory values, such as serum albumin and total lymphocyte count, may help identify the patient's nutritional status. Serum albumin contributes to the amino acid pool for protein synthesis and is required to maintain oncotic pressure in the vascular system. When there is inadequate dietary intake of protein, the serum albumin level decreases. Albuminemia decreases the oncotic pressure, resulting in tissue edema, which further compromises wound healing. The total lymphocyte count is a reflection of immune competence. Normally the total lymphocyte count should be greater than 1700. If it drops below 900, the patient will become anergic and can be expected to do poorly.

Early identification of malnutrition and subsequent intervention can alter the healing trajectory in patients with wounds.[14] A nutritional plan should be comprehensive and individualized. Since there is no such thing as a standard patient, there can be no such thing as a standard formula.[15] Nutritional support of patients with wounds includes participation of the dietitian, physician, nurse, pharmacist, patient, and family. Principles of nutritional therapy include a) a multidisciplinary approach, b) early and regular assessment of nutritional status, c) goal setting, and d) meeting the patient's metabolic needs.[14]

Studies in various clinical settings confirmed that patients with serum albumin levels lower than 3.5 g/dl are at higher risk for morbidity and mortality, greater duration of hospital stay, higher costs, more time on a ventilator, and greater use of antibiotics than patients whose albumin is higher than 3.5g/dl. Serum albumin commonly is used as an index to identify the nutritional status of patients. While some studies found that hypoalbuminemia was associated with pressure ulceration,[16,17] others found no such relationship.[18,19] A retrospective that explored association between serum albumin and pressure ulcer healing found that baseline serum albumin concentrations equal to or less than 2.0 g/dl had little prognostic value for pressure ulcer healing.[20]

Nutrition intervention begins with a nutritional assessment which serves as a basis for planning. See Chapter 6 for factors to include in nutritional assessment. A suggestion for staging nutritional intervention is given in Table 7.1.

Table 7.1 Staging Nutritional Intervention

Level I

1. Estimate nutritional needs.
2. Monitor ability to self-feed; consider use of finger foods, adaptive utensils, refeeding programs, increased time, or feeding assistance.
3. Pay attention to food preferences and tolerances; optimize the eating environment by individualizing meal times and patterns as much as possible; ensure good food quality and variety.
4. Monitor food and fluid intake.
5. Consider an interdisciplinary assessment of chewing and swallowing ability.
6. Add medical nutritional products to supplement intake.
7. Limit use of unsupplemented liquid diets or other restrictive diets.
8. Routinely reassess nutritional status and response to nutrition intervention.
9. Document and reevaluate the plan of care.

Level II

1. Institute tube feedings to meet nutritional needs if this is compatible with overall goals of care.
2. Take precautions to prevent pulmonary aspiration and other complications.
3. Monitor nutritional intake through counting calories.
4. Routinely reassess nutritional status and response to nutrition intervention.
5. Document and reevaluate the plan of care.

Used with permission of Ross Products Division, Abbott Laboratories, Columbus, Ohio, from Campbell SM: *Pressure Ulcer Prevention and Intervention: A Role for Nutrition,* May 1994, pp 14-15.

Treatment, including feeding, must incorporate overall patient goals. If the patient is on an air-fluidized bed, there is some evidence that air-fluidized therapy may reduce protein requirements and increase fluid requirements. Patients on air-loss therapy should have continued nutritional assessments.[21] Feeding tubes often are placed in malnourished patients with the hope of improved pressure ulcer healing. Finucane found that routine use of tube feedings to prevent or treat pressure sores is not clearly supported by data.[10] More research is needed to identify markers that predict healing and to establish the relationship between nutrition and pressure ulcer healing.

Pressure ulcer care

Local pressure ulcer care involves wound debridement, wound cleansing, appropriate dressing materials, and selected adjuvant therapy.[22]

Debridement

Wound healing is optimized and potential for infection decreased when all necrotic tissue, exudate, and metabolic wastes have been removed from the wound.[23,24] Devitalized tissue is a source for bacterial overgrowth. Necrotic tissue may present itself as moist yellow or gray tissue that is in the process of separating from viable tissue. If this moist, necrotic tissue becomes dry, it presents itself as thick, hard, leathery black eschar.[1] Areas of necrotic or devitalized tissue may mask underlying fluid collections and/or abscesses.

Debridement of nonviable tissue is considered the most important factor in the management of contaminated wounds. Wound healing cannot take place until necrotic tissue is removed. The various methods of debridement are classified as (a) sharp (b) mechanical, (c) chemical, and (d) autolytic. The clinician should select the debridement method most appropriate to the type of wound, the amount of necrotic tissue, the condition of the patient, the setting, and the clinician's and caregiver's experience. Various debridement modalities can be combined to increase effectiveness.[23-24]

Sharp debridement

The most rapid and efficient method of debridement is sharp surgical debridement. Sharp debridement involves the use of a cutting tool, such as a scalpel, scissor, or laser, to remove macroscopically identified necrotic tissue from the wound bed. Sharp debridement is imprecise and also may remove some viable tissue. Caution should be used on patients who have low platelet counts or who are taking anticoagulants.

A scalpel can be used to separate the edges of eschar from the necrotic wound bed. Scissors can be used to snip black, brown, gray or yellow necrotic tissue from the pressure ulcer. If the patient has cellulitis that is advancing, sharp debridement of devitalized tissue is urgent.[22] The main benefit of sharp debridement is the rapidity with which dead tissue can be removed. A physician, physician's assistant, physical therapist, or advanced practice nurse determines the need for this type of debridement.[25] State laws and community standards determine the requirements for performing this procedure.[24,25]

Mechanical debridement

Mechanical debridement removes dead tissue by applying a mechanical scrubbing force or use of wet-to-dry dressings (see "Gauze dressings" later in this chapter). Mechanical debridement is nonselective, can harm healthy granulation tissue or epithelial cells, and may be painful.[22,24] Superficial wounds or wounds with small amounts of necrotic tissue can be more effectively treated with other debridement techniques.

Chemical debridement

Chemical debridement with enzymatic agents is a selective method of debridement. The various types of enzymes target specific necrotic tissues, such as protein, fibrin, and collagen. The type of enzyme chosen depends on the type of necrotic tissue in the wound. Enzymes are generally categorized into 1) proteolytics 2) fibrinolytics, and 3) collagenases. Necrotic fibrins and proteins are located in the wound bed more superficially than devitalized collagen.[24]

During the inflammatory process of wound healing, one of the more important enzymes released is endogenous collagenase. Because collagen comprises at least 75% of the dry weight of skin, the role of endogenous collagenase can be considered one of the rate-limiting steps in tissue remodeling.[23] Chemical debridement of wounds can be initiated with topical enzymatic agents that attack natured and denatured collagen in necrotic tissue. The enzyme collagenase is derived from *Clostridium histolyticum*. Four double blind studies[26-29] reported the debriding efficacy of collagenase when compared with placebo. Two studies[26,29] demonstrated that collagenase can solubilize undenatured collagen and facilitate debridement of stubborn necrotic tissue. Within the physiologic pH range of 6-8, the enzyme collagenase is effective in dissolving and liquefying necrotic wound debris. Enzymes can be inactivated with topical anti-infective agents containing heavy metals or acidic solutions that alter the pH. Debilitated patients should be closely monitored for systemic bacterial infections with the use of enzymatic debridement.

Autolytic debridement

Autolysis makes use of the body's own ezymes to digest devitalized tissue. Autolytic debridement can be initiated by applying moisture-retentive dressings to the wound bed. These dressings allow endogenous enzymes in the wound fluid to liquefy necrotic tissue selectively. The wound fluid contains macrophages and neutrophils that digest and solubilize necrotic tissue. Autolytic debridement is the most selective form of debridement but requires an extended time to remove devitalized tissue.[23,24] Autolytic debridement generally is not associated with pain.

Pressure ulcer cleansing

Optimal wound healing cannot proceed until all foreign material is removed from the wound. The purpose of wound cleansing is to remove inflammatory material on the wound surface. This can be done with pressure irrigations. Wound irrigation has two components: a cleansing solution and a mechanical means of delivering the solution to the wound bed.[22,30]

Selecting the cleansing agent

The most common, cost effective wound cleansing solution is isotonic saline (0.9% sodium chloride).[22] Multiple commercial skin and wound cleansers also are available. Skin cleansers never should be used on open wounds. There is a major difference in toxicity between wound cleansers and skin cleansers. Tests that directly compare the toxicity of cleansing solutions can provide useful information on their relative safety. Two studies[31,32] ranked many of the commercial wound cleansers based on their relative toxicity to white blood cells. The extent of dilution required to provide viability and phagocytic efficiency of white blood cells was used as the basis of an index of toxicity. The toxicity index for wound and skin cleansers is displayed in Table 7.2.[22,30]

Table 7.2 Toxicity Index for Wound and Skin Cleansers

Test Agent	Toxicity Index[a]
Shur Clens®	1:10
Biolex™	1:100
Saf Clens™	1:100
Cara Klenz™	1:100
Ultra Klenz™	1:1,000
Clinical Care™	1:1,000
Uni Wash®	1:1,000
Ivory Soap® (0.5 percent)	1:1,000
Constant Clens™	1:10,000
Dermal Wound Cleanser	1:10,000
Puri-Clens™	1:10,000
Hibiclens®	1:10,000
Betadine® Surgical Scrub	1:10,000
Techni-Care™ Scrub	1:100,000
Bard™ Skin Cleanser	1:100,000
Hollister™	1:100,000

[a]The dilution required to maintain white blood cell viability and phagocytic efficiency.
Source: Foresman, Payne, Becker, et al., 1993.

This toxicity index does not mean to imply that the toxic solutions should be diluted and then used for wound cleansing. The recommendation is not to use them on open wounds. The cleansing capacity of any cleansing solution should be balanced against its potential to damage essential macrophage and fibroblast cells of the wound tissue.

Selecting the irrigation technique

Wounds need to be irrigated with enough force to enhance cleansing without traumatizing the wound bed. Hydraulic forces generated by a stream of fluid can flush debris from a wound surface. To be effective, the irrigation force must be greater than the adhesion forces holding the debris to the wound bed.[33] Various methods of wound irrigation have been reported. Cleansing the wound with a steady stream from a piston syringe is more beneficial than cleansing the wound with a bulb syringe or gravity drip. A bulb syringe delivers pressure at less than 1 pound per square inch (psi) and is an insufficient cleansing method. A water-pic delivers pressure at 50-70 psi, is needlessly traumatizing, and should be avoided. An ideal pressure for flushing necrotic tissue from a wound is 8 psi.[34]

Several studies have demonstrated that increasing the pressure of the irrigating stream enhanced removal of bacteria and soil from wounds.[33,34] In one study, 335 patients who presented to the emergency department with traumatic wounds less than 24 hours old were randomly assigned for wound cleansing. The control group received irrigation with a standard bulb syringe that delivered an irrigation stream of 0.05 psi to the wound bed. The experimental group received irrigation with a 12-cc syringe and 22-gauge needle that delivered an irrigation stream of 13 psi to the wound. There was a statistically significant decrease in both wound inflammation and wound infection for wounds cleansed with the syringe and needle irrigation system as compared to wounds cleansed with the bulb syringe.[35] At follow up, 27.8% of the wounds in the bulb syringe group were inflamed, and 6.9% were infected. In the syringe and needle group, 16.8% of the wounds were inflamed, and 1.3% were infected.[35]

Increasing the pressure of an irrigation stream can increase the cleansing efficiency of the irrigation process to a point. Too high an irrigation pressure can cause trauma to the soft tissue.[36,37] Fluid dispersion into wound tissue was significantly greater for a 70 psi irrigation stream than for an 8 psi irrigation stream.[36] When a single orifice tip was used to irrigate wounds in dogs, there was extensive penetration of the irrigation fluid into the tissue, especially when the pressure was increased above 30 psi.[37] With a multijet tip shower head, irrigating fluid was not forced into the surrounding tissue. When the experimental wounds were contaminated, the dispersion of irrigating fluid was not associated with dispersion of bacteria into the wound tissue[36] or the development of bacteremia.[38] However, the trauma induced by the high-pressure irrigation did make the wounds more susceptible to the development of infection.[36]

Clinical practicalities of selecting an irrigation method

One way to produce a pressurized irrigation stream is to deliver the irrigant from a syringe through a needle or catheter. Use of a 35-ml syringe and a 19-gauge needle will deliver a stream of irrigant to the wound surface at 8 psi.[39] Although this is an effective irrigation pressure, needles used for wound lavage can become contaminated with blood, exudate, and other body fluids. A major concern is transmission of hepatitis B, non-A, non-B hepatitis and human immunodeficiency virus.[40] To reduce danger from needle sticks to care providers, alternatives to using a needle were investigated. One viable alternative is a 19-gauge angiocatheter attached to a 35-cc syringe. The vinyl tubing of the angiocatheter delivers the right amount of pressure and eliminates unnecessary use of a needle. The use of a syringe, angiocatheter, and bottle of saline is an expensive but effective clinical method of irrigating wounds.

At Harper Hospital, as part of a quality improvement initiative, an alternative cost effective wound irrigation method was selected. A 250-cc soft plastic bottle of sterile normal saline was paired with a Baxter screw cap with irrigating tip. When squeezed with full force, this irrigation system delivers an irrigating stream with impact pressures of approximately 4.5-5 psi. The compliance with wound cleansing and infection control policies has improved since adoption of this method, and nurses appreciate the user-friendly approach. This system of wound irrigation has become part of the Harper Skin/Wound Care Protocol at less cost than previous wound irrigation techniques. One bottle provides adequate cleansing solution for irrigating a large wound or enough solution for three dressing changes per 24 hours on a smaller wound. The bottle and cap are discarded 24 hours after opening. As with any pressurized irrigation method, clinicians should be aware of splashback and use appropriate precautions. Table 7.3, produced for the AHCPR Guideline on Pressure Ulcer Treatment, is reproduced here to assist clinicians in selecting equipment with appropriate irrigation pressures.[22]

Table 7.3 Irrigation Pressures

Device	Irrigation Impact Pressure (psi)
Spray Bottle-Ultra Klenz™[a] (Carrington Laboratories, Inc., Dallas, TX)	1.2
Bulb Syringe[a] (Davol Inc., Cranston, RI)	2.0
Piston Irrigation Syringe (60-ml) with catheter tip (Premium Plastics, Inc., Chicago, IL)	4.2
Saline Squeeze Bottle (250-ml) with irrigation cap (Baxter Healthcare Corp., Deerfield, IL)`4.5	
Water Pik® at lowest setting (#1) (Teledyne Water Pik, Fort Collins, CO)	6.0
Irrijet® DS Syringe with tip (Ackrad Laboratories, Inc., Cranford, NJ)	7.6
35-ml syringe with 19-gauge needle or angiocatheter	8.0
Water Pik® at middle setting (#3)[b] (Teledyne Water Pik, Fort Collins, CO)	42.0
Water Pik® at highest setting (#5)[b] (Teledyne Water Pik, Fort Collins, CO)	>50.0
Pressurized Cannister-Dey-Wash™ [b] (Dey Laboratories, Inc., Napa, CA)	>50.0

[a]These devices may not deliver enough pressure to adequately cleanse wounds.
[b]These devices may cause trauma and drive bacteria into wounds. They are not recommended for cleansing of soft-tissue wounds.
Source: Beltran, Thacker, and Rodeheaver, 1994.

Whirlpool cleansing

Whirlpool baths have been used for wound cleansing since their development by French surgeons during World War I. The vigorous whirling and agitation of the water contributes to its cleansing action. Neiderhuber, Stribley and Koepke[41] demonstrated the use of a whirlpool bath to remove bacteria from a contaminated surface. Cultures of the feet were taken before and after treatment to assess efficacy of whirlpool cleansing. The results showed that water temperature had no effect on the removal of bacteria from the plantar surface of the foot. Bacterial load was optimally reduced with an immersion time of 20 minutes. Agitation was a better technique than spraying or soaking alone in the removal of bacteria. The best technique was a combination of agitation followed by spraying with clean water to remove the remaining contaminated water from the feet. This technique left a surface that was 95% freer of bacteria than at the start of treatment. These findings were supported in a repeated measures study by Bohannon,[42] who found that a 20-30 minute whirlpool treatment, followed by more than 30 seconds of rinsing with maximum force tolerated, removed more than four times as many bacteria from a venous stasis ulcer as whirlpool alone.

Feedar and Kloth[43] described hydrotherapy in the form of whirlpool treatments to cleanse chronic open wounds of dirt, foreign contaminants, and toxic residue. They recommended twice-daily whirlpool treatments in conjunction with interim wound dressings to facilitate debridement of necrotic tissue. The turbulence of the water is thought to assist in removing surface debris. The authors cautioned that the use of whirlpool with even moderate water agitation can damage granulation tissue and migrating epidermal cells. Once a wound has been cleansed of foreign debris, the benefits of the whirlpool are outweighed by its potential to harm regenerating tissue. Therefore, for clean wounds, the use of a whirlpool bath is not recommended.

Maintaining a moist wound environment

The role of humidity has been shown to be of prime importance in affecting both the rate of epithelialization and the amount of scar formation.[44] Studies investigating the mechanisms of re-epithelialization have shown that a moist—not a dry—environment provides the optimum condition for healing. When wounds are left uncovered and allowed to dry, epidermal cells must migrate under dry crusts or scabs and over the fibrous tissue below. Conversely, under semioccluded or occluded conditions in which the surface of the wound remains moist, epidermal cells are able to migrate more readily, and hence epithelialization is more rapid[45] (see Figure 4.2).

A wound bed is kept hydrated with the use of appropriate dressings. Moisture-retentive dressings prevent wound desiccation and promote granulation tissue.[46] If the wound bed is exposed to the air, it will dehydrate and cellular death will occur.[46]

Open wounds, such as pressure ulcers, require dressings that protect and maintain their physiological integrity. Ideally, the dressing will keep the wound surface moist without accumulation of excessive fluids that macerate the skin and allow bacterial proliferation. Some of the occlusive dressings designed to keep wounds moist have caused concern about the possibility of promoting bacterial growth under the dressing. However, studies have shown that these dressings may protect wounds from pathogenic bacteria.[47-50]

Purpose of wound dressings

Many diverse materials have been used to treat wounds through the ages. Historically, they range from hot oils and waxes to animal membranes and feces.[51] Currently, there are many dressing materials available for care of chronic wounds, such as pressure ulcers. The basic purpose of the dressing must be considered before one is selected. Functions of a dressing are: (a) to protect the wound from contamination, (b) to protect the wound from trauma, (c) to provide compression if bleeding or swelling is anticipated, (d) to apply medications, and (e) to absorb drainage or debride necrotic tissue. The condition of the wound bed and the desired function will determine the type of dressing that is used. The pressure ulcer must be evaluated and a treatment plan determined before the most suitable dressing can be selected. Clinicians should choose dressing techniques that will ensure that the wound bed is kept moist and the surrounding intact skin is kept dry.[1,22] See Table 7.4 for properties of commonly used dressing materials, along with indications, advantages, and disadvantages.[52]

Types of dressings

There is no single dressing that can provide an optimum environment for all wounds. Each type of dressing product has its advantages and disadvantages.[53] Types of dressings, their characteristics, and their functions are discussed below. This is followed by a review of the scientific literature on various types of dressings used specifically on pressure ulcers.[54]

Gauze dressings

Gauze dressings are made of cotton or synthetic fabric that is absorptive and permeable to water, water vapor, and oxygen. Gauze may be used dry, moist, or impregnated with petrolatum, antiseptics, or other agents. It is made in varying weaves and with different size interstices. It may be used in special dressing techniques.

Dry gauze

The purpose of a dry dressing is protection from trauma and infection. On a primarily closed wound, the dressing is placed on the wound dry, and removed dry. On an open wound, dry dressings should only be used when there is excessive exudate. The gauze wicks the excess fluid from the ulcer. The dressing is changed as needed to control the exudate.[1]

Wet-to-dry saline gauze

Wet-to-dry saline gauze dressings are used for debridement of necrotic tissue in the wound bed. Saline-moistened gauze is wrung until it is just damp. It is opened and

Table 7.4 Properties of Commonly Used Dressing Materials

Dressing Category	Examples	Indications
Polyurethane films	Op-Site, Tegaderm, Bioclusive, Blisterfilm, Ensure-it, Accuderm, Uniflex, Opraflex, etc.	Protection of partial thickness red wounds Cover dressing for hydrophillic powder and paste preparations and hydrogels
Hydrocolloids	DuoDerm, J&J Ulcer Dr., Comfeel, Restore, Intact, Intrasite, Tegasorb, etc.	Protection of superficial and small, deep red wounds Autolytic debridement of small, noninfected yellow wounds[*]
Hydrogel sheets	Vigilon, Geliperm, Elastogel, Cutinova, etc.	Protection of superficial and moderately deep red wounds Autolytic debridement of small, noninfected yellow or black wounds[*] Delivery system for topical antimicrobial creams (increases penetration)
Hydrophillic beads, powders, and pastes	Bard Absorption dressing, Hydrogran, Hollister Exudate, Absorber, Duoderm granules, Comfeel Powder, Envisan, Debrisan, etc.	Cleansing of draining yellow wounds Protection of deep draining and nondraining red wounds (except Envisan and Debrisan) Autolytic debridement of noninfected black wounds[*] (except Envisan and Debrisan)
Gel pastes	Carrington Gel, Geliperm, Intrasite, Biolex, etc.	Protection of red wounds Autolytic debridement of noninfected yellow or black wounds[*]
Foams	Lyofoam, Epi-Lock, Allevin, Cutinova Plus, etc.	Protection of red wounds Dressing tracheostomy and drain sites
Impregnated dressings	Adaptic, Xeroform, Aquaphor, Scarlet Red, Vaseline Gauze, etc.	Protection of superficial infected and noninfected red wounds; "contact layer" for primarily closed wounds
Cotton and gauze dressings	Wet to dry ⟶	Mechanical debridement of yellow wounds
	Wet to damp ⟶	Mechanical debridement of red/yellow wounds
	Continuous dry ⟶	Heavily exudating red wounds
	Continuous moist ⟶	Protection of red wounds Autolytic debridement of yellow or black wounds[*] Delivery of topical meds

[*]Use with caution in critically ill patients who are leukopenic or have poor wound perfusion. Avoid in patients with clinically infected wounds.

Advantages	Disadvantages	Considerations
Transparent; good adhesion; waterproof; reduces pain; minimizes friction forces to wound; time saving; easy to store	Adhesive injury to intact and new skin; nonabsorbent; some products difficult to apply; variable barrier function; can promote wound infection	Protect wound margins; avoid in wounds with infection, copious drainage, or tracts; change only if dressing leaks
Absorbent; nonadhesive to healing tissue; good barrier; waterproof; reduce pain; easy to apply; time saving; easy to store	Nontransparent; may soften and lose shape with heat or friction; odor and brown drainage on removal (melted dressing material)	Frequency of changes will depend on amount of exudate (change as needed for leakage); avoid in wounds with infection or tracts
Absorbent; nonadhesive; reduces pain; compatible with topicals; good conformity; easy to store	Poor barrier; semi-transparent; requires cover dressing to secure; can promote growth of *Pseudomonas* and yeast; expensive	Avoid in infected wounds; change every 8 hrs or as needed for leakage
Good "filler" for deep wounds; absorbs large amounts of exudate; rapid cleansing of yellow wounds; cost effective; helps control odor	Occasional pain on application; requires cover dressing; dressing material leaks out with position change if outer dressing not sealed; difficult to remove from tracts and deep pockets	Partially fill wound cavities to allow for expansion; avoid in wounds with fistulas or deep tracts; monitor electrolytes if copious drainage
Good "filler" for small deep red wounds, easy to apply	Requires cover dressing; expensive; variable absorbency	Same as hydrogels
Insulates wound; provides some padding; nonadherent; easy to use; easy to store	Poor absorbency; poor barrier; nontransparent; requires sealing of edges with tape; poor conformability to deep wounds	Change every 24 hrs or as needed for leakage; avoid in draining wounds with viscous exudate
Nonadherent (if gauze cover dressing used); antibacterial if medicated; easy to use; easy to store	Some products will adhere to wound if allowed to dry out; poor barrier if nonmedicated	Change at least every 24 hrs (if nonadherent); if adherent, allow to separate spontaneously
Readily available; good mechanical debridement if properly used; cost effective "filler" for large wounds; effective delivery of topicals if kept moist	Delayed healing if used improperly; pain on removal (wet to dry); labor intensive	Use rolled gauze for packing large wounds (ensures complete removal); pack loosely (tight packing delays healing); use wide mesh gauze for debriding; use fine mesh for protection; do not use cotton-filled materials on wound surface

placed on the wound surface moist and allowed to dry until it adheres to the necrotic tissue in the wound bed. It is then pulled away from the wound, removing debris adherent to the interstices of the dressing. This method of debridement is nonselective and may damage new tissue growth when the dressing is removed from the wound.[1] Mulder[55] suggests that an open mesh 100% cotton nonwoven gauze sponge is effective in debriding nonviable tissue with minimal damage to viable tissue.

Continuously moist saline gauze

Continuously moist saline gauze dressings are used to keep the wound bed moist when frequent inspection of the wound bed is necessary. The purpose of this type of dressing is to keep the wound bed moist to allow for the proliferation of new tissue and epithelial migration. It is used for wounds that do not contain large amounts of necrotic tissue. This dressing should be placed in the wound moist, and be remoistened or changed frequently enough to keep the wound tissue continuously moist. Care must be taken that the moist gauze dressing is placed in the wound bed only and not on the surrounding intact skin. Constant moisture on skin will cause it to macerate. A thin layer of petrolatum or hydrocolloid may be placed on the surrounding intact skin to protect it from the moist dressing.

Effect of gauze dressings

The effect of gauze dressings on pressure ulcers was examined in nine controlled studies.[54] In all, gauze was used to treat 403 subjects with 591 ulcers. Two studies[56,57] used wet-to-dry saline gauze, one study[58] used wet-to-dry Dakin's solution on gauze, and one study[59] used povidone-iodine, a saline wash, and dry gauze dressings. Five investigators[60-64] used continuously moist saline gauze dressings as the control treatment. Two controlled trials[59,65] compared dry wound healing techniques to moist wound healing. Kurzuk-Howard[65] compared heat lamp treatments to film dressings. Saydak[59] compared dry gauze dressings to an absorptive powder dressing on bilateral Stages II and III pressure ulcers in 11 subjects. These studies showed a significantly better rate of healing with the moist wound healing treatment than with dry gauze. In the wet-to-dry gauze studies,[56-59] gauze was compared with various moist wound healing alternatives. Results of these studies suggested that moist wound healing outperformed wet-to-dry gauze dressings. Five controlled trials[60-64] compared moist saline gauze with other types of moist wound healing. No significant differences in healing rates were found between moist saline gauze and other moist wound healing alternatives. Based on this literature, moist wound healing methods performed better than dry gauze. Moist wound healing techniques also performed better than wet-to-dry gauze. Pressure ulcers treated with moist saline gauze healed at a rate similar to other moist wound healing techniques.

Five controlled trials[60-64] measured nursing time to care for patients treated with gauze dressings versus other types of dressings. These studies agreed that it takes significantly more nursing time to care for a patient's pressure ulcers when saline gauze dressings are used rather than hydrocolloid or transparent film dressings. The difference in nursing time is related to the number of required dressing changes for hydrocolloid or film dressings as compared to gauze dressings.

Polyurethane film

Polyurethane film dressings are synthetic, semipermeable, transparent, and adhesive. They allow free flow of oxygen through the pores in the dressing. They allow water vapor to pass from the wound to the air, but they are impermeable to bacteria and to the particles in the environment. These dressings enhance epithelial migration by preventing a scab from forming.[66] Polyurethane dressings have adhesive backings that allow them to adhere to dry skin. Some film dressings adhere to the base of the ulcer and, when removed, strip away new epidermis. On skin surface areas at risk for abrasion, polyurethane film can be used prophylactically to decrease the amount of friction between the patient's skin and the bedsheets. It also may be used to protect the skin from fecal and urinary incontinence.[1]

Film dressings are effective for treating pressure ulcers. Ten studies—three controlled trials and seven case series—reported the use of film dressings for pressure ulcer treatment.[54] In controlled trials, film was studied on 106 subjects with 139 pressure ulcers. In case series, 240 subjects with 351 pressure ulcers were treated with film dressings. The case series reported that 65%-100% of the ulcers healed or improved and 6%-14% of the ulcers enlarged while using film dressings. Nearly all of the trials used infected ulcers as an exclusion criterion for the study. A number of investigators reported that some film dressings would not remain adherent[67-69] in the sacral region, particularly near the anus. In three trials, film was compared to different control treatments: Seburn[56] compared film to wet-to-dry saline gauze, Kurzuk-Howard[65] compared film to dry wound treatment with a heat lamp, and Oleske[63] compared film to moist saline gauze. In the wet-to-dry gauze versus film trial, 44 subjects with 77 pressure ulcers were evaluated. Film was found to improve healing and decrease cost for Stage II ulcers, but no difference was found in either cost or healing rates for Stage III ulcers. Patients who had intact sensation reported less pain with film dressings.[56] In the study that compared film dressings with moist saline gauze for uninfected superficial pressure ulcers, no differences in ulcer healing were noted between the two groups.[63]

There appears to be relatively little risk of wound infection using film dressings.[54] When film is compared with other treatment, film dressings appeared to result in faster healing and lower cost than wet-to-dry ulcer techniques for Stage II ulcers but not for Stage III ulcers. The effectiveness of film dressings was no different than other moist wound healing techniques. Additionally, film dressings resulted in a significant savings in nursing time compared to techniques employing saline gauze.[54]

Hydrocolloids

Hydrocolloid dressings are adhesive, moldable wafers made of carbohydrate-based materials, usually with a waterproof backing. Usually, they are impermeable to oxygen, water, and water vapor.[22,54] These dressings contain hydroactive particles that interact with moisture to form a gel. They adhere to the dry, surrounding, undamaged skin to contain the wound exudate and prevent wound contamination. The wound is kept bathed in serous exudate. This enhances healing and enables removal of the dressing without adherence to the newly formed epithelium.[70] It is important that dressings do not adhere to wound surfaces because epithelial cells that have migrated may be torn away with each dressing change. Some researchers believe that interactive dressings need to have a porous backing to allow for a more controlled evaporation of wound exudate. If they have an occlusive backing, they should not be used on clinically infected wounds.

A total of 19 studies examined the effects of hydrocolloid dressings on pressure ulcers.[54] Approximately 531 subjects with more than 650 ulcers participated in the studies. Of the 19 reports, 11 were controlled studies and 8 were case series. Four studies[60-62,64] compared a hydrocolloid dressing with moist saline gauze, and one study[58] compared hydrocolloid with wet-to dry Dakin's gauze dressings. Three studies[71-73] compared one hydrocolloid to another, and three studies[74-76] compared a hydrocolloid dressing to assorted other ulcer treatments.

All studies demonstrated that hydrocolloids were an effective dressing for Stages II, III, and IV pressure ulcers. The rate of ulcer healing varied with initial ulcer depth and the length of the study. One study,[77] which included only deep Stages III and IV ulcers, reported that 38% of the ulcers healed during the course of therapy. Another short study with only 8 days of treatment revealed that 22% of the ulcers completely healed. The remaining studies showed that 50%-100% of ulcers healed or improved during their course of treatment with hydrocolloid dressings. The percentage of ulcers that worsened during hydrocolloid treatment ranged from 0% to 31%. Patients with debilitating cancer[78] or diabetes[79] seemed more likely to have their ulcers worsen. Gourse suggested that deeper ulcers were more likely to worsen with hydrocolloid dressing treatment.[58]

Controlled trials did not provide evidence to support the claim that hydrocolloid dressings were more likely to cause wound infection than the control treatments. However, it should be noted that most of the controlled trials *excluded* subjects whose ulcers, at initial assessment, were clinically judged to be infected. Sheridan[78] and Neill[62] studied wound bacterial counts. Neill found that the growth of *Candida albicans* and alpha streptococcus increased during hydrocolloid treatment.[62] In contrast to the hydrocolloid-treated ulcers, Neill found an increased growth of *Pseudomonas aeruginosa* and *Providentia stuartii* in ulcers treated with wet-to-moist saline gauze. In the Neill study, *Candida albicans* was the only organism more likely to be found in hydrocolloid-treated ulcers when compared with wet-to-damp saline gauze ulcers.[62] Sheridan reported either resolution of bacterial colonization during hydrocolloid treatment or a change in organism pattern to normal skin flora.[78] Gourse, who initially did not exclude clinically infected ulcers, reported that one subject became bacteremic, presumably from the pressure ulcer, while being treated with a hydrocolloid dressing.[58]

One controlled trial[60] and three case series[77,80,81] reported on pain control with hydrocolloid dressings. Alm reported that neither the moist saline gauze nor the hydrocolloid dressing treatments were associated with significant pain.[60] The three case series reported that a significant number of patients reported less pain or discomfort with hydrocolloid dressings compared with previous treatments.

The cost of hydrocolloid dressings versus control treatments was reported in several studies.[58,61,62,64,82] Of these trials, four[61-64] measured, rather than estimated, nursing time. All four studies noted that treatment with hydrocolloid dressings saved a significant amount of nursing time when compared with saline gauze treatment.

One study[64] compared hydrocolloid dressings with moist saline gauze in a prospective, randomized controlled trial of 39 subjects in an 80-bed long-term-care facility. There was no statistical difference in healing between the hydrocolloid and continuously moist saline gauze. There was a significantly lower cost with the use of hydrocolloid over moist saline gauze. However, since unsterile supplies were used for the saline gauze dressings, sterile supply use would inflate these costs and probably decrease the cost differential between moist saline gauze and hydrocolloid.

Gels/hydrogels

Hydrogel dressings are water-based, nonadherent, polymer-based dressings with some absorptive properties. These dressings maintain a moist environment and may be used with a topical medication if indicated. One property of gel dressings is the ability to cool the wound by as much as 5°. This may increase comfort for patients with painful wounds.[1] Not all hydrogels behave in the same manner. A recent laboratory study was undertaken to examine the fluid-handling properties of four hydrogel dressings.[83] Three of the dressings were likely to be fluid-donating agents, while one of the dressings had a dual ability to donate or absorb liquid, depending on the moisture content of the substrate to which it was applied. In the future, gel dressings may be able to "read" the moisture content of a wound and deliver or absorb the necessary amount of fluid to maintain an ideal environment. Also, it is possible that these dressings can become carriers for growth factors and biologically active molecules.

Currently, gels/hydrogels appear to be effective for treating pressure ulcers. The relative benefits of gels/hydrogels over other types of moist wound healing techniques for pressure ulcer treatment remain to be determined. Data examined on the effectiveness of gels/hydrogels for pressure ulcer treatment come from three studies: one controlled trial[76] and two case series.[54,85] These three studies assessed 122 subjects with 196 pressure ulcers. From 77% to 90% of ulcers treated with gel or hydrogel healed or improved during treatment. From 3% to 4% of the ulcers treated with hydrogel deteriorated. No infections were reported. No analysis on pain control was reported. The single controlled trial showed no overall statistical difference between gel and hydrocolloid dressings. Most of the ulcers in both groups either healed or improved.[76]

Foam dressings

Foam dressings are made from a spongelike polymer that may or may not be adherent. Foam may be impregnated or coated with other materials. It has some absorptive properties. Foam dressings create a moist environment and provide thermal insulation of the wound. If it has hydrophilic dressing properties, this will allow for some absorption of wound drainage. Topical medication may be used in combination with foam dressings.[1]

Two case series[86,87] used foam dressings on 20 subjects with 37 pressure ulcers. Foam dressings, like film and hydrocolloid dressings, appeared to provide a moist wound healing environment and needed to be changed only when leakage of wound exudate occurred. From 48% to 60% of ulcers healed with foam dressing treatment. From 58% to 94% of the ulcers either healed or improved during treatment with foam dressings. In this small group of subjects, no infections, ulcer enlargement, or other complications were reported. However, it cannot be extrapolated that these complications are less likely to occur than with hydrocolloid or film dressings because the number of patients reported is small.[54]

Alginate dressings

Alginate dressings are made from a naturally occurring polysaccharide found in brown seaweed. The principal constituent is alginic acid, converted to mixed calcium and sodium salts. This dressing is a nonwoven twisted fiber rope or fibrous mat. The mat is placed in the wound and held in place with a secondary dressing. As the dressing absorbs wound fluid, it forms a soft hydrogel. The dressing is capable of absorbing up to 20 times its own weight in exudate, and its primary use is on moderately to heavily exudating wounds.[1]

Data examining the use of alginates were taken from three case series[88-90] on approximately 35 subjects.[54] In this group of subjects, alginate dressings appeared to allow healing in deep exudative pressure ulcers. Subjective evaluations reported that dressings were effective for exudate control, odor control, and pain control. Alginates appeared to be associated with minimal pain on dressing changes and less pain than historical control treatments. No studies with cost comparisons were found, and no controlled trials were found comparing alginates to other strategies for treating pressure ulcers in humans.[54]

Pastes, powders, and beads

Paste, powder, and bead dressing materials are formulated primarily to fill wound cavities. They usually have properties that allow absorption of wound exudate, which then converts the dressing to a gelatinous mass. The gelled agent then can be irrigated from the wound. Hydrophilic beads or paste can be inserted into a wound cavity. One gram of hydrophilic beads can absorb up to 4 grams of water. The granules do not digest bacteria or necrotic tissue, but they draw bacteria away from the wound bed. The wound and dressing debris then is removed by irrigation.[1]

Three controlled trials[57,59,75] studied the use of paste or powder on 54 subjects with 88 pressure ulcers.[54] Complete healing occurred in 0%-52% of the ulcers, and 52%-64% of ulcers either healed or improved. When compared to dry gauze dressings, an absorptive dressing made of powder mixed with water resulted in significantly better ulcer healing.[59] One small study[57] showed no difference in healing between wet-to-dry saline gauze and copolymer starch, and another study[75] showed no difference between paste and hydrocolloid dressings. No wound infections occurred with either type of dressing materials.

Selecting dressings

Some dressings claim to have enhanced capabilities or lower complication rates than other types of dressings. Controlled studies are needed to support such claims (see Table 12.8).[91] Also, a single study probably is insufficient evidence to allow claims of enhanced performance of one dressing over another.[54]

There remains the mistaken belief that dressings heal wounds. This encourages clinicians to try multiple dressings without consideration of other factors that are of even greater importance. To assist nurses with selection of appropriate dressing materials, skin/wound care decision-making flowcharts were developed at Harper Hospital. Based on a model published by Sween Corporation,[92] multiple wound care flowcharts were customized for products carried at Harper Hospital (see Appendices). These flowcharts have improved and standardized the care of specific types of wounds.

Bacterial management

Infection is a major concern in the care of a patient with a pressure ulcer. Bacteria normally cover the body surface and the gut; however, when skin is damaged and the immune system is compromised, these same bacteria can become virulent. Acute wounds generally are more susceptible to bacterial invasion than chronic wounds. All chronic wound surfaces are colonized with bacteria. It is only when conditions are favorable that infection occurs. Number and type of organism, wound type, and general condition of the patient affect the patient's ability to resist infection. The patient's clinical response is taken into account when diagnosing infection.[93] The most common sites for infection are the lungs, urinary tract, skin, and abdomen. All sites must be evaluated when the patient presents with a fever and high white blood cell count because bacteria is most likely the cause.[94,95] When infection of an ulcer is suspected, a culture should be obtained. The AHCPR Pressure Ulcer Treatment Guideline recommends that quantitative bacterial cultures also be obtained when clean ulcers are not healing. Open wounds do not have to be sterile to heal. However, pressure ulcer healing may be impaired when the bacterial count in an ulcer exceeds 10^5 organisms per gram of tissue.[96,97] The most accurate method of determining bacterial load is by tissue biopsy or by fluid from needle aspiration.[98,99] But not all facilities have the capability or the laboratory facilities to obtain tissue with a scalpel or punch biopsy. Nor do they have the laboratory facilities to process the tissue. Use of a swab technique for obtaining a specimen cannot be relied on to accurately document the bioburden in the tissues because the swabbing is done in a variety of ways.[100] However, according to Stotts,[100] if a standardized technique is used, a quantitative swab technique can accurately document the bioburden in pressure ulcers. The technique for obtaining the specimen should reflect bacteria in the tissue rather than from the surface of the wound. The results of the swab culture must give more than just presence or absence of bacteria. Reports on the bioburden must be presented in a quantitative or semiquantitative manner for the information to be useful.[100]

Techniques for obtaining a wound culture are as follows:

Tissue biopsy technique
1. Cleanse wound or skin surface with antimicrobial solution and allow to dry.
2. Obtain tissue by punch biopsy or scalpel.
3. Send the tissue to the laboratory for preparation and analysis.
4. Results are reported as number of organisms per gram of tissue.

Needle aspiration procedure
1. Cleanse intact skin with antimicrobial solution and allow to dry.
2. Using a 10ml. syringe and a 22 gauge needle, with 0.5ml. of air in the syringe, the needle is inserted through the intact skin. Suction is created by briskly withdrawing the plunger to the 10-cc mark. Move the needle backward and forward at different angles for two to four explorations. Gently return the plunger to the 0.5 mark.
3. Withdraw and cap the needle. Transport the fluid to the laboratory.
4. Results are reported as the number of organisms per gram of tissue.

Quantitative swab procedure
1. Cleanse wound surface with non-antimicrobial solution.
2. Rotate the end of a sterile cotton-tipped applicator stick while a 1-cm area of the open wound is swabbed for 5 seconds. Use sufficient pressure on the swab to express fresh tissue fluid.
3. Break the swab tip into a sterile tube containing transport media and transport to the laboratory.
4. Results are expressed either as the number of organisms per swab or in a semiquantitative manner, such as scant, small, moderate, and large (1+ to 4+) bacterial growth.[100]

If a pressure ulcer is infected, antimicrobial therapy should begin as soon as possible.[101] Antibiotic selection is based on the most likely etiologic pathogen, the known antimicrobial susceptibility pattern for the suspected organism, the efficacy of the drugs, potential adverse effects, and cost. Antibiotics are biologically derived products that have a specific method of inhibiting microbial function. Lineaweaver[102,103] studied the toxicity of bacitracin, neomycin, and kanamycin on human fibroblasts. McCauley et al[104] studied the effects of silver sulfadiazine on human fibroblasts. It appears that silver sulfadiazine exerts its toxic effects on bacteria through heavy metal poisoning. It is thought that this same heavy metal poisoning accounts for the toxic effects on human fibroblasts. A significant reduction in cell proliferation occurred when dermal fibroblasts were exposed to silver sulfadiazine. These findings may explain the clinical observation of delayed wound healing with the use of silver sulfadiazine. The effect of various topical agents on bacterial counts and on the viability of healthy tissue is not clear. Also, the emergence of allergy, sensitivity and resistant organisms following the use of topical treatments is of concern.

Topical antimicrobials

Topical antimicrobial agents include both antibiotics and antiseptics. Many practitioners believe that it is necessary to disinfect a chronic ulcer with topical antimicrobials. However, the use of antimicrobials on open wounds is highly controversial, and the results of several studies report adverse effects.[102,105,106] Patients with chronic wounds may develop allergies to topical agents, such as bacitracin and neomycin.[107,108] Patients on these medications should be monitored for sensitivity. The AHCPR Pressure Ulcer Treatment Guideline recommends initiating a 2-week trial of topical antibiotics for clean pressure ulcers that are resistant to healing or are continuing to produce exudate after 2 to 4 weeks of optimal care.[22] Research studies show topical antibiotics are effective in reducing the bacterial levels in pressure ulcers to 10^5 organisms per gram of tissue.[99] Topical antibiotics should be used only on wounds that exhibit local signs of infection and on clean ulcers that show no signs of healing, and their usage should be limited because prolonged use may create resistant organisms.[105,106,109]

Antiseptics

Antiseptics are highly reactive chemicals that indiscriminately destroy cell function. Lineaweaver[102,103] studied the toxicity of four antiseptic solutions: povidone-iodine, acetic acid, sodium hypochlorite, and hydrogen peroxide. All of the antiseptics were 100% cytotoxic to fibroblasts. Only hydrogen peroxide did not retard healing of open skin wounds. The study concluded that povidone-iodine was harmful to the tissues and delayed wound healing. The use of antiseptics to decrease the bacterial count in open wounds is contraindicated. Antiseptics indiscriminately damage tissue, interfere with tissue function, increase injury, and delay wound healing. In one study, the use of povidone-iodine inhibited tissue defenses and made them more prone to infection.[102] Pressure ulcers are contaminated with bacteria, but the wound can protect itself against bacteria if natural defenses are not inhibited. If only saline is used, tissue defenses can protect the body against the development of infection unless the patient is immunocompromised. It is recommended that only physiological agents, such as saline, be used to allow the tissue defenses to control the infection. Pressure ulcers should be managed by aggressive attention with conservative agents.

Studies have reported that approximately 25% of nonhealing pressure ulcers have underlying osteomyelitis.[110,111,112] Obtaining a bone biopsy is recommended to diagnose osteomyelitis.[111,113] One study[111] recommends obtaining a white blood count, erythrocyte sedimentation rate, and plain X-ray. If all three of these tests are positive, the positive predictive value for osteomyelitis is 69%. Bone scans may produce false positive results; however, a negative bone scan will rule out the diagnosis.[101] Treatment for osteomyelitis is long-term intravenous antibiotics.

Operative repair

Operative repair is an option for Clean Stage III and Stage IV ulcers that do not respond to optimal care.[22] With surgical intervention, skin closure and tissue coverage is rapid. Criteria need to be standardized to determine patient eligibility. Before operative repair, certain factors need to be weighed: the patient's medical stability, nutritional status, and ability to tolerate the operative procedure/postoperative recovery as well as the likelihood that an operation will improve the patient's functional status. Included in the discussion are patient concerns regarding quality of life, personal preferences, treatment goals, risk of recurrence, and anticipated rehabilitative outcomes.[114,115,116]

Operative procedures indicated for pressure ulcer repair include one or more of the following: direct closure, skin grafting, skin flaps, musculocutaneous flaps, and free flaps.[22] Selection of a specific reconstructive technique is individualized for each patient. The location of the ulcer, prior ulceration and/or surgery, and the patient's mobility status, daily habits, and other associated medical problems are factored into the decision.

A good perioperative program includes comprehensive pre-operative assessment and planning for postoperative care and followup. Since patients often enter the hospital on the operative day, it is helpful if the nurse can meet with the patient prior to admission for postoperative teaching. Patients are informed of factors within their control that may impair wound healing, including smoking, diet, activity, and pressure relief. Nurses should help patients develop postoperative plans to reduce risk factors and increase the chance of operative success. The patient's commitment to participating in success of the program often can be determined at this time.

Surgical repair of the pressure ulcer may include skin grafts and/or muscle flaps. A muscle rotation flap consists of lifting nearby healthy tissue from the fascia[117] and rotating the tissues to cover the defect caused by the pressure ulcer. Blood vessels that are carried over in the muscle flap nourish the tissues. This type of wound closure is beneficial for ulcers that have large amounts of missing tissue because the muscle adds padding to dissipate pressure. It may be necessary to skin graft the donor site if a large tissue defect is caused by the rotation. It is often necessary to smooth the bony prominence to prevent recurrence of the problem.[117]

Postoperative care for patients is crucial to the success of the operation. In any situation where skin grafts or muscle rotation flaps are used, nursing care focuses on maintaining circulation and preventing infection. At the time of a muscle flap operation, wound drains are placed to remove air, serum, or fluid that collects beneath the flap. These drains should be checked to ensure that they are functioning properly. Hematoma formation seriously compromises circulation and may result in flap necrosis. Flap circulation is assessed carefully, and measures are taken to assist in protecting the healing tissue.[118]

After the operation, patients are kept immobile. The use of an air-fluidized or low-air-loss bed for about 2 weeks postoperatively allows the patient to lie on the flap without undue pressure. Caution should be used when turning the patient from side to side, even when using a specialty bed to avoid tension on the suture line and friction and shear on the flap during repositioning. Special nursing care after a rotation flap operation consists of using extra personnel to move the patient in order to reduce the risk of shear on the new graft. Changing the patient's position requires lifting the body to reposition. Under no circumstances should the patient be allowed to slide across the bed. Protection of the grafted blood supply is critical for the first 14 days until the new capillaries are formed in the flap. The graft area should be inspected routinely for pallor or cyanosis indicating tissue ischemia. A healthy flap looks like the patient's normal skin. Color changes should be reported to the surgeon immediately. Activity that increases pressure on the flap must be avoided. This includes the use of a bedpan if it places pressure on the newly grafted area. The patient can defecate onto a plastic pad until the graft is healed enough to tolerate brief periods of pressure.[117] Fecal contamination can be avoided by using constipating medications and a low-fiber diet.[117,119] Controlled bowel evacuation is accomplished with scheduled suppository insertion.

In addition to maintaining circulation, nursing care focuses on measures to prevent infection. Because the vascular reserve of a flap is never normal, infection must be prevented at all costs. While the vasculature may be able to cope with the normal metabolic needs, the added burden of an inflammatory reaction may predispose the flap to necrosis. Infection at the graft site may result in loss of all or part of the graft. Because infection threatens the viability of the flap, the incision areas are cleansed carefully. Crusts and dried areas should be removed from the incision lines with sterile cotton-tipped applicators and sterile saline. Regular cleansing of the flap incisions should continue until all the sutures are removed. Steps can be taken throughout all phases of hospitalization to promote healing and prevent infection in skin grafts and flaps used primarily to close pressure ulcers.

As the flap heals, activity is increased. Approximately 2 weeks after the operation, the patient begins sitting for progressively longer periods of time. After each sitting period, the flap is inspected by the caregiver or by the patient using a mirror. There should be no redness or pallor at the operative site. Ongoing management of the repaired wound emphasizes education about pressure reduction and routine skin inspection.

Operative repair is only the beginning of a long-term recovery and maintenance process. Recurrence rates for pressure ulcers after operative repair vary, but the results of surgical correction often are dependent on patient selection.[120] Risk factors for recurrence include noncompliance and carelessness.[121,122] Pressure ulcers may recur because of patient behavior or from inadequate access to assistance and equipment that would allow continuous prevention of ulcers.[123] Perioperative patient education programs are necessary regardless of the operative method chosen. Long-term follow-up is essential to determine adherence to recommended protocols.

Adjunctive therapy

It is difficult for practitioners to remain abreast of all the new wound care technology and products being introduced to the marketplace as the science of wound healing evolves. Several adjunctive therapies have emerged for the treatment of pressure ulcers. These include growth factors, electrical stimulation, hyperbaric oxygen, cultured epithelium, and ultrasound therapy. Research supporting these therapies is limited. Electrical stimulation is the only adjunctive therapy recommended in the AHCPR Clinical Practice Guideline.[22] Selected adjunctive therapies are discussed below.

Growth factors

In the past, the rate of wound healing was set by nature, and there was little one could do except to create optimal conditions to assist the body's own healing mechanisms. Advances have been made in the understanding of wound repair as topical growth factor research continues. Growth factors are purported to promote new granulation tissue and the growth of new skin to cover the wound.[1] There are many types of growth factors, including platelet-derived growth factors, fibroblast growth factors, transforming growth factor beta, transforming growth factor alpha, interleukins, and epidermal growth factors, among others. Growth factors appear to act within a network of interacting growth factors. It is the combination of factors that produces the biologic response.

The effect of growth factors is due to their interaction with cells at the local level to stimulate or accelerate the repair of chronic, nonhealing wounds.[124] In the use of platelet-derived growth factors, blood is drawn from the patient and sent to a laboratory, where platelet growth factors are extracted and suspended in a solution. The solution is dispensed to the patient and self-administered to the wound topically.[124] The growth factor solution is believed to stimulate initial wound healing, but the underlying cause of the ulcer must be treated to prevent recurrence of the wound. The rate of healing varies with the disease underlying the ulceration.[125] This treatment is usually accompanied by other wound treatment, such as nutritional supplementation, wound debridement, and compression and non-weight bearing if the ulcer is in the lower leg or of venous origin.[126]

Improvements have been reported in chronic wounds treated with growth factors. Currently there are not enough outcome studies documenting the benefits of growth factors on pressure ulcers. However, preliminary growth factor research shows encouraging results on pressure ulcer healing.[127] There still are a number of unanswered concerns: (a) too few clinical trials with demonstrated clinical efficacy, (b) the lack of FDA standards against which the effects of growth factors will be measured, (c) the need to demonstrate lack of side effects, such as tissue overgrowth resulting in excessive scarring, and (d) the need to determine dosages and methods of delivering the growth factors to the wound. It may be that different growth factors will be beneficial at different phases of wound healing. It is anticipated that continued growth factor research will more fully explain the action of growth factors in healing wounds.

Electrical stimulation

Traditionally, electrical stimulation was used for conditions treated by physical therapists, such as muscle spasms and injuries, but there is an increasing interest in this method of treatment for accelerating closure of chronic wounds. A variety of electrotherapy modalities are cited in the literature. Clinical trials have shown that a course of treatment with electrotherapy enhanced the healing rate of pressure ulcers unresponsive to conventional therapy.[128-134] Three types of electrical waveforms have been applied to wound healing: low-intensity direct current, high-voltage pulsed current, and pulsed electrical stimulation.[135] Certain physiologic changes occur at the tissue and cellular level in a wound exposed to exogenous electrical stimulation.

Diapulse is a form of electrical stimulation that has been studied in wound healing. It produces pulsed high-frequency high peak power electromagnetic energy. Energy is delivered in 65 microsecond bursts at settings of 80 to 600 pulses per second with a wattage range from 293 to 975 peak watts. Energy is induced through a 9-inch treatment head. The treatment is noninvasive and can be applied through clothing and surgical dressings.[131] The biological effects produced by Diapulse that enhance wound healing include increased blood flow, stimulation of collagen formation, and phagocytosis. Low-intensity pulsed direct current is thought to enhance the growth of fibroblasts and keratinocytes. One study found a significant improvement in healing of Stage II pressure ulcers in spinal cord-injured men, suggesting that this may be a cost-effective treatment.[128]

Hyperbaric oxygen

Hyperbaric oxygen (HBO) therapy is the administration of 100% oxygen under pressure greater than one atmosphere.[136] HBO may be administered in a monoplace chamber that accommodates a single patient or in a multiplace chamber that accommodates more than one patient. Within the chamber, oxygen is inspired and the atmospheric pressure gradually is increased to dissolve oxygen in the plasma at a higher concentration than would be dissolved at sea level. By supersaturating the hemoglobin, a greater supply of oxygen is provided to the tissues.

Hyperbaric oxygen therapy was used first in the 1930s to treat the decompression sickness of undersea divers. Rapid ascent, particularly from deep dives, causes nitrogen gas bubbles to form in a diver's intravascular compartment. The nitrogen bubbles interfere with coagulation, and the bubbles can become large enough to obstruct blood vessels resulting in problems ranging from a dull ache to stroke or cardiovascular collapse. Hyperbaric oxygen treatment decreases the size of nitrogen bubbles, oxygenates the ischemic tissue, and reduces the nitrogen gradient.[136] Hyperbaric oxygen therapy also has been shown to be effective for carbon monoxide poisoning as it is the most rapid way of displacing carbon monoxide bound to hemoglobin.[137]

Research demonstrating the effectiveness of hyperbaric oxygen therapy for wound healing has been less well documented. The immune system, vascular tone, and wound healing all are affected by oxygen. It has been proposed that intermittent hyperbaric oxygen treatments stimulate the oxidative functions of wound healing, providing greater availability of oxygen to fibroblasts, leukocytes, and endothelial cells.[138] Conditions that reduce oxygen supply, such as anemia and chronic pulmonary conditions, decrease metabolic functions. Increasing the oxygen level allows restoration of these activities.[139] A tissue pO_2 of at least 30 mm Hg is necessary for normal oxidative function. Partial pressures of O_2 lower than this are seen in damaged or infected tissues. Raising the pO_2 at the tissue level will restore immune function needed to resist infection and support wound healing.[138,140] Wound healing is optimal when there are alternate periods of oxygenation and ischemia.[141] Intermittent periods of relative hypoxia stimulate granulation tissue formation.

HBO is thought to be most effective in wounds that can demonstrate an increase in tissue oxygen tension. Topical hyperbaric oxygen is not recommended for treatment of pressure ulcers as it does not increase tissue oxygen tension beyond the superficial dermis.[22] Wounds that are poorly perfused due to arterial insufficiency require surgical intervention to restore blood flow to the tissue. Oxygen, even under pressure, cannot get to tissues that have insufficient arterial inflow.

Hyperbaric oxygen treatment requires specialized equipment and highly trained personnel. Most patients with chronic wounds are unlikely to have access to this treatment unless a nearby facility has an HBO chamber already in place for treatment of decompression and carbon monoxide poisoning. More research is needed to find out whether the effects of HBO on chronic wounds are worth the time and expense required. According to Hunt,[142] the rationale for hyperbaric oxygen therapy is well established, but because studies of chronic wounds are difficult to conduct, efficacy of HBO in humans has not yet been shown.

Cultured epithelium

The use of cultured epithelium in wound management is likely to increase significantly over the next decade. Cell culture techniques have been developed that permit the successful cultivation of cells in vitro to produce viable epithelial sheets. Applications include the successful treatment of skin ulcers. Long-term results in burn wounds appear to be comparable to split-thickness skin grafting. This modality cannot be recommended for pressure ulcers since no controlled studies are available.[143]

Ultrasound

Ultrasound therapy is the use of high frequency sound waves generated by oscillation of a crystal in a transducer. The oscillation can be produced continuously or in a pulsed interrupted mode. Ultrasound is available with thermal and nonthermal effects. The passage of the sound wave across the cell wall is thought to cause a change in diffusion rate and cell membrane permeability and thereby influence wound healing. In one clinical study,[144] the use of ultrasound was associated with an accelerated rate of the inflammatory phase of wound healing.[145] More research is needed to support the use of ultrasound in treatment of pressure ulcers.

Evaluating outcomes of care

All pressure ulcers should be reevaluated weekly.[146] There appears to be sufficient evidence to suggest that weeks of ineffective treatment can be avoided if appropriate clinical assessments are done at least once a week.[22,146,147] Given optimal care, the pressure ulcer should show signs of healing within 2 weeks. If the ulcer does not show progress, the entire plan of care must be revisited. Gorse[58] and Xakellis[64] demonstrated that exudative ulcers take longer to heal than nonexudative ulcers. Since wound exudate has been associated with a slower healing, a dressing should be used that abosorbs excessive exudate. One study showed that most full-thickness ulcers can heal in 6 to 7 weeks. Of these full-thickness ulcers, none of the baseline characteristics were predictive of healing. However, differences in the patient characteristics were substantial. Patients who were mentally alert healed 33 days earlier than patients who were confused or disoriented. Similar differences were seen as a function of the patient's mobility, where the more mobile patients healed earlier. Also, at baseline, a patient's nutritional status had a significant effect on time to healing. Nutrition remained an independent predictor of time to healing after 2 weeks. Another predictor of time to healing was the percentage of reduction in ulcer size after 2 weeks of treatment.[146]

Healing of partial-thickness pressure ulcers can be determined clinically by observing epithelialization. Epithelial maturation occurs approximately 10 to 14 days after resurfacing.[148] Epithelial migration, cell division, and differentiation constitute epidermal healing. At this time, the visual appearance is that of blending into the surrounding undamaged epidermis.

According to Brown-Etris,[148] expected outcomes or wound healing markers for full-thickness pressure ulcers include the following:
- Removal of eschar.
- Reduction of surrounding tissue erythema, edema, induration if present.
- Initiation of granulation tissue ingrowth and reduction of slough, necrotic tissue, and debris.
- Wound margin undermining becomes more evident.
- Shift from purulent and malodorous exudate to serous exudate. A less offensive odor will continue if necrotic tissue autolysis is occurring.
- Surface area (length and width) increases.
- Granulation tissue base is well established. Depth reduction begins. Signs of wound contraction are subtle. Surface area begins to reduce.
- Surrounding erythema, edema, and induration decrease.
- Exudate is serous or serosanguinous without odor.
- Wound margin attachment begins as evidenced by reduction in measurable undermining.
- Granulation tissue ingrowth has occurred.

Table 7.5 CareMap: Full-Thickness Pressure Ulcer

In the CareMap below, the first column represents the areas of interest or indicators. The second column includes the areas for assessment and suggested interventions. The information in the other four columns represent the expected outcomes. Variances from these outcomes require alteration in the management plan. Identification of variances early in the treatment saves time and resources.

Care paths should be clear and specific, include management actions, and define treatment outcomes within a timeframe. The care path suggested below is not all-inclusive and not institution-specific. It does not address pressure ulcer prevention and pressure ulcer healing with complications. It is intended as a suggestion for developing and refining a useful path to predict pressure ulcer healing. While there are pathways for diagnostic related groups (DRGs) and disease-specific problems, there is no pathway developed to address pressure ulcer healing within a timeframe.

INDICATOR	INITIAL ASSESSMENT	OUTCOME WITHIN 24 HOURS

Physiologic/Anatomic	1. Measure PU
	2. Objectify characteristics
	3. Set goals
	4. Determine interventions
		1. Interventions in place
		  a. debride
		  b. dressings
		  c. pressure reduction
		  d. pain management

Nutrition	1. Obtain baseline data (diet, weight +IBW, alb.) 2. Ask food preferences 3. Determine ability to obtain food 4. Consult dietitian 5. Develop plan, and teach dietary information	1. Patient able to state foods necessary for healing 2. Patient able to identify how food will be obtained and prepared
Activity	1. Assess ability to move 2. Assess motivation and desire to move 3. Assess availability of assistive devices 4. Consult PT, OT	1. Patient moving according to plan 2. Correct use of assistive devices
Cognitive/Emotional	1. Assess knowledge for PU prevention, protection 2. Assess motivation and desire	1. Patient able to state goals and interventions
Social	1. Assess living arrangements 2. Identify social support	
Pressure reduction	1. Assess current pressure reduction techniques used (mattress overlay, wheelchair, WC cushion, chair cushion, sliding board, trapeze) 2. Teach repositioning	1. Pressure-reducing devices in use 2. Repositioning occurs on schedule 3. Pressure is relieved over all bony prominences

OUTCOME WITHIN 7 DAYS	OUTCOME WITHIN 14 DAYS	OUTCOME WITHIN 21 DAYS
1. Drainage decreased 2. Necrosis decreased 3. Odor decreased 4. No infection present 5. Granulation present in ulcer 6. Epithelium at borders	1. Size of PU decreased (diameter, depth) 2. No necrosis 3. Ulcer crater filling with granulation tissue 4. Epithelial migration moving from borders inward	1. Size decreased by 25% 2. Ulcer bed covered with granulation 3. Epithelial migration moving from borders inward, or completely covering ulcer
1. Dietary plan in place 2. Diet is balanced	1. Dietary plan effective 2. Albumin WNL (>3.0) 3. Weight stable 4. Access to food	1. Dietary plan is a part of patient's lifestyle 2. Albumin WNL 3. Weight stable
1. Activities consistent with therapeutic regimen 2. Mobility increased		1. Activities for pressure reduction are incorporated into lifestyle and routine 2. Mobility increased
	Behaviors reflect new knowledge	Behaviors to reduce risk continue
	Support consistent	Support consistent
1. No new reddened areas 2. No broken skin 3. Complete pressure relief over any existing ulcers	1. No new reddened areas 2. No broken skin 3. Complete pressure relief over any existing ulcers	1. No new reddened areas 2. No broken skin 3. Complete pressure relief over any existing ulcers

- Epithelialization is evident, particularly where margin attachment and granulation ingrowth have occurred.
- Wound margin attachment and granulation tissue in-growth is complete; exudate production decreases.
- Wound contraction and resurfacing are complete.

Wound stage does not change throughout the course of healing. New, dissimilar tissue replaces the original tissue. Wound healing is measured by the indicators above.[148]

Tracking variances from expected outcomes

Based on studies of time to healing, it is logical to "map" optimal care and then track variances from these expected outcomes. If pressure ulcer reassessment should be done weekly and progress toward healing should be seen within 2 weeks, a logical course of care emerges (see Table 7.5). Case management of patients with pressure ulcers involves optimizing care, charting progress toward healing, and controlling variances with aggressive intervention.[149-154]

Summary

The wound healing sequence follows an expected course if the intrinsic and extrinsic conditions are optimal. Routine wound cleansing should be accomplished with a minimum of chemical and mechanical trauma. The benefits of obtaining a clean wound must be weighed against the potential cleansing trauma to the wound bed. Wound healing is inhibited by the indiscriminate use of antiseptics. Optimum healing is promoted by allowing the body's own healing mechanisms to occur. Dressings provide an immediate environment that can support or impede wound healing. There is no significant difference in pressure ulcer outcomes among the dressings that support moist wound healing. All products that go on or into a wound should be nontraumatic. Careful monitoring of the wound healing process without too much interference seems to serve the patient and the wound best. Factors that promote optimum healing, such as protection from trauma or provision of a moist environment, should be supported. Whenever possible, the body should be allowed to heal itself. New techniques for wound care must stand up to scientific scrutiny before their impact upon wound management is realized.

References

1. Maklebust, J., and Sieggreen, M. *Pressure Ulcers: Guidelines for Prevention and Nursing Management*, 1st ed. West Dundee, Ill.: S-N Publications, 1991.

2. Maklebust, J., et al. "Pressure Relief Capabilities of the Sof-Care Bed Cushion and the Clinitron Bed," *Ostomy/Wound Management* 21:32-41, 1988.

3. Gendron, F. " `Burns' Occurring During Lengthy Surgical Procedures," *Journal of Clinical Engineering* 5(1):19-26, 1980.

4. Hoyman, K., and Gruber, N. "A Case of Interdepartmental Cooperation: Operating Room-Acquired Pressure Ulcers," *Nursing Administration Quarterly* (Special Report: Clinical Implications for Quality), 12-17, 1992.

5. Kemp, M.G., et al. "Factors that Contribute to Pressure Ulcers in Surgical Patients," *Research in Nursing and Health* 13:293-301, 1990.

6. Vermillion, C. "Operating Room-Acquired Pressure Ulcers," *Decubitus* 3(1): 26-30, 1990.

7. Souther, S.G., et al. "Pressure, Tissue Ischemia, and Operating Table Pads," *Archives of Surgery* 107: 544-547, 1973.

8. Stewart, T.P. "Another Opinion on Interface Pressures," *Decubitus* 2(3): 9-10, 1989.

9. Krouskop, T.A., and Garber, S. "Tissue Interface Confusion, *Decubitus* 2(3): 9, 1989.

10. Finucane, T.E. "Malnutrition, Tube Feeding and Pressure Sores: Data Are Incomplete," *JAGS* 43(4): 447-451, 1995.

11. Breslow, R.A. "Nutrition and Air-Fluidized Beds: A Literature Review," *Advances in Wound Care* 7(3): 57-62, 1994.

12. Long, C.L., et al. "A Physiologic Basis for the Provision of Fuel Mixtures in Normal and Stressed Patient," *J Trauma* 30: 1077-1086.a, 1990.

13. National Research Council. "Recommended Dietary Allowances," ed 10. Washington, D.C.: National Academy Press, 1989.

14. Stotts, N.A., and Washington, D.F. "Nutrition: A Critical Component of Wound Healing," *AACN* 1(3): 585-594, 1990.

15. Kaminski, M.V., and Blumeyer, T.J. "Metabolic and Nutritional Support of the Intensive Care Patient," *Critical Care Clinics* 9(2): 363-376, 1993.

16. Allman, R., et al. "Pressure Sores Among Hospitalized Patients," *Ann Intern Med* 105: 337-342, 1986.

17. Pinchofsky-Devin, G., and Kaminski, M. "Correlation of Pressure Sores and Nutritional Status," *J Am Ger Soc* 34: 435-440, 1986.

18. Stotts, N. "Nutritional Parameters at Hospital Admission as Predictors of Pressure Ulcer Development in Elective Surgery," *JPEN* 11(3): 298-301, 1987.

19. Berlowitz, D., and Wilking, S. "The Short-Term Outcome of Pressure Sores," *J Am Ger Soc* 38: 748-752, 1990.

20. Hill, D.P., et al. "Serum Albumin Is a Poor Prognostic Factor for Pressure Ulcer Healing in Controlled Clinical Trials," *Wounds* 1994.

21. Breslow, R.A., et al. "The Importance of Dietary Protein in Healing Pressure Ulcers," *JAGS* 41(4): 357-362, 1993.

22. Bergstrom, N., et al. *Treatment of Pressure Ulcers.* Clinical Practice Guideline, No. 15. Rockville, Md.: U.S. Department of Health and Human Services. Public Health Service, Agency for Health Care Policy and Research. AHCPR Publication No. 95-0652. December, 1994.

23. Rodeheaver, G.T., et al. "Wound Healing and Wound Management: Focus on Debridement," *Advances in Wound Care* 7(1): 22-36, 1994.

24. Feedar, J.A. "Products that Facilitate Wound Healing," *Topics in Geriatric Rehabilitation* 9(4): 58-81, 1994.

25. Troyer-Caudle, J. "Debridement: Removal of Non-viable Tissue" *Ostomy/Wound Management* 39 (6): 24-32, 1993.

26. Boxer, A.M., et al. "Debridement of Dermal Ulcers and Decubiti with Collagenase," *Geriatrics* 24(7): 75-86, 1969.

27. Rao, D.B., et al. "Collagenase in the Treatment of Dermal and Decubitus Ulcers," *Journal of the American Geriatrics Society* 23(1): 22-30, 1975.

28. Lee, L.K., and Ambrus, J.L. "Collagenase Therapy for Decubitus Ulcers," *Geriatrics* 30(5): 91-98, 1975.

29. Varma, A.O., et al. "Debridement of Dermal Ulcers with Collagenase," *Surgery, Gynecology & Obstetrics* 136(2): 281-282, 1973.

30. Rodeheaver, G.T., and Maklebust, J. "Wound Cleansing," in Bergstrom, N., and Cuddigan, J. (Eds.). *Treatment of Pressure Ulcers.* Clinical Practice Guideline. Guideline Technical Report, No. 15. Rockville, Md.: U.S. Department of Health and Human Services. Public Health Service, Agency for Health Care Policy and Research. AHCPR Publication No. 95-xxxx. December, 1994.

31. Foresman, P.A., et al. "A Relative Toxicity Index for Wound Cleansers," *Wounds* 5(5): 226-231, 1993.

32. Burkey, J.L., et al. "Differential Methodology for the Evaluation of Skin and Wound Cleansers," *Wounds* 5(6): 284-291, 1993.

33. Madden, J., et al. "Application of Principles of Fluid Dynamics to Surgical Wound Infection," *Current Topics in Surgical Research* 3: 85-93, 1971.

34. Rodeheaver, G.T., et al. "Mechanical Cleansing by High-Pressure Irrigation," *Surgery, Gynecology & Obstetrics* 141(3): 357-362, 1975.

35. Longmire, A.W., et al. "Wound Infection Following High Pressure Syringe and Needle Irrigation," *American Journal of Emergency Medicine* 5(2): 179-181, 1987.

36. Wheeler, C.B., et al. Side effects of High Pressure Irrigation," *Surgery, Gynecology & Obstetrics* 143(5): 775-778, 1976.

37. Carlson, H.C., et al. "Effect of Pressure and Tip Modification on the Dispersion of Fluid Throughout Cells and Tissues During the Irrigation of Experimental Wounds," *Oral Surgery* 32(2): 347-355, 1971.

38. Gross, A., et al. Effectiveness of Pulsating Water Jet Lavage in Treatment of Contaminated Crush Wounds," *American Journal of Surgery* 124(3): 373-377, 1972.

39 Stevenson, T.R., et al. "Cleansing the Traumatic Wound by High Pressure Irrigation," *JACEP* 5(1): 17-21, 1976.

40. Krasinski, K., et al. "Effects of Changing Needle Disposal Systems on Needle Puncture Injuries," *Infection Control* 8: 59-62, 1987.

41. Neiderhuber, S., et al. "Reduction of Skin Bacterial Load with Use of Therapeutic Whirlpool," *Physical Therapy* 55(5): 482-486, 1975.

42. Bohannon, R.W. "Whirlpool Versus Whirlpool Rinse for Removal of Bacteria from a Venous Stasis Ulcer," *Physical Therapy* 62(3): 304-308, 1982.

43. Feedar, J.A., and Kloth, L.C. "Conservative Management of Chronic Wounds," in Kloth, L.C., et al., eds. *Wound Healing: Alternatives in Management.* Philadelphia: F.A. Davis, 1990.

44. Field, C.K., and Kerstein, M.D. "Overview of Wound Healing in a Moist Environment," *American Journal of Surgery* 167, No. 1A (Suppl): 2S-6S, 1994.

45. Winter, G.D., and Scales, J.T. "Effect of Air Drying and Dressings on the Surface of a Wound," *Nature* 197: 91-92, 1963.

46. Alvarez, O.M., et al. "The Effect of Occlusive Dressings on Collagen Synthesis and Re-Epithelialization of Superficial Wounds," *Journal of Surgical Research* 35(2): 142-148, 1983.

47. Hutchinson, J.J., and McGuckin, M. "Occlusive Dressings: A Microbiologic and Clinical Review," *American Journal of Infection Control* 18(4): 257-268, 1990.

48. Hutchinson, J.J., and Lawrence, J.C. "Wound Infection under Occlusive Dressings," *Journal of Hospital Infection* 17: 83-94, 1991.

49. Mertz, P.A., et al. "Occlusive Wound Dressings to Prevent Bacterial Invasion and Wound Infection," *Journal of the American Academy of Dermatology* 12(4): 662-668, 1985.

50. Varghese, M.C., et al. "Local Environment of Chronic Wounds under Synthetic Dressings," *Archives of Dermatology* 122: 52-57, 1986.

51. Turner, T. "The Development of Wound Management Products," *Wounds* 1(30): 155-171, 1989.

52. Cuzzell, J. "Choosing a Wound Dressing: A Systematic Approach," *AACN Clinical Issues* 1(3): 566-577, 1990.

53. Resnick, B. "Wound Care for the Elderly," *Geriatric Nursing* 14(1): 26-29, 1993.

54. Xakellis, G., and Maklebust, J. "Dressings Used for Treatment of Pressure Ulcers," in Bergstrom, N., and Cuddigan, J. (Eds.). *Treatment of Pressure Ulcers.* Clinical Practice Guideline. Guideline Technical Report, No. 15. Rockville, Md.: U.S. Department of Health and Human Services. Public Health Service, Agency for Health Care Policy and Research. AHCPR Publication No. 95-xxxx. December, 1994.

55. Mulder, G.D. "Evaluation of Three Nonwoven Sponges in the Debridement of Chronic Wounds," *Ostomy/Wound Management* 41(3): 62-67, 1995.

56. Seburn, M.D. "Pressure Ulcer Management in Home Health Care," *Archives of Physical Medicine and Rehabilitation* 67(10): 726-729, 1986.

57. Fowler, E., and Goupil, D.L. "Comparison of Wet-to-Dry Dressing and a Copolymer Starch in the Management of Debrided Pressure Sores," *Journal of Enterostomal Therapy* 11(1): 22-25, 1984.

58. Gourse, J.G., and Messner, R.L. "Improved Pressure Sore Healing with Hydrocolloid Dressings," *Archives of Dermatology* 123(6): 766-771, 1987.

59. Saydak, S.J. "A Pilot Test of Two Methods for the Treatment of Pressure Sores," *Journal of Enterostomal Therapy* 17(3): 139-142, 1990.

60. Alm, A., et al. "Care of Pressure Sores: A Controlled Study of the Use of a Hydrocolloid Dressing Compared with Wet Saline Gauze Compresses," *Acta Derm Venereol* (Stockholm) 149, Supplement: 1-10, 1989.

61. Colwell, J.C., et al. "A Comparison of the Efficacy and Cost of Two Methods of Managing Pressure Ulcers," *Decubitus* 6(4): 28-36, 1992.

62. Neill, K.M., et al. "Pressure Sore Response to a New Hydrocolloid Dressing," *Wounds* 1(3): 173-185, 1989.

63. Oleske, D.M., et al. "A Randomized Clinical Trial of Two Dressing Methods for the Treatment of Low Grade Pressure Ulcers," *Journal of Enterostomal Therapy* 13(3): 90-98, 1986.

64. Xakellis, G.C., and Chrischilles, E.A. "Hydrocolloid Versus Saline Gauze Dressings in Treatment of Pressure Ulcers: A Cost-Effective Analysis," *Archives of Physical Medicine and Rehabilitation* 73: 463-469, 1992.

65. Kurzek-Howard, G., et al. "Decubitus Ulcer Care: A Comparative Study," *Western Journal of Nursing Research* 7(1): 58-79, 1985.

66. Barnett, A., et al. "Comparison of Synthetic Adhesive Moisture Vapor Permeable and Fine Mesh Gauze Dressings for Split Thickness Skin Graft Donor Sites," *Am J of Surg* 145(3): 379-381, 1993.

67. Ahmed, M.C. "Opsite for Decubitus Care," *American Journal of Nursing* 82(1): 61-64, 1982.

68. Goren, D. "Use of Omiderm in Treatment of Low-Grade Pressure Sores in Terminally Ill Cancer Patients," *Cancer Nursing* 12(3): 165-169, 1989.

69. Lingner, C., et al. "Clinical Trial of a Moisture Vapor Permeable Dressing on Superficial Pressure Sores," *Journal of Enterostomal Therapy* 11(4): 147-149, 1984.

70. Bolton, L., and van Rijswijk, L. "Wound Dressings: Meeting Clinical and Biological Needs," *Dermatology Nursing* 3(3): 146-160, 1991.

71. Dobrzanski, S., et al. "Granuflex Dressings in Treatment of Full Thickness Pressure Sores," *Professional Nurse* 5(11): 594-599, 1990.

72. Myers, R.B., et al. "Report of a Multicenter Clinical Trial on the Performance Characteristics of Two Occlusive Hydrocolloid Dressings in the Treatment of Noninfected Partial-Thickness Wounds," *Journal of Enterostomal Therapy* 15(4): 158-161, 1988.

73. Watts, C., and Shipes, E. "A Study to Compare the Overall Performance of Two Hydrocolloid Dressings on Partial Thickness Wounds," *Ostomy/Wound Management* 21: 28-31, 1988.

74. Boykin, A., and Winland-Brown, J. "Pressure Sores: Nursing Management," *Journal of Gerontological Nursing* 12(12): 17-21, 1986.

75. Brod, M., et al. "A Randomized Comparison of Poly-hema and Hydrocolloid Dressings for Treatment of Pressure Sores," *Archives of Dermatology* 26(7): 969-970, 1990.

76. Darkovich, S.L., et al. "Biofilm Hydrogel Dressing: A Clinical Evaluation in the Treatment of Pressure Ulcers," *Ostomy/Wound Management* 29: 47-60, 1990.

77. van Rijswijk, L. "Full Thickness Pressure Ulcers: Patient and Wound Healing Characteristics," *Decubitus* 6: 16-23, 1993.

78. Sheridan, C.A., and Jackson, B.S. "Clinical Safety and Efficacy Evaluation of a Hydroactive Hydrocolloid Dressing in the Care of Cancer Patients," *Journal of Enterostomal Therapy* 16(5): 213-219, 1989.

79. McGowen, C.A. "Management of Pressure Ulcers Using DuoDerm Hydroactive Dressings." Unpublished research, Convatec.

80. Tudhope, M. "Management of Pressure Ulcers with a Hydrocolloid Occlusive Dressing: Results in Twenty-Three Patients," *Journal of Enterostomal Therapy* 11(3): 102-105, 1984.

81. Yarkony, G.M., et al. "Pressure Sore Management: Efficacy of a Moisture Reactive Occlusive Dressing," *Archives of Physical Medicine and Rehabilitation* 65: 597-600, 1984.

82. Brady, S.M. "Management of Pressure Sores with Occlusive Dressings in a Select Population," *Nursing Management* 18(8): 47-50, 1987.

83. Thomas, S.T., and Hay, P. "Fluid Handling Properties of Hydrogel Dressings," *Ostomy/Wound Management* 41(3): 54-59, 1995.

84. Fowler, E., and Papen, J.C. "A New Hydrogel Wound Dressing for the Treatment of Open Wounds: Gel-syte Wound Care Dressing Evaluation," *Ostomy/Wound Management* 37: 39-45, 1991.

85. Gross, H.A., et al. "Evaluation of Carrington Wound Products on Healing of Pressure Ulcers in a Long Term Care Facility," Carrington Laboratories, Dallas, TX, January 16, 1990.

86. Carr, R.D., and Lalagos, D.E. "Clinical Evaluation of a Polymeric Membrane Dressing in the Treatment of Pressure Ulcers," *Decubitus* 3(3): 38-42, 1990.

87. Fowler, E., and Papen, J.C. "Clinical Evaluation of a Polymeric Membrane Dressing in the Treatment of Dermal Ulcers," *Ostomy/Wound Management* 35: 35-44, 1991.

88. Chapuis, A., et al. "The Use of a Calcium Alginate Dressing in the Management of Decubitus Ulcers in Patients with Spinal Cord Lesions," *Paraplegia* 28(4): 269-271, 1990.

89. Fowler, E., and Papen, J.C. "Evaluation of an Alginate Dressing for Pressure Ulcers," *Decubitus* 4(3): 47-53, 1991.

90. McMullen, D. "Clinical Experience with a Calcium Alginate," *Dermatology Nursing* 3(4): 216-220, 1991.

91. Xakellis, G.C., and Maklebust, J. "Template for Pressure Ulcer Research," *Advances in Wound Care* 8(1): 46-53, 1995.

92. Diebold, E., et al. *Wound-Care Algorithms.* Mankato, Minn.: Sween Corporation, 1993.

93. Thomson, P.D., and Smith, D.J. "What Is Infection?" *American Journal of Surgery* 167(1ASuppl): 78-11, 1994.

94. Wasserman, M., et al. "Utility of Fever, White Blood Cells, and Differential Count in Predicting Bacterial Infections in the Elderly," *J Am Ger Soc* 37: 537-541, 1989.

95. Yoshikawa, T.T. Antimicrobial Therapy for the Elderly Patient," *J Amer. Geriatr. Soc.* 38: 1353-72, 1990.

96. Daltry, D.C., et al. "Investigation into the Microbial Flora of Healing and Non-healing Decubitus Ulcers," *J Clin Pathol* 34(7): 701-705, 1981.

97. Lyman, I.R., et al. "Correlation between Decrease in Bacterial Load and Rate of Wound Healing," *Surg Gynecol Obst* 130(4): 616-621, 1970.

98. Garner, J.S., et al. "CDC Definitions for Nosocomial Infections," *Am J Infect Control* 16(3): 128-140, 1988.

99. Robson, M.C. "Plastic Surgery in Quantitative Bacteriology: Its Role in the Armamentarium of the Surgeon," in Heggers, J.P., and Robson, M.C., eds. Boca Raton, Fla.: CRC Press, 71-84, 1991.

100. Stotts, N.A. "Determination of Bacterial Burden in Wounds. NPUAP Proceedings," *Advances in Wound Care* 8(4): 46-52, 1995.

101. Alvarez, O.M. "Pressure Ulcers: Critical Considerations in Prevention and Management," *Clinical Materials* 8: 209-222, 1991.

102. Lineaweaver, W., et al. "Cellular and Bacterial Toxicities of Topical Antimicrobials," *Plastic Reconstruct Surg* 75: 94-96, 1985.

103. Lineaweaver, W., et al. "Topical Antimicrobial Toxicity," *Archives of Surgery* 120: 267-270, 1985.

104. McCauley, R.L., et al. "In Vivo Toxicity of Topical Antimicrobial Agents to Human Fibroblasts," *Journal of Surgical Research* 46(3): 267-274, 1989.

105. Teepe, R.G.C., et al. "Cytotoxic Effects of Topical Antimicrobial and Antiseptic Agents on Human Keratinocytes in Vitro," *Journal of Trauma* 35(1): 8-19, 1993.

106. Hirschman, J.V. "Topical Antibiotics in Dermatology," *Arch Dermatolo* 124: 1691-1694, 1988.

107. Johnson, A.R., et al. "Comparison of Common Topical Agents for Wound Treatment: Cytotoxicity for Human Fibroblasts in Culture," *Wounds* 1(3): 186-192, 1989.

108. Schechter, J.F., et al. "Anaphylaxis Following the Use of Bacitracin Ointment: Report of a Case and Review of the Literature," *Arch Dermatol* 120(7): 909-911, 1984.

109. Leaper, D.J. "Prophylactic and Therapeutic Role of Antibiotics in Wound Care," *American Journal of Surgery* 167(1A suppl): 15S-20S, 1994.

110. Allman, R.M. "Epidemiology of Pressure Sores in Different Populations," *Decubitus* 2(2): 30-33, 1989.

111. Lewis, V.L., et al. "The Diagnosis of Osteomyelitis in Patients with Pressure Sores," *Plast Reconstru Surg* 81(2): 229-232, 1988.

112. Sugarman, B. "Osteomyelitis in Spinal Cord Injury," *Arch Phys Med Rehabil* 65(3): 52-59, 1984.

113. Sugarman, B. "Pressure Sores and Underlying Bone Infection," *Arch Intern Med* 147(30): 553-555, 1987.

114. Goldberg, N.H. "Outcomes in Surgical Intervention. NPUAP Proceedings," *Advances in Wound Care* 8(4): 69-70, 1995.

115. Rintala, D.H. "Quality of Life Considerations. NPUAP Proceedings," *Advances in Wound Care* 8(4): 71-82, 1995.

116. Lawrence, W.T. "Clinical Management of Nonhealing Wounds," in Cohen, I.K., et al., eds. *Wound Healing: Biochemical and Clinical Aspects.* Philadelphia: W.B. Saunders Co., 1992.

117. Black, J.M., and Black, S.B. "Surgical Management of Pressure Ulcers," *Nurs Clinics North America* 22(2): 429-438, 1987.

118. Lyons, R. "Promoting Healing of Skin Flaps and Grafts," *AORN J* 35(6): 1174-1183, 1982.

119. Rubayi, S., et al. "Myocutaneous Flaps: Surgical Treatment of Severe Pressure Ulcers," *AORN* 52(1): 40-52, 1990.

120. Evans, G.R.D., et al. "Surgical Correction of Pressure Ulcers in an Urban Center: Is It Efficacious?" *Advances in Wound Care* 7(1): 40-46, 1994.

121. Disa, J.J., et al. "Efficacy of Operative Cure in Pressure Sore Patients," *Plastic Reconstructive Surgery* 89(2): 272-278, 1992.

122. Morgan, J.E. "Recurrence of Pressure Ulcers: A Study of Five Cases," *JAMA* 236(21): 2430-2431, 1976.

123. Mandrekas, A., and Mastorakos, D.P. "The Management of Decubitus Ulcers by Musculocutaneous Flaps: A Five- Year Experience," *Ann Plastic Surgery* 28(2): 167-174, 1992.

124. Fylling, C.P. "Comprehensive Wound Management with Topical Growth Factors," *Ostomy/Wound Management* 22:62-71, 1989.

125. McMahon, M. "Nursing Experience Using Growth Factors in Nonhealing Wound Repair," *Journal of Gerontological Nursing* 20(9): 49-52, 1994.

126. Steed, D., et al. Clinical Trial with Purified Platelet Releasate," *Prog Clin Biol Res* 365: 103-113, 1991.

127. Pierce, G.F., et al. "Tissue repair processes in healing chronic pressure ulcers treated with recombinant platelet-derived growth factor bb," *American Journal of Pathology* 145 (6): 1399-1410, 1994.

128. Feedar, J.A., et al. "Chronic Dermal Ulcer Healing Enhanced with Monophasic Pulsed Electrical Stimulation," *Phys Therapy* 71(9): 639-649, 1991.

129. Feedar, J.A. "Physical Therapy Modalities to Augment Wound Healing," *Topics in Geriatric Rehabilitation* 9(4): 43-57, 1994.

130. Gentzkow, G.D., et al. "Improved Healing of Pressure Ulcers Using Dermapulse, a New Electrical Stimulation Device," *Wounds* 3(5): 158-170, 1991.

131. Itoh, M., et al. "Accelerated Wound Healing of Pressure Ulcers by Pulsed High Peak Power Electromagnetic Energy (Diapulse)," *Decubitus* 4(1): 24, 1991.

132. Salzberg, C.A., et al. "The Effects of Non-thermal Pulsed Electromagnetic Energy (Diapulse) on Wound Healing of Pressure Ulcers in Spinal Cord-Injured Patients: A Randomized, Double-blind Study," *Wounds* 7(1): 11-16, 1995.

133. Wood, J.M., et al. "A Multicenter Study on the Use of Pulsed Low-Intensity Direct Current for Healing Chronic Stage II and Stage III Decubitus Ulcers," *Archives Dermatology* 129: 999-1009, 1993.

134. Kloth, L., and Feedar, J. "Acceleration of Wound Healing with High Voltage Monophasic, Pulsed Current," *Physical Therapist* 58: 503-508, 19...

135. Frantz, R. "Electrical Stimulation," in Bryant, R.A., ed. *Acute and Chronic Wounds: Nursing Management.* St. Louis: Mosby, 308-311, 1992.

136. Davis, J.C., et al. "Hyperbaric Medicine: Patient Selection, Treatment, Procedures, and Side Effects," in Davis, J.C., and Hunt, T.K., eds. *Problem Wounds: The Role of Oxygen.* New York: Elsevier Science Publishing Co. Inc., 1988.

137. Kindwall, E.P. "Carbon Monoxide and Cyanide Poisoning," in Davis, J.C., and Hunt, T.K., eds. *Problem Wounds: The Role of Oxygen.* New York: Elsevier Science Publishing Co. Inc., 1988.

138. Whitney, J.D. "The Influence of Tissue Oxygen and Perfusion on Wound Healing," *AACN, Clinical Issues* 1(3): 578-584, 1990.

139. Uhl, E., et al. "Hyperbaric Oxygen Improves Wound Healing in Normal and Ischemic Skin Tissue," *Plastic and Reconstructive Surgery* 93(4): 835-841, 1994.

140. Hammarlund, C., and Sundberg, T. "Hyperbaric Oxygen Reduced Size of Chronic Leg Ulcers: A Randomized Double-Blind Study," *Plastic and Reconstructive Surgery* 93(4): 829-833, 1994.

141. Grim, P.S., et al. "Hyperbaric Oxygen Therapy," *JAMA* 263(16): 2216-2220, 1990.

142. Hunt, T.K. "Discussion. Hyperbaric oxygen reduced size of chronic leg ulcers: A randomized double-blind study," *Plastic and Reconstructive Surgery* 93(4): 1994.

143. Margolis, D.J., and Lewis, V.L. "A Literature Assessment of the Use of Miscellaneous Topical Agents, Growth Factors, and Skin Equivalents for the Treatment of Pressure Ulcers," *Dermatological Surgery* 21: 145-148, 1995.

144. Sussman, C.A. "The Role of Physical Therapy in Wound Care," in Krasner, D., ed. *Chronic Wound Care: A Clinical Source Book for Healthcare Professionals.* King of Prussia, Pa.: Health Management Publications, Inc., 1990.

145. Dyson, M. "The Role of Ultrasound in Wound Healing," in Kloth, L.C., et al., eds. *Wound Healing: Alternatives in Management.* Philadelphia: F.A. Davis, 1990.

146. van Rijswijk, L., and Polansky, M. "Predictors of Time to Healing Deep Pressure Ulcers," *Wounds* 6(5): 159-165, 1994.

147. van Rijswijk, L. "Reassessment Frequency for Pressure Ulcers," *Advances in Wound Care* 8(4): 1-19, 1995.

148. Brown-Etris, M. "Measuring Healing in Wounds. NPUAP Proceedings," *Advances in Wound Care* 8(4): 53-58, 1995.

149. Wood, R.G., et al. "Managed Care: The Missing Link in Quality Improvement," *Journal of Nursing Care Quality* 6(4): 55-65, 1992.

150. Gartner, M.B. "Care Guidelines: Journey Through the Managed Care Maze," *JWOCN* 22(3): 118-121, 1995.

151. Van Buskirk, M.C., and Vanderbuilt, D. "Evaluating Patient Care by the Use of a Ketoacidosis Caremap in an Intensive Care Unit Setting," *Journal of Nursing Care Quality* 9(3): 59-68, 1995.

152. Tallon, R.W. "Critical Paths for Wound Care," *Advances in Wound Care* 8(1): 26-34, 1995.

153. Allman, R.M. "Outcomes in Prospective Studies and Clinical Trials," *Advances in Wound Care* 8(4): 61-64, 1995.

154. Tallon, R.W. "Hospital Critical Paths," Abstract, Personal communication, 1995.

CHAPTER 8

Care Planning for Pressure Ulcer Management

After instituting a systematic approach for assessing the degree of pressure ulcer risk, an institutional protocol should be developed to guide the caregiver in planning individual care. Most nurses plan care based on the patient's nursing diagnoses. Nursing diagnoses are patient problems that nurses treat independently.[1-2] Examples of independent nursing interventions include assisting with activities of daily living, patient teaching, and promoting mobility.[1] Nurses independently assess the degree of patient risk for developing pressure ulcers. Patients at risk for pressure ulcers have a nursing diagnosis titled "high risk for impaired skin integrity." Patients with pressure ulcers have a nursing diagnosis titled "impaired skin integrity" or "impaired tissue integrity." Nursing diagnostic statements include a second phrase that indicates the etiology of the problem. The pressure ulcer problem and the etiology are connected by a "related to" clause. Examples of nursing diagnostic statements include "Impaired tissue integrity: dermal ulcer related to prolonged sacral pressure and fecal incontinence" and "High risk for impaired skin integrity related to immobility and poor nutritional status." Nursing interventions are then directed toward resolving these clearly defined problems.[1-2] Standardized care plans for impaired skin integrity nursing diagnoses have been published in the literature.[3]

Many times, nurses ask for a "recipe" for pressure ulcer care. If the ideal treatment were known, the pressure ulcer problem could be solved. To date, there is no recipe or ideal treatment. Figure 8.1 is a decision tree to aid in determining local wound care.

The Pharmacy and Therapeutics (P&T) and Pressure Ulcer Committees at Harper Hospital entered a collaborative project to increase the quality and decrease the cost of topical pressure ulcer treatment. Members of the Pressure Ulcer Committee developed decision-tree skin/wound care flowcharts to guide the staff nurses caring for patients. Physicians, pharmacists, and nurses on the P&T Committee approved the flowcharts as a standard hospital protocol. Physicians now write an order for "Skin and Wound Care Protocol," and nurses then use the flowcharts to independently order products from either pharmacy or central supply. Prior to implementation, hospital-wide education of physicians, physician assistants, nurses, physical therapists, pharmacists, and others interested in skin/wound care products took place. It was emphasized that the flowcharts represented only topical treatment and not total care required. Harper Skin/Wound Care Flowcharts include those for Skin Care, Surgical Wounds, Leg Ulcers, Pressure Ulcers, Debridement, Peri-wound Skin, and Attach-

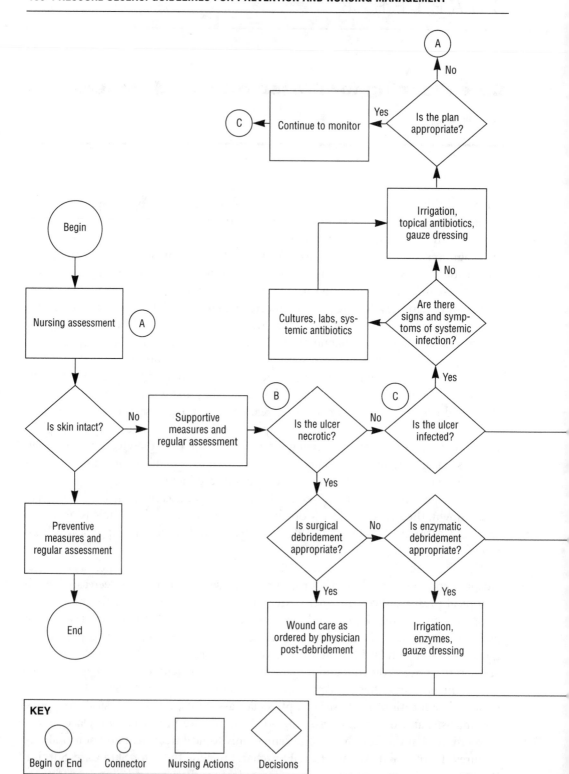

Figure 8.1 Pressure ulcers: a decision tree for local wound care

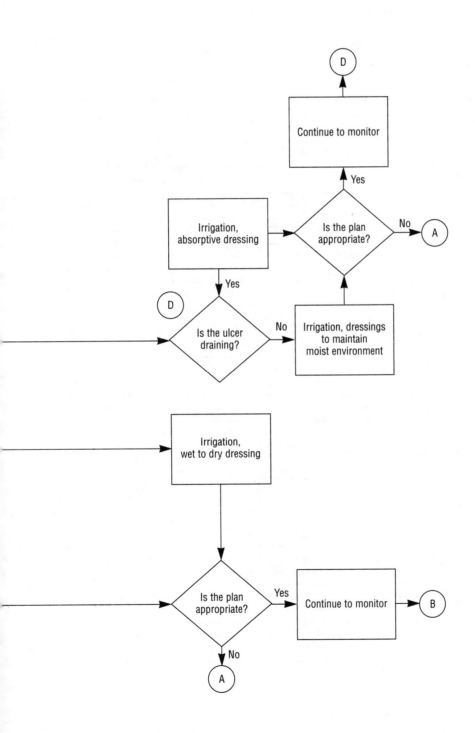

Table 8.1 Documenting Pressure Ulcer Outcomes

❑ Nursing Diagnosis ❑ Collaborative Problem ❑ Date Resolved

❑ High risk for impaired skin integrity re:
  ❑ Immobility ❑ Incontinence ❑ Malnutrition

❑ Impaired skin integrity re:
  ❑ Pressure ❑ Shear ❑ Friction ❑ Excess Wetness

OUTCOME CRITERIA	DAY:___ DATE:___ Signature	DAY:___ DATE:___ Signature	DAY:___ DATE:___ Signature
Absence of nonblanchable erythema over bony prominences. Skin well moisturized. Norton score >16. Achieved: Date _____	❑ Met	❑ Met	❑ Met
Absence of perianal irritation/denuded skin. Achieved: Date _____	❑ Met	❑ Met	❑ Met
Ulcer base moist, beefy red over entire surface with evidence of new skin growth at border of wound bed. Achieved: Date _____	❑ Met	❑ Met	❑ Met
Skin surrounding ulcer not indurated (hard), inflamed, warm, or painful to touch. Achieved: Date _____	❑ Met	❑ Met	❑ Met
Pt/so verbalize rationale for repositioning, pressure relief, adequate nutrition, good hygiene, and treatment regimen. Achieved: Date _____	❑ Met	❑ Met	❑ Met

ment of Products Without Tape (see the Appendices). The flowcharts are a form of treatment map for cleansing, debridement, and topical treatment of specified wound types. The products named within the boxes represent products used at Harper Hospital at the time the flowcharts were developed. The P&P numbers within the boxes refer to the corresponding policy and procedure for that item (for more information on policies and procedures, see Chapter 9).

The care plans on the following pages were developed for use at Harper Hospital.[4] Health care agencies may use the care planning section of this text to develop their own institution's specific guidelines or standard care plans. Nursing care orders for an individual patient then can be selected from the sample care plans, depending on the pressure ulcer risk factors, the characteristics of the pressure ulcer, and environmental setting.

(Text continues on page 164)

Table 8.2 GUIDELINES FOR PRESSURE ULCER MANAGEMENT

ASSESSMENT	PLAN		EVALUATION
Nursing Diagnosis/ Risk Factors	Nursing Care Orders	Key Rationale for Nursing Care Orders	Expected Outcome
High-risk for impaired skin integrity related to specific external and/or internal risk factors	I. Assess pressure ulcer risk on admission, daily, and when condition changes A. Assess patient's general health status	Prevention begins with identifying patients at risk for developing pressure ulcers.	Intact skin with absence of non-blanchable erythema.
	1. Age	Aging process is associated with arteriosclerotic change in vessels, loss of subcutaneous tissue, and decreased skin elasticity.	
	2. Nutrition	Poor nutrition, as evidenced by unintentional weight loss, iron-deficiency anemia, hypoproteinemia, and vitamin deficiency, predisposes patients to tissue breakdown and is detrimental to wound healing.	
	3. Mobility	Pressure for prolonged periods of time can lead to tissue destruction from anoxia.	
	4. Sensory deficits	Sensory deficits may include absent or decreased awareness of pain and pressure. Sensory deficits may be due to physical impairment or altered mental status.	
	5. Presence of excessive moisture	Moist skin at pressure points may lead to maceration. Macerated skin is easily rubbed away by friction.	

(continued)

Table 8.2 GUIDELINES FOR PRESSURE ULCER MANAGEMENT *(continued)*

ASSESSMENT	PLAN		EVALUATION
Nursing Diagnosis/ Risk Factors	Nursing Care Orders	Key Rationale for Nursing Care Orders	Expected Outcome
	a. Bowel incontinence b. Bladder incontinence c. Diaphoresis	Moisture from perspiration or incontinence of urine/feces also reduces the resistance of skin to bacteria. Bacteria and toxins in the stool increase the risk of skin breakdown.	
	d. Excess lotion	Extra lotion adds excess moisture, which can macerate the skin.	
	e. Bed protectors/"blue pads" next to the skin	"Blue pads" hold moisture next to the skin. They are not absorbent and serve only as bed protectors.	
	6. Diabetes mellitus	Diabetics often have neuropathy, impaired circulation, and poor wound healing.	
	7. Infection	Infection increases the metabolic rate.	
	B. Assess for areas of blanchable and non-blanchable erythema, especially over bony prominences and pressure points.	Blanchable erythema indicates temporary ischemia or temporarily interrupted blood flow. Reactive hyperemia is the first response to temporary ischemia. It is characterized by a bright red flush caused by excessive blood flow to the area following a temporarily arrested blood flow. The flush should not last more than one-half to three-fourths the ischemic time. Nonblanchable erythema indicates redness of the skin that does not pale when gentle pressure is applied. Nonblanchable erythema indicates tissue damage that is not yet ulcerated and is classified as a stage I pressure ulcer.	
Nursing Diagnosis/ Knowledge Deficit	Nursing Care Orders	Key Rationale for Nursing Care Orders	Expected Outcome
Knowledge deficit: pressure ulcer prevention techniques as evidenced by inability of patient/significant other to state or demonstrate techniques of prevention	I. Assess patient's/significant other's understanding of factors that contribute to pressure ulcers.	Level of knowledge and motivation must be assessed in order to develop teaching plan.	Verbalization or demonstration of pressure ulcer prevention techniques, e.g., • correct positioning • movement • skin care • nutrition • early recognition of tissue damage

Table 8.2 GUIDELINES FOR PRESSURE ULCER MANAGEMENT *(continued)*

ASSESSMENT	PLAN		EVALUATION
Nursing Diagnosis/ Knowledge Deficit	Nursing Care Orders	Key Rationale for Nursing Care Orders	Expected Outcome
	II. Teach patient/significant other appropriate measures to prevent pressure ulcers.		
	A. Nutrition	Adequate nutrients maintain positive nitrogen balance, which increases the quality of the soft tissue.	
	B. Full-Body repositioning	Relieves pressure from major bony prominences.	
	C. Small shifts in body weight	Relieves pressure on bony prominences in extremities.	
	D. Active/passive range of motion (ROM)	Prevents joint contractures. Helps prevent deconditioning.	
	E. Skin care	Use of fundamental principles of cleansing, moisturizing, and protecting is essential to healthy skin.	
	F. Skin protection from urine and/or feces	Prevents skin breakdown from maceration or chemical irritation.	
	G. Early recognition of tissue damage	Alerts caregiver to avoid turning patient onto areas of nonblanchable erythema.	
Nursing Diagnosis/ Pressure	Nursing Care Orders	Key Rationale for Nursing Care Orders	Expected Outcome
High-risk for impaired skin integrity related to pressure from immobility	I. Encourage highest degree of mobility and activity for patient.	Occlusion of blood vessels due to pressure from lack of normal movement is the basic cause of pressure ulcers. Flow is blocked by pressure on vessel from underlying bony prominences and compressing surfaces.	Intact skin with absence of non-blanchable erythema.
		Severe or prolonged interrupted blood flow will stop nutrients/O_2 from getting to cell and metabolites/CO_2 from leaving cell, thus leading to cell destruction.	Patient repositions self or is repositioned as condition indicates.
	A. Ambulate as ordered and tolerated.	Increased activity and mobility facilitate circulation and increase the sense of well-being.	
	B. Provide assistive devices to increase independent movement.	The greatest risk for the development of pressure ulcers exists when the patient is unable to move.	
	1. Bedbound: trapeze, siderails	Assists patient to increase independent mobility.	
	2. Impaired ambulatory: canes, walkers, hand rails	Assists patient to increase independent activity.	

(continued)

Table 8.2 GUIDELINES FOR PRESSURE ULCER MANAGEMENT *(continued)*

ASSESSMENT	PLAN		EVALUATION
Nursing Diagnosis/ Pressure	Nursing Care Orders	Key Rationale for Nursing Care Orders	Expected Outcome
	C. Use active and passive ROM as appropriate	Physiotherapy relieves pressure, promotes circulation, and decreases risk for joint contracture.	
	II. Change patient's position when in bed at least every 2 hours around the clock unless there is a medical contraindication as stated in the physician's orders. Shift patient's position every 15 minutes while chair sitting.	The critical time period for tissue changes due to pressure is between 1 and 2 hours, after which irreversible changes can occur. Patients having one or more predisposing factors may need more frequent turning. Low pressure for a long period of time is more detrimental than high pressure for a short period of time. Moderate pressure within normal physiological limits can cause tissue damage if repeated too frequently.	
	A. Use the 30-degree, laterally inclined position for bed patients whenever possible.	This position eliminates pressure from the sacrum and trochanter simultaneously.	
	B. Position pillows to relieve pressure over bony prominences.	The patient is supported above the surface of the bed with free space between the bony prominence and the bed.	
	C. Encourage proper posture in a chair.	Slouching in a chair and improper footstool height can increase pressure on bony prominences.	
	Limit chair sitting time to 1 hour.	Tissue compression is highest in the sitting position.	
	D. Supplement full-body repositioning with minor shifts in body weight.	Small shifts in body weight are known to reduce the incidence of pressure ulcers.	
	E. Post "turn clock" or repositioning schedule at bedside.	Alerts caregiver to recommended position changes and appropriate time intervals for turning.	
	III. Increase comfort and reduce mechanical sources of irritation.		
	A. Apply 2-inch convoluted foam mattress for comfort, e.g., eggcrate.	Thin foam mattress overlays do not adequately reduce pressure but provide comfort only.	
	B. Keep linen smooth.	Wrinkles and foreign objects in the bed/chair may produce pressure and/or friction.	
	C. Remove foreign objects from bed/chair.		
	IV. Select pressure-reducing devices/measures as appropriate.		

Table 8.2 GUIDELINES FOR PRESSURE ULCER MANAGEMENT *(continued)*

ASSESSMENT	PLAN		EVALUATION
Nursing Diagnosis/ Pressure	Nursing Care Orders	Key Rationale for Nursing Care Orders	Expected Outcome
	A. Obtain pressure-dispersing mattress or sleep surface.		
	1. Use air mattress overlay that reduces pressure below capillary closing pressure.	To maintain capillary blood flow	
	2. Use only one sheet and one lift sheet between the patient and the mattress.	Excessive linen interferes with pressure dispersion.	
	B. Suspend heels to relieve pressure, e.g., pillow under calf, eggcrate under Achilles tendon, Vascular Boot.	Vascular Boots relieve pressure by suspending the heels. However, Vascular Boots should not be used in patients who have "foot drop." If there is fixed plantar flexion, the heel will not be in proper position for pressure relief.	
	C. Obtain pressure-reducing chair cushion.	To maintain capillary blood flow. Tissue compression is highest in the sitting position.	
	D. Do not use rubber or inflatable rings, e.g., donuts.	Donuts have a propensity to impede circulation. The donut relieves pressure in one area but increases pressure in the surrounding areas.	
	E. Limit time on bedpan.	The bedpan causes pressure and impedes circulation.	
	F. Avoid massage over bony prominences and hyperemic areas.	Massage over reddened areas may cause breaking of capillaries and traumatize skin. Vigorous massage angulates and tears the vessels.	
Nursing Diagnosis/ Shear	Nursing Care Orders	Key Rationale for Nursing Care Orders	Expected Outcome
High-risk for impaired skin integrity related to shearing forces	I. Carefully assist the patient into a sitting position. Avoid sliding patient across bed surface.	Shearing forces damage soft tissue by causing an opposite but parallel sliding motion of the layers of tissue underneath skin surfaces. This regulates in torn, angulated, and/or compressed blood vessels.	Intact skin with absence of non-blanching erythma. Patient is repositioned to minimize shearing forces in reclining and sitting positions.
	II. Limit Fowler's or high-Fowler's positions in high-risk patients.	When the head of the bed is raised 30 degrees or more, a greater compression force is placed on the posterior sacral tissues. Additional weight from the upper body is transferred to the tissues via the spinal column	
	III. Encourage low semi-Fowler's position when in bed.		

(continued)

Table 8.2 GUIDELINES FOR PRESSURE ULCER MANAGEMENT *(continued)*

ASSESSMENT	PLAN		EVALUATION
Nursing Diagnosis/ Shear	Nursing Care Orders	Key Rationale for Nursing Care Orders	Expected Outcome
	Position the patient upright while in chair. Limit the use of a geriatric chair. Use pressure-reducing chair cushion while sitting.	and sacrum. The body tends to slide downward to the foot of the bed; thus, increased compression and shearing forces are exerted upon the posterior sacral tissues, increasing risk for tissue breakdown.	
	Limit chair sitting time to 1 hour.	Tissue compression is highest in the sitting position.	
	Position hips and knees on an even plane to distribute pressure evenly over back of thighs.	This body alignment will decrease ischial pressure and shear while chair sitting. Elevating knees higher than hips transfers pressure to ischial tuberosities.	
	IV. Avoid use of "knee gatch."	Pressure behind the knees may reduce the blood flow to the lower extremities, thereby increasing risk for tissue ischemia.	
Nursing Diagnosis/ Shear	Nursing Care Orders	Key Rationale for Nursing Care Orders	Expected Outcome
High-risk for impaired skin integrity related to friction	I. Lift patient carefully when positioning, using a lift sheet.	Friction can cause abrasion by rubbing away outer layers of skin. Use of lift or draw sheet will minimize friction on skin.	Intact skin with absence of abrasion. Patient will be positioned and/or moved to avoid frictional forces.
	II. Encourage patient to assist as much as possible when moving in bed. Obtain over-head trapeze if indicated.	Use of trapeze facilitates self-care in positioning. Lifting buttocks from bed may reduce friction.	
	III. Use long sleeves and cotton/wool socks to prevent friction over elbows or heels.	These devices decrease friction but do not relieve pressure.	
	Avoid devices, such as heel and elbow protectors, that require strapping tightly around an extremity.	Any device that is secured with a tight strap impedes blood flow and increases the risk of pressure ulcer formation.	
	IV. May use a sheepskin pad under back/buttocks to decrease friction.	A genuine sheepskin minimizes friction but does not relieve pressure. Sheepskin may retain body heat and lead to increased perspiration. Synthetic orlon pile does not have properties that reduce pressure or friction.	

Table 8.2 GUIDELINES FOR PRESSURE ULCER MANAGEMENT *(continued)*

ASSESSMENT	PLAN		EVALUATION
Nursing Diagnosis/ Nutrition-Fluid	Nursing Care Orders	Key Rationale for Nursing Care Orders	Expected Outcome
High-risk for impaired skin integrity related to inadequate nutritional and/or fluid intake	I. Obtain patient's dietary history.	Provides baseline data.	Intact skin with absence of non-blanchable ery-thema. Patient maintains stable body weight. Serum albumin level will be 3.0 or greater.
	II. Assess patient's nutritional status.	Poor general nutrition is frequently associated with loss of weight and muscle atrophy. The reduction in subcutaneous tissue and muscle reduces the mechanical padding between the skin and underlying bony prominences and increases susceptibility to pressure ulcers. Poor nutrition also leads to decreased resistance to infection and interferes with wound healing.	
	III. Consult dietitian if patient has problems with nutrition.	Nutritional deficit is a known risk factor for the development of pressure ulcers.	
	A. Body weight:		
	1. Weigh on admission.	Initial weight provides baseline data.	
	2. Weigh 2 times/week.	Weight loss or gain serves as a guide for nutritional/fluid status.	
	B. Dietary intake:	Adequate calories do not necessarily reflect a healthy diet.	
	1. Specify amounts and types of foods.		
	2. Indicate calorie count if indicated.	Calorie count with the amount and quality of the dietary intake provides objective data.	
	3. Supplement feedings if indicated. Request vitamin supplement if indicated.	Commercial liquid formula may be easily tolerated by patients and usually is well absorbed by the gut.	
	C. Factors limiting intake:	Patient may be able to increase oral intake if limiting factors are decreased.	
	1. Ability to feed self		
	2. Physical impairment		
	3. Dentition		
	4. Nothing-by-mouth status		
	5. Nausea/vomiting		
	6. Psychosocial factors		

(continued)

Table 8.2 GUIDELINES FOR PRESSURE ULCER MANAGEMENT *(continued)*

ASSESSMENT	PLAN		EVALUATION
Nursing Diagnosis/ Nutrition-Fluid	Nursing Care Orders	Key Rationale for Nursing Care Orders	Expected Outcome
	D. Monitor lab values:	Hemoglobin (Hbg) and serum albumin may be indicators of general nutritional status.	
	1. Hemoglobin	Hgb is needed to transport O_2 to cell.	

	2. Albumin
	  a. 3.0-3.5 indicates mild protein malnutrition.
	  b. 2.5-3.0 indicates moderate protein malnutrition.
	  c. <2.5 indicates severe malnutrition.
		Protein is necessary for new tissue synthesis.
		Serum albumin level is a gross indicator of protein available for use in the body. Albumin levels may be decreased due to inadequate protein intake or loss of protein from a draining ulcer.	

	3. Serum transferrin	Because it reflects a more specific and more current nutritional status, serum transferrin level may be indicated.	
	4. Total lymphocyte count <1,800/mm^3	Lymphocyte count reflects the body's ability to mobilize an inflammatory response.	
	E. Edema	Decreased colloid osmotic pressure due to low levels of albumin will result in edema. Edema interferes with the supply of nutrients to the cell and exerts pressure on the vasculature, making edematous tissue fragile and prone to breakdown.	
	IV. Assess patient's fluid history including oral intake and urine output.		Urine output approximates fluid intake.
	V. Assess patient's current fluid status.		

	A. Fluid overload:
	  1. Sacral edema
	  2. Lower extremity edema
		Fluid collects in the most dependent body part.	

	3. Pulmonary edema	Fluid overload in a patient with compromised cardiopulmonary status will result in pulmonary edema.	
	B. Fluid deficit:	Dehydration may lead to hypovolemia, causing decreased oxygenation to the tissue. It also may lead to cracking of the skin and increased susceptibility to breakdown.	

Table 8.2 GUIDELINES FOR PRESSURE ULCER MANAGEMENT *(continued)*

ASSESSMENT	PLAN		EVALUATION
Nursing Diagnosis/ Nutrition-Fluid	Nursing Care Orders	Key Rationale for Nursing Care Orders	Expected Outcome
	1. Poor skin turgor	Skin turgor may be an inaccurate indicator of dehydration in the elderly due to normal loss of subcutaneous tissue and decrease in skin elasticity with age.	
	2. Dry mucous membranes		
	3. Dry tongue		
	VI. Consult with physician and dietitian for individualized assessment of fluid/nutritional status.	Fluid intake of 2,000 ml in 24 hours will maintain tissue hydration. Fluid intake may be contraindicated in some patients.	
Assessment Process/ Actual Pressure Ulcer	Nursing Care Orders	Key Rationale for Nursing Care Orders	Expected Outcome
	I. Assess pressure ulcer characteristics.	Use a clockwise orientation to describe location of ulcer characteristics. The patient's head signifies the 12 o'clock position.	
	A. Assess dimensions of ulcer base in centimeters.	Initial measurements serve as baseline data and provide a basis for comparison of healing or deterioration of tissue.	
	1. Length		
	2. Width		
	3. Depth		
	4. Undermining		
	5. Sinus tracts or fistulae		
	6. Tunneling		
	B. Color		
	C. Granulation		
	D. Epithelialization		
	E. Drainage	Exudative wounds take longer to heal.	
	F. Necrosis		
	1. Slough		
	2. Eschar		
	G. Odor		
	H. Wound margins		
	II. Assess surrounding intact skin		
	A. Surrounding erythema		
	B. Induration		
	C. Maceration		

(continued)

Table 8.2 GUIDELINES FOR PRESSURE ULCER MANAGEMENT *(continued)*

ASSESSMENT	PLAN		EVALUATION
Assessment Process/ Staging	Nursing Care Orders	Key Rationale for Nursing Care Orders	Expected Outcome
	III. Analyze stage of pressure ulcer(s). Determine stage.		
Stage I Pressure Ulcer:			
Nonblanchable erythema of intact skin—the heralding lesion of skin ulceration.			
Stage II Pressure Ulcer:			
Partial-thickness skin loss involving epidermis and/or dermis. The ulcer is superficial and presents clinically as an abrasion, blister, or shallow crater.			
Stage III Pressure Ulcer:			
Full-thickness skin loss involving damage or necrosis of subcutaneous tissue, which may extend down to but not through underlying fascia. The ulcer presents clinically as a deep crater with or without undermining of adjacent tissues.			
Stage IV Pressure Ulcer:			
Full-thickness skin loss with extensive destruction, tissue necrosis, or damage to muscle, bone, or supporting structures (e.g., tendon, joint capsule, etc.).			
Closed Pressure Ulcer:			

Table 8.2 GUIDELINES FOR PRESSURE ULCER MANAGEMENT *(continued)*

ASSESSMENT	PLAN		EVALUATION
Assessment Process/ Staging	Nursing Care Orders	Key Rationale for Nursing Care Orders	Expected Outcome
A large, bursa-like cavity lined by chronic fibrosis extending to deep fascia or bone. There is drainage through a small sinus tract.			
	IV. Determine presence of individual risk factors that may affect the healing process.	Specific risk factors vary in individuals. The plan of care is directed toward compensating for the risk factors.	
	V. Determine goal of care.	The goal for the patient directs the plan of care.	
	VI. Develop an individualized plan of care based on goal of care, characteristics of pressure ulcer, and presence of related risk factors.		
	VII. Communicate the importance of providing consistent care throughout the course of treatment.	Consistency is the key to effectiveness. A treatment regimen cannot be critically evaluated unless all caregivers implement the plan in the same manner.	

STAGE I PRESSURE ULCERS

Nursing Diagnosis/ Stage I Pressure Ulcer	Nursing Care Orders	Key Rationale for Nursing Care Orders	Expected Outcome
Impaired tissue integrity: Stage I Pressure Ulcer			
Nonblanchable erythema of intact skin: ulceration.	I. Reduce individual risk with special emphasis on relief of pressure. Avoid pressure to area.	Risk assessment applies to every individual with a pressure ulcer.	Intact skin with absence of nonblanchable erythema.
	II. Assess and record skin characteristics. Document changes.	Change in pressure areas can develop rapidly and will require appropriate changes in care plan. Measurements should be done at least weekly and documented in the nursing progress notes.	
	III. Keep area clean:		
	A. Use plain water. Soap should be avoided.	Commercial soaps contain alkalies, which dry the surface layer of the skin.	

(continued)

Table 8.2 GUIDELINES FOR PRESSURE ULCER MANAGEMENT *(continued)*

ASSESSMENT	PLAN		EVALUATION
Nursing Diagnosis/ Risk Factors	Nursing Care Orders	Key Rationale for Nursing Care Orders	Expected Outcome
	B. Consult with pharmacist for special cleansing agents that do not alter skin pH.	Use cleansing agents only if needed.	
	C. Use emollients judiciously if skin is dry.	Dry skin can lead to cracking, which alters the body's first line of defense. Excessive use of emollients can lead to maceration.	
	IV. May apply transparent film or Hydrocolloid over reddened bony prominence. Frequency of dressing change determined by nursing judgment.	Dressing reduces friction by acting as a protective layer over skin.	
	V. Avoid massage over bony prominences.	Massage of soft tissue over the area of hyperemia is contraindicated because it may facilitate further breakdown of tissue.	

STAGE II PRESSURE ULCERS

Nursing Diagnosis/ Stage II Pressure Ulcer	Nursing Care Orders	Key Rationale for Nursing Care Orders	Expected Outcome
Impaired tissue integrity: Stage II Pressure Ulcer			
Partial-thickness skin loss involving epidermis and/or dermis. The ulcer is superficial and presents clinically as an abrasion, blister, or shallow crater.	I. Reduce individual risk with special emphasis on relief of pressure. Avoid pressure to involved area.	Risk assessment applies to every individual with a pressure ulcer.	Progressive healing is evidenced by increasing amounts of epithelium.
	A. Assess and document dimensions of ulcer base in centimeters. 1. Length 2. Width 3. Depth 4. Undermining 5. Sinus tracts or fistulae 6. Tunneling B. Color C. Granulation D. Epithelialization	Change in pressure areas can develop rapidly and will require appropriate changes in care plan. Measurements should be done at least weekly and documented in the nursing progress notes.	

Table 8.2 GUIDELINES FOR PRESSURE ULCER MANAGEMENT *(continued)*

ASSESSMENT	PLAN		EVALUATION
Nursing Diagnosis/ Risk Factors	Nursing Care Orders	Key Rationale for Nursing Care Orders	Expected Outcome
	E. Drainage		
	F. Necrosis		
	1. Slough		
	2. Eschar		
	G. Odor		
	H. Wound margins		
	II. Assess surrounding intact skin		
	A. Surrounding erythema		
	B. Induration		
	C. Maceration		
	III. Cleanse ulcer with nor- mal saline.	Cleansing is necessary because broken skin is an interruption in the body's first line of defense against infection.	
	IV. Cover pressure ulcer with a dressing that maintains a moist envi- ronment over the ulcer.	Wound healing occurs best in a moist environment. Maintenance of adequate wound hydration minimizes scab formation so that epithelial migration can proceed unimpeded.	
	A. Semipermeable polyurethane dress- ing	Semipermeable polyurethane dressings maintain a moist envi- ronment because they are per- meable to water vapor and oxy- gen yet act as a barrier to fluid and bacterial ointments.	
	B. Hydrocolloid dressing	Interacts with wound fluid to form a moist protective gel that allows for moist wound healing while remaining adherent to intact skin.	
	C. Moist normal saline dressing over ulcer base only	Moisture mechanically softens tissue while it absorbs and reduces drainage. Maceration of intact skin surrounding the ulcer could lead to further breakdown.	
	V. Never use drying agents/treatments, e.g., heat lamps, Maalox, Milk of Magnesia.	Wound healing is delayed in a dry environment, which pro- motes scab formation and impedes epithelial migration. Heat increases demand for O_2 and is injurious to ischemic tis- sues. The skin has a normal acidic pH. Antacids change the skin pH and alter the skin flora.	

(continued)

Table 8.2 GUIDELINES FOR PRESSURE ULCER MANAGEMENT *(continued)*

STAGE III PRESSURE ULCERS

ASSESSMENT	PLAN		EVALUATION
Nursing Diagnosis/ Stage III Pressure Ulcer	Nursing Care Orders	Key Rationale for Nursing Care Orders	Expected Outcome
Impaired tissue integrity: Stage III Pressure Ulcer			
Full-thickness skin loss involving damage or necrosis of subcutaneous tissue, which may extend down to but not through underlying fascia. The ulcer presents clinically as a deep crater with or without undermining of adjacent tissues.	I. Reduce individual risk with special emphasis on relief of pressure. Avoid pressure to involved area.	Risk assessment applies to every individual with a pressure ulcer.	Progressive healing is evidenced by decreasing dimensions of ulcer base and the presence of granulation tissue.
	A. Assess and document dimensions of ulcer base in centimeters. 1. Length 2. Width 3. Depth 4. Undermining 5. Sinus tracts or fistulae 6. Tunneling	Change in pressure areas can develop rapidly and will require appropriate changes in care plan. Measurements should be done at least weekly and documented in the nursing progress notes.	
	B. Color		
	C. Granulation	Indicates new blood vessel growth.	
	D. Epithelialization	Indicates new skin growth.	
	E. Drainage		
	F. Necrosis 1. Slough 2. Eschar	Indicates dead tissue in wound.	
	G. Odor		
	H. Wound margins		
	II. Assess surrounding intact skin		
	A. Surrounding erythema	Indicates inflammation.	
	B. Induration	Indicates chronic venous congestion.	
	C. Maceration		
	III. Aspirate blister to decrease fluid pressure.	The blister acts as a protective barrier against infection and provides a moist medium for epithelialization.	
	IV. If blister is broken, gently cleanse with normal saline.	Cleansing is necessary because broken skin is an interruption in the body's first line of defense against infection.	

Table 8.2 GUIDELINES FOR PRESSURE ULCER MANAGEMENT *(continued)*

ASSESSMENT	PLAN		EVALUATION
Nursing Diagnosis/ Stage III Pressure Ulcer	Nursing Care Orders	Key Rationale for Nursing Care Orders	Expected Outcome
	V. Cover ulcer base with a dressing that maintains a moist environment over the ulcer.	Wound healing occurs best in a moist environment. Maintenance of adequate hydration minimizes scab formation so that epithelial migration can proceed unimpeded.	
	A. Semipermeable polyurethane dressing	Semipermeable polyurethane dressings maintain a moist environment because they are permeable to water vapor and oxygen but impermeable to fluids and bacteria.	
	B. Hydrocolloid dressing	Allows for moist wound healing while remaining adherent to intact skin. Because of its ability to absorb fluid, it may be effective for draining, noninfected wounds. Should not be used for clinically apparent infection.	
	C. Moist, normal saline dressing over ulcer base only	Maceration of intact skin surrounding the ulcer could lead to further breakdown.	
	VI. Do not cover a wound cavity with an occlusive dressing.	Open wounds must be allowed to drain to the surface to avoid abscess formation.	
	VII. Never use drying agents/treatments, e.g., heat lamps, Maalox, Milk of Magnesia.	Wound healing is delayed in a dry environment that promotes scab formation and impedes epithelial migration. Antacids alter the protective acid mantle of the skin.	

STAGE III PRESSURE ULCER/STAGE IV PRESSURE ULCER

Nursing Diagnosis/ Stage III/IV Pressure Ulcer without Necrosis or Infection	Nursing Care Orders	Key Rationale for Nursing Care Orders	Expected Outcome
Impaired tissue integrity: Stage III Pressure Ulcer without Necrosis or Infection Full-thickness skin loss involving damage or necrosis of subcutaneous tissue, which may extend down to but not through underlying fascia.	I. Reduce individual risk with special emphasis on pressure relief. Avoid any pressure to involved area.	Risk assessment applies to every individual with a pressure ulcer.	Progressive healing as evidenced by presence of granulation tissue and progressive decrease in diameter and depth.

(continued)

Table 8.2 GUIDELINES FOR PRESSURE ULCER MANAGEMENT *(continued)*

ASSESSMENT	PLAN		EVALUATION
Nursing Diagnosis/ Stage III/IV Pressure Ulcer without Necrosis or Infection	Nursing Care Orders	Key Rationale for Nursing Care Orders	Expected Outcome
And/or	A. Assess and document dimensions of ulcer base in centimeters.	Change in pressure ulcers can develop rapidly and will require appropriate changes in care plan.	
Impaired tissue integrity:			
Stage IV Pressure Ulcer without Necrosis or Infection	1. Length		
	2. Width		
	3. Depth		
Full-thickness skin loss with extensive destruction, tissue necrosis, or damage to muscle, bone, or supporting structures.	4. Undermining	Indicates extension of ulcer that cannot be visualized.	
	5. Sinus tracts or fistulae	Indicates connection of deep ulcer to surface tissue.	
	6. Tunneling		
	B. Color		
	C. Granulation	Indicates new blood vessel growth.	
	D. Epithelialization	Indicates new skin growth.	
	E. Drainage		
	F. Necrosis	Indicates dead tissue in wound.	
	1. Slough		
	2. Eschar		
	G. Odor		
	H. Wound margins		
	II. Assess surrounding intact skin		
	A. Surrounding erythema	Indicates inflammation.	
	B. Induration	Indicates chronic venous congestion.	
	C. Maceration		
	III. Develop wound management plan:		
	A. Irrigate wound with normal saline. Use enough irrigation pressure to cleanse wound without causing trauma.	Irrigation with normal saline may assist in removing dead cells and reducing the bacterial count. Safe, effective irrigation pressures range from 4-15 psi. Forceful irrigation greater than 15 psi should not be used.	
	B. Examine sinus tracts and undermined areas of wound for retained dressing materials.	Use of a dressing with cotton filler is contraindicated for wound packing, as the filling may act as a foreign substance and retard healing.	
	C. Fill wound loosely with dressing materials.		

Table 8.2 GUIDELINES FOR PRESSURE ULCER MANAGEMENT *(continued)*

ASSESSMENT	PLAN		EVALUATION
Nursing Diagnosis/ Stage III/IV Pressure Ulcer without Necrosis or Infection	Nursing Care Orders	Key Rationale for Nursing Care Orders	Expected Outcome
	1. Nondraining ulcer: Use dressings such as: Plain gauze Impregnated gauze • saline • gel • vaseline • bismuth Foam	Moist dressings provide a physiological environment for formation of granulation tissue. A wound is filled to reduce dead space, decreasing the risk of abscess formation. Packing should not be so tight as to compress tissue and interfere with circulation.	
	2. Draining ulcer: Use absorptive dressings such as: Dry gauze Alginates Hydro-gels pastes powders Beads	Heavily exudative wounds heal more slowly than non-exudative wounds. Absorption of exudate will prevent maceration of the intact skin.	
	D. Cover wound with secondary dressing.	The dressing helps to protect the wound.	
	E. Consult pressure ulcer resource persons to determine suitability of a moisture- retentive dressing.	These dressings provide a moist physiological environment for formation of granulation tissue but may be contraindicated in certain situations. A wound care specialist can determine appropriate use.	
	V. Evaluate plan of care and institute changes as appropriate.	Change in the pressure ulcer may necessitate revision of the plan of care.	

STAGE III NECROTIC PRESSURE ULCER/ STAGE IV NECROTIC PRESSURE ULCER

Nursing Diagnosis/ Stage III/IV Necrotic Pressure Ulcer	Nursing Care Orders	Key Rationale for Nursing Care Orders	Expected Outcome
Impaired tissue integrity: Stage III Necrotic Pressure Ulcer			
Full-thickness skin loss involving damage or necrosis of subcutaneous tissue, which may extend down to but	I. Reduce individual risk with special emphasis on pressure relief. Avoid any pressure to involved area.	Risk assessment applies to each individual with a pressure ulcer.	Pressure ulcer is clean as evidenced by absence of slough or eschar.

(continued)

Table 8.2 GUIDELINES FOR PRESSURE ULCER MANAGEMENT *(continued)*

ASSESSMENT	PLAN		EVALUATION
Nursing Diagnosis/ Stage III/IV Necrotic Pressure Ulcer	Nursing Care Orders	Key Rationale for Nursing Care Orders	Expected Outcome
not through underlying fascia. And/or Impaired tissue integrity: Stage IV Necrotic Pressure Ulcer Full-thickness skin loss with extensive destruction, tissue necrosis, or damage to muscle, bone, or supporting structures.	A. Assess dimensions of ulcer base in centimeters. 1. Length 2. Width 3. Depth 4. Undermining	Changes in pressure ulcer can develop rapidly and will require appropriate changes in plan of care. Indicates extension of ulcer that cannot be visualized.	
	5. Sinus tracts or fistulae 6. Tunneling	Indicates connection of deep ulcer to surface tissue.	
	B. Color		
	C. Granulation	Indicates new blood vessel growth.	
	D. Epithelialization	Indicates new skin growth.	
	E. Drainage		
	F. Necrosis 1. Slough 2. Eschar	Indicates dead tissue in wound. Moist dead tissue. Dry dead tissue. Depth cannot be determined until eschar is removed.	
	G. Odor		
	H. Wound margins		
	II. Assess surrounding intact skin		
	A. Surrounding erythema	Indicates inflammation.	
	B. Induration	Indicates chronic venous congestion.	
	C. Maceration		
	IV. Cleanse Pressure Ulcer		
	A. Irrigate wound forcefully with normal saline every 8 hours or with each dressing change.	Irrigation under pressure reduces bacterial count and removes debris from the wound.	
	B. Consult with a physician regarding use of whirlpool.	The agitation of the water assists in softening and removing wound debris.	
	V. Debride necrotic tissue: Surgical debridement		
	A. Consult with physician or wound care specialist regarding surgical debridement if eschar or necrosis is present.	Surgical debridement is the most effective method of removing necrotic tissue.	

Table 8.2 GUIDELINES FOR PRESSURE ULCER MANAGEMENT *(continued)*

ASSESSMENT	PLAN		EVALUATION
Nursing Diagnosis/ Stage III/IV Necrotic Pressure Ulcer	Nursing Care Orders	Key Rationale for Nursing Care Orders	Expected Outcome
	B. Mechanical debridement with gauze dressing		
	1. Apply moist-to-dry dressing using normal saline.	As the gauze dries, it sticks to the necrotic tissue. When the dressing is removed, it debrides the wound by tearing away the adherent material non-selectively. Pulling the dressing from the wound may be painful.	
	C. Debride the necrotic tissue Chemical debridement using enzymes		
	1. Consult with physician or wound care specialist regarding:		
	a. Surgical debridement or eschar and large amounts of slough prior to chemical debridement.	Debridement time is decreased if eschar and large amounts of slough are first removed.	
	b. Crosshatching of eschar with a scalpel.	Enzymatic action occurs only on the surface of the wound. Crosshatching of eschar allows for penetration of the enzymatic debriding agent into and through the eschar.	
	2. Irrigate wound as appropriate for each enzymatic agent.	Irrigation rinses away debris and should be done at least daily, as most enzymatic debriding agents lose their effectiveness within 24 hours. The irrigation solution should not interfere with the action of the enzymatic agent. Whirlpool can also provide effective wound irrigation.	
	3. Apply the enzymatic debriding agent only to necrotic tissue.	Some enzymatic debriding agents may damage healthy tissue.	
	4. Apply a dressing as directed for the selected enzymatic debriding agent.	The dressing should be applied so the enzyme is in contact with necrotic tissue. Some enzymatic agents require a moist dressing, while others require a dry dressing.	
	5. Collaborate with physician or wound specialist regarding	Enzymatic debriding agents may irritate healthy tissue.	

(continued)

Table 8.2 GUIDELINES FOR PRESSURE ULCER MANAGEMENT *(continued)*

ASSESSMENT	PLAN		EVALUATION
Nursing Diagnosis/ Stage III/IV Necrotic Pressure Ulcer	Nursing Care Orders	Key Rationale for Nursing Care Orders	Expected Outcome
	discontinuation of enzy- matic agent when wound is no longer necrotic and healthy granulation base is present.		
	D. Debride necrotic tis- sue. Autolytic debridement: With moisture-reten- tive dressings	Within a moist environment, the body produces lytic enzymes that selectively separate necrotic tissue from healthy tissue.	
	1. Consult with a wound care special- ist regarding:		
	a. Hydrocolloid dressings		
	b. Film dressings	Film acts as a barrier to fluid, stool, environmental contami- nants; permeable to oxygen, and moisture vapor; keep wound base moist.	
	c. Moist saline gauze dressings		
	d. Gel dressings		
	e. Foam		
	2. Cleanse wound as directed.		
	3. Dry surrounding tis- sue.		
	4. Apply dressing. Change as directed.	Dressings vary in time to remain in place for effective debride- ment.	

STAGE III INFECTED PRESSURE ULCER/
STAGE IV INFECTED PRESSURE ULCER

Nursing Diagnosis/ Stage III/IV Infected Pressure Ulcer	Nursing Care Orders	Key Rationale for Nursing Care Orders	Expected Outcome
Impaired tissue integrity: Stage III Infected Pressure Ulcer Stage III infected pressure ulcer related to bacterial invasion of sur- rounding tissue as evidenced by cel- lulitis, systemic	I. Reduce individual risk with special emphasis on relief of pressure. Avoid pressure to involved area. A. Assess dimensions of ulcer base in centime- ters.	Risk assessment applies to each individual with a pressure ulcer. Changes in pressure ulcers can develop rapidly and will require appropriate changes in care plan.	Absence of local/systemic signs of infection as evidenced by swelling, heat, and tenderness.

Table 8.2 GUIDELINES FOR PRESSURE ULCER MANAGEMENT *(continued)*

ASSESSMENT	PLAN		EVALUATION
Nursing Diagnosis/ Stage III/IV Infected Pressure Ulcer	Nursing Care Orders	Key Rationale for Nursing Care Orders	Expected Outcome
signs of infections, and/or purulent drainage	1. Length 2. Width 3. Depth	Measurements should be done at least weekly and documented on the care plan.	
And/or Impaired tissue integrity:	4. Undermining	Indicates new extension of ulcer that cannot be visualized.	
Stage IV Infected Pressure Ulcer	5. Sinus tracts or fistulae	Indicates connection of deep ulcer to surface tissue.	
Stage IV infected pressure ulcer related to bacterial invasion of sur- rounding tissue as evidenced by cel- lulitis, systemic signs of infection, and/or purulent drainage	6. Tunneling B. Color C. Granulation	Indicates new blood vessel growth.	
	D. Epithelialization	Indicates new skin growth.	
	E. Drainage		

	F. Necrosis
	  1. Slough
	  2. Eschar
		Indicates dead tissue in wound.	

	G. Odor		
	H. Wound margins		
	II. Assess surrounding intact skin.		
	A. Surrounding erythema	Indicates inflammation.	
	B. Induration	Indicates chronic venous con- gestion.	
	C. Maceration		
	III. Assess for signs of local infection in sur- rounding tissue:	Erythema, heat, induration, and pain may be evidence of tissue response to bacterial invasion.	
	A. Redness		
	B. Heat		
	C. Induration		
	D. Edema		
	E. Pain		
	F. Purulent drainage		
	IV. Assess for signs of sys- temic infection:		
	A. Elevated temperature B. Changes in WBC	Elevation in body temperature and an abnormal rise in white blood cell count (WBC) may be signs of systemic infection. Body temperature should be carefully monitored after surgical wound debridement, as bacteria may enter the bloodstream at this time.	
	C. Confusion	Acute confusion may be an indi- cation of sepsis.	

(continued)

Table 8.2 GUIDELINES FOR PRESSURE ULCER MANAGEMENT *(continued)*

ASSESSMENT	PLAN		EVALUATION
Nursing Diagnosis/ Stage III/IV Infected Pressure Ulcer	Nursing Care Orders	Key Rationale for Nursing Care Orders	Expected Outcome
	V. Notify the physician if there are signs of local or systemic infection.	A deep wound culture or tissue biopsy may be indicated.	
	VI. Implement a wound management plan in collaboration with a physician or wound care specialist.		
	A. Irrigate wound with normal saline with each dressing change.	Irrigation dilutes the bacterial count and removes debris. Saline is physiologic and is the irrigating solution of choice.	
	B. Apply topical antibiotics if ordered, e.g. silvadene	The use of antiseptics is controversial. Iodophors may be toxic to fibroblasts and interfere with wound healing. Allergic reactions can be seen with Iodophors. The use of topical antibiotics is controversial. There is no scientific evidence that they will decrease the bacterial count in the tissue surrounding the wound. Topical antibiotics may be used to decrease the bacterial count in the wound itself prior to surgical repair of the ulcer.	
	C. Absorb purulent wound drainage using:		
	1. Coarse mesh gauze dressing.	Dressings absorb drainage and prevent crust formation, which could interfere with healing.	
	2. Moisture-retentive dressings with absorptive properties.		
	a. Dry gauze	Dry gauze absorbs drainage.	
	b. Alginates	Absorptive. For use in highly exudating wounds. Not for use in mildly exudating or dry wounds. Dressing becomes hard if allowed to dry.	
	c. Pastes d. Powders e. Beads	Pastes, powders, and beads interact with wound fluid forming a protective gel. The absorbent action draws microorganisms and debris away from the wound, decreasing bacterial contamination and inflammation.	
	3. Retained starch-based dressings must be removed prior to reapplication.		

Table 8.2 GUIDELINES FOR PRESSURE ULCER MANAGEMENT *(continued)*

CLOSED PRESSURE ULCER

ASSESSMENT	PLAN		EVALUATION
Nursing Diagnosis/ Closed Pressure Ulcer	Nursing Care Orders	Key Rationale for Nursing Care Orders	Expected Outcome
Impaired tissue integrity: Closed Pressure Ulcer			
Closed pressure ulcer related to prolonged pressure as evidenced by drainage from small sinus tract	I. Reduce individual risk with special emphasis on relief of pressure. Avoid pressure to involved area.	Risk assessment applies to all persons with ulcers.	
	II. Assess bony prominences for drainage from small sinus tracts.	The patient may be unaware of a closed pressure ulcer.	
	III. Consult physician if there are draining lesions.	Surgical intervention may be necessary.	
	IV. Assess for signs of local infection in surrounding tissue:	Erythema, heat, induration, and pain may be evidence of tissue response to bacterial invasion.	
	A. Redness		
	B. Heat		
	C. Induration		
	D. Edema		
	E. Pain		
	F. Purulent drainage		
	V. Assess for signs of systemic infection:		
	A. Elevated temperature	Elevation in body temperature and an abnormal rise in WBC may be signs of systemic infection. Body temperature should be carefully monitored after surgical wound debridement, as bacteria may enter the bloodstream at this time.	
	B. Changes in WBC		
	C. Confusion	Acute confusion may be an indication of sepsis.	
	VI. Notify the physician if there are signs of local or systemic infection.		

Today, many agencies use standard care plans with daily checklists to decrease documentation time. Less importance is placed on documenting interventions and more importance placed on patient outcomes. In light of this, documentation forms in a critical pathway format were developed to track patient progress toward expected outcomes of care. The documentation forms give expected outcomes for patients at high risk for impaired skin integrity: pressure ulcers and for patients with impaired skin integrity: pressure ulcers. Nursing documentation reflects daily progress toward these outcomes. If the outcome is met, nurses check the box only; if the outcome is not met, an explanation is written in the box. Progress can be tracked and care altered to improve clinical outcomes. This pathway is a precursor to a critical path, which will give accompanying treatment and expected outcome timelines.[5] An example of a pathway for documenting pressure ulcer outcomes is shown in Table 8.1. For an example of pressure ulcer care using the Harper Hospital documentation format, see the case study in the Appendices.

References

1. Alfaro, R. *Applying Nursing Diagnosis and Nursing Process: A Step-by-Step Guide*, 3rd ed. Philadelphia: J.B. Lippincott, 1995.
2. Carpenito, L.J. *Nursing Diagnosis: Application to Clinical Practice*, 6th ed. Philadelphia: J.B. Lippincott, 1995.
3. Trelease, C.C. "Developing Standards for Wound Care," *Ostomy/Wound Management* 20:46-56, 1989.
4. Maklebust, J., and Sieggreen, M.Y. *Pressure Ulcers: Guidelines for Prevention and Nursing Management*. West Dundee, Ill.: S-N Publications, 1991.
5. Ducharme, M.A., and Maklebust, J. "Nursing Diagnosis in an Acute Care Setting." *Proceedings of the 11th Annual Conference for the Classification of Nursing Diagnoses*. Philadelphia: NURSECOM, 1995.

CHAPTER 9

Developing Institutional Policies and Procedures

A program for pressure ulcer management must begin with the development of institutional policies that govern the care of patients in that agency. Authorities in an agency approve institutional policies, and these policies determine the actions of its employees. A policy may include professional standards, patient care plans, procedures, and protocols that are implemented by the staff who work there (see definitions in Table 9.1).

The employees of an agency may be asked to assist in writing institutional protocols and procedures. Generally, the protocol format is standard and may include the title, purpose, desired patient outcome, personnel affected, steps of the procedure, and rationale, if necessary. Appropriate documentation is indicated, references are given, authors are credited, and approving signatures and titles are included.

The following section provides examples of pressure ulcer policies and procedures from Harper Hospital. Agencies may adapt the format to develop policies and procedures that are specific to their own institutions.

Table 9.1 Policy and Procedure Definitions

Policy: statement governing a course of action

Procedure: steps required to complete a task

Protocol: actions prescribed to manage a problem

Standard: statement defining rules, conditions, or actions

Standard Care Plan: predetermined written plan for managing care

Standard of Care: indicator that defines expected patient care

Standard of Practice: indicator that defines expected nursing action

Table 9.2 Universal Precautions/Isolation

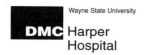

Wayne State University
Harper
Hospital

POLICY NO.___256___

NURSING PATIENT SERVICES

TITLE: UNIVERSAL PRECAUTIONS/ISOLATION

A. UNIVERSAL PRECAUTIONS

1. Universal precaution standards apply to all healthcare workers who could have potential contact with blood or other potentially infectious body fluids as a result of their job duties.

2. Gloves are worn when anticipating contact with blood, other body fluids, mucous membranes, or nonintact skin. Gloves must be changed after contact with each patient.

3. Handwashing is done immediately after gloves are removed. Hands and other surfaces should be washed immediately and thoroughly if contaminated with blood or other body fluids.

4. Mask and Protective Eyewear are not routinely necessary but are used during procedures likely to generate droplets of blood or other body fluids and to prevent exposure of the mucous membranes of the mouth, nose, and eyes.

5. Gowns are used during procedures likely to generate splashes of blood or other body fluids and to prevent soiling of clothes.

6. Sharp Instruments (e.g., used needles) are not recapped, purposely bent or broken, removed from disposable syringes, or otherwise manipulated by hand. This includes needles used for blood cultures. Needles are not changed before placing the specimen in the bottles. Disposable syringes, needles, sutures, scalpels, etc. are placed in puncture-resistant containers designed for this purpose as close to the point of use as possible.

7. Blood and blood-contaminated body fluid specimens are handled as potentially infectious material and are bagged in clear plastic bags before being transported. Bags are not required for blood tubes transported by means of blood trays. The Pneumatic Tube System policy and procedure is followed for specimens transferred by the pneumatic tube system. Specimens are sent in a tube with a foam insert. See references.

(continued)

Table 9.2 Universal Precautions/Isolation (continued)

TITLE: UNIVERSAL PRECAUTIONS/ISOLATION   POLICY NO. <u>256</u>

8. Universal precaution equipment is located either in each patient room in the universal precaution bin, specified drawers in the intensive care units, or the medication room in the psychiatric units, as well as the department treatment rooms and crash carts.

B. ISOLATION

1. Isolation protocol is followed according to the Universal Precaution and Isolation policy in the Infection Control Manual.

2. Epidemiology is notified of patients placed in AFB and Respiratory Isolation.

3. The order for a specific isolation is entered into HOWIE for a computerized isolation sign which is placed on the patient's door.

4. A private room is required.

5. All personnel entering the room follow the prescribed practices outlined on the posted isolation sign.

6. The isolation bin may be obtained from SRD if needed.

REFERENCES:

OSHA Enforcement Policy and Procedures for Occupational Exposure to Tuberculosis, October, 1993.
OSHA Final Blood Borne Pathogen Rule: Federal Register, December, 1991.
Universal Precaution and Isolation Policy, Infection Control Manual.
Pneumatic Tube System Use, Administrative Policy and Procedure 1.14, October, 1993.
Administrative Policy Manual.

AUTHORS:

Flanagan, E.., RN, BSN, CIC, Epidemiology Coordinator, February, 1995.
Pone, J., RN, ADN, Administrative Manager, Medical Patient Services, February, 1995.

APPROVAL:

Shirley L Green   5/2/95
Shirley L. Green   Date
Vice President Patient Services

Table 9.3 Skin Care

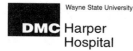 Wayne State University
Harper
Hospital

PROCEDURE NO.____150____

NURSING PATIENT SERVICES

TITLE: SKIN CARE

POLICY:
Each patient has systematic skin assessment and care consisting of: inspection, cleaning, hydration, and protection.

EQUIPMENT:
Mild Soap or detergent
Moisturizers
Barrier agent (e.g., aluminum paste)
Absorbent materials
Film dressing
Powder
Positioning products (cushions, wedge pillows, trapeze)

PROCEDURE	RATIONALE/EMPHASIS
A. INSPECTION 1. Inspect skin during admission assessment. 2. Evaluate skin integrity, color, temperature, texture, and turgor. 3. Reassess the skin. Frequency of reassessment is determined by the patient's level of risk.	Ongoing assessment of the skin can be done at time of physical assessment, bathing, changing dressings, exercise routines, or other patient care activities. Risk factors include weight loss, inactivity, immobility, incontinence, decreased LOC and/or malnutrition (decreased albumin).

(continued)

Table 9.3 Skin Care *(continued)*

TITLE: SKIN CARE	PROCEDURE NO. 150

PROCEDURE	RATIONALE/EMPHASIS
B. CLEANSING 1. Cleanse skin when needed.	The purpose of skin cleansing is to remove foreign materials, bacterial contaminants, and the residues of skin secretions.
2. Select mild soap or detergent for individual use.	The ideal soap or detergent will remove only the skin contaminants and will preserve the natural lipids and oils of the skin. Excessive cleansing or use of harsh cleansers lead to skin drying.
3. Minimize any force or friction during cleansing. 4. Avoid chemical additives in soaps or detergents such as colorants, fragrances, and conditioners.	Chemical agents may lead to skin irritation or sensitization.
C. HYDRATION 1. Apply topical moisturizing agents to dry skin.	Decreased skin hydration/dry skin is associated with fissuring and cracking of the skin.

D. PROTECTION FROM EXCESSIVE MOISTURE
1. Avoid excessive moisture on skin (urine, stool, perspiration, wound drainage) by either of these methods:
  a. Use urinary or fecal pouch to manage incontinence.
  b. Use a barrier agent to protect skin from excessive moisture.
	Skin that is moist or wet is more susceptible to injury from friction, more easily abraded, more readily penetrated by irritating solutions and promotes higher microbial growth.

Table 9.3 Skin Care *(continued)*

TITLE: SKIN CARE   PROCEDURE NO.___150___

PROCEDURE	RATIONALE/EMPHASIS
2. Use an absorbent material under the patient to absorb fluid. Avoid the use of plastic and paper protectors.	Absorbent products wick moisture away from the skin. Absorbent products are composed of at least two layers. The layer that contacts the skin is usually a permeable material that quickly dries. The second layer is hydrophilic material that has a high capacity to absorb fluid.

E. PROTECTION FROM FRICTION, SHEAR, AND PRESSURE

PROCEDURE	RATIONALE/EMPHASIS
1. Avoid prolonged elevation of the head of the bed >30° if the patient is able to tolerate other positions.	Shear injury occurs when the head of the bed is raised. The torso has a tendency to slide downward while the skin of the sacrum remains fixed between the skin and the bed linen.
2. Avoid massage over bony prominence and reddened or broken areas of skin.	Massage over bony prominence may cause maceration and tearing of underlying tissue.
3. Lift patient when repositioning. Avoid dragging skin across bed linens.	Frictional trauma to the skin occurs when the skin, while under load, is moved across a coarse surface such as bed linen.
4. Use a film dressing or powder on areas of skin susceptible to friction forces.	Material that can be placed on the skin to reduce its coefficient of friction will reduce the potential for friction injury.

(continued)

Table 9.3 Skin Care *(continued)*

TITLE: SKIN CARE   PROCEDURE NO. 150

PROCEDURE	RATIONALE/EMPHASIS
5. Provide and teach patient to use overhead trapeze to assist in moving about in bed unless medically contraindicated.	Lifting prevents friction injury.
6. Use positioning wedges or pillows.	External support will assist position changes.
7. Suspend heels while in bed.	Since heels are the hardest area to bridge for pressure relief, special attention is needed to prevent pressure on heels while patient is in bed.
8. Use wheelchair/chair cushion when in sitting position.	Ischial tuberosities are at increased risk for pressure when in sitting position.
9. Avoid the use of donuts and products fashioned in the shape of donuts.	Products that curcumscribe the pressure ulcer or bony prominence compromise the skin circulation around the area of concern.
10. Teach patient to do small shifts in body weight at regular intervals.	Shifts in body weight provide intermittent relief of pressure.

DOCUMENTATION:

Non ICU/CCU:
Nursing Care Plan: As intervention for nursing diagnosis or collaborative problem.
Nursing Procedures/Treatments Sheet: Chart skin care given and condition of skin.
Progress Notes: Progress toward expected outcome.

Table 9.3 Skin Care *(continued)*

TITLE: SKIN CARE   PROCEDURE NO.___150___

ICU/CCU:
24 Hour Flow Sheet.
Progress Notes: Progress toward expected outcome.

REFERENCES:

Agency for Health Care Policy and Research. (1992). Clinical Practice Guidelines, Number 3, Publication No. 92-0047. *Pressure ulcers in adults: Prediction and prevention.* U.S. Department of Health and Human Services.

Kramer, D., & Honig, P.J. (1988). Diaper dermatitis in the hospitalized child. *Enterostomal Therapy*, 15: (4), 164-170.

Leyden, J.J. (1984). Cornstarch, candida albicans, and diaper rash. *Pediatric Dermatology*, 1:(4), 322-5.

Leyden, J.J., Katz, S., Stewart, R., & Kligman, A.M. (1977). Urinary ammonia and ammonia producing microorganisms in infants with and without diaper dermatitis. *Archives Dermatology*, 113: (12), 1679-80.

Maklebust, J. (1991). Impact of AHCPR pressure ulcer guidelines on nursing practice, *Decubitus.*

Maklebust, J., & Sieggreen, M. (1991). *Pressure ulcers: Guidelines for prevention and nursing management*, West Dundee, IL: S-N Publication.

Shipes, E., & Stanley, I. (1981). Effects of a liquid copolymer skin barrier for preventing skin-problems. *Ostomy Management*, 4: 19-23.

Shipes, E., & Stanley, I. (1983). A study of a liquid copolymer skin barrier for preventing and alleviating perineal irritations in incontinent patients. *Journal of Urological Nursing*, 2: (3), 32-34.

Zimmera, R.E., Lawson, K.D., & Calvert, C.J. (1986). The effects of wearing diapers on skin. *Pediatric Dermatology*, 3 (2), 95-101.

AUTHORS:

Maklebust, J., RN, MSN, CS, Case Manager, Surgical Patient Services, March, 1995.
Seiggreen, M., RN, MSN, CS, Case Manager, Critical Care/Cardiology Patient Services, March, 1995.

APPROVAL:

_____*Shirley L. Green*_____ 5/2/95_____
Shirley L. Green   Date
Vice President Patient Services

Table 9.4 Wound Culture: Aerobic and Anaerobic

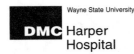

Wayne State University

Harper
Hospital

PROCEDURE NO. 165

NURSING PATIENT SERVICES

TITLE: WOUND CULTURE: AEROBIC AND ANAEROBIC

GENERAL INFORMATION: Tissue or fluid obtained from a site is superior to a swab specimen. Swabs of chronic wounds are not recommended. All chronic wounds are colonized.

POLICY:
   1. Physician order is required.
   2. Cultures should be obtained before starting antibiotic therapy.

PERSONNEL: RN, LPN, NT, NA

EQUIPMENT:
   Aerobic specimen collector - Culturette II and/or Anaerobic specimen
      collector-Vacutainer
   4x4 sponges
   Clean gloves
   Paper tape
   Impervious bag
   250 mL bottle of normal saline
   Iodophor solution
   Baxter irrigation tip

PROCEDURE	RATIONALE/EMPHASIS
A. PREPARATION	
1. Wash hands. Use no-touch technique to remove old dressings.	To prevent further contamination of the wound.
2. Discard soiled dressings in impervious bag.	
3. Wash hands.	
4. Apply clean gloves and assess wound for origin of drainage.	To examine the wound bed for depth of undermined areas.

Table 9.4 Wound Culture: Aerobic and Anaerobic *(continued)*

TITLE: WOUND CULTURE: PROCEDURE NO.___165___
     AEROBIC AND ANAEROBIC

PROCEDURE	RATIONALE/EMPHASIS
5. Notify physician for further clarification if no drainage is present.	Do not culture dry wounds. Swabs of dry wounds and sinus tracts are inaccurate and of little value.
6. Irrigate the wound area with sterile water or normal saline irrigation solution.	To remove loose necrotic material and surface contaminants which colonize the wound and result in an inaccurate polymicrobial culture. Avoid the use of bacteriostatic solutions for wound irrigation, such as water/normal saline for injection, because it will prevent recovery of pathogens.
7. Cleanse wound periphery, unless contraindicated, with sterile water or normal saline irrigation solution. An iodophor solution or 70% alcohol may be used around a small wound opening.	Cleansing the wound periphery will prevent contamination of the swab when obtaining the specimen. Do not allow the disinfectant solution to touch the wound surface being cultured because it will weaken/kill the desired pathogen to be cultured.
8. Dry wound periphery area gently with sterile 4x4 sponge using sterile gloved hand.	
9. Remove gloves.	

B. AEROBIC CULTURE

1. Remove the swab from the aerobic specimen collector, being careful to touch only the top of the cap.	Do not touch swab.
2. If possible obtain a tissue specimen of the healthiest tissue in the wound.	

(continued)

Table 9.4 Wound Culture: Aerobic and Anaerobic *(continued)*

TITLE: WOUND CULTURE: PROCEDURE NO.＿＿165＿
    AEROBIC AND ANAEROBIC

PROCEDURE	RATIONALE/EMPHASIS
3. If unable to get a tissue specimen, press the swabs against the wound margin or ulcer base using sufficient force to cause fresh exudate to thoroughly moisten swab.	Surface swabs are of little value. Avoid creating a fresh blood flow which will dilute the specimen.
4. Avoid contaminating the swabs with organisms from the skin and adjacent tissues.	To decrease the chance of a polymicrobial culture.
5. Place the swabs back into the specimen collector. Crush the ampule at the base and force the swabs into the transport medium.	To preserve the pathogens by preventing the swabs from drying out.
6. Attach a stamped label to specimen container.	
7. Transport specimen to the lab within 1 hour.	Prolonged time results in death of representative pathogens or allows other pathogens to multiply (microbial overgrowth).

C. ANAEROBIC CULTURE

PROCEDURE	RATIONALE/EMPHASIS
1. Clean area around wound with iodophor solution. Remove drainage or crusts. Allow to dry.	Superficial wounds or abscesses and sinus tracts are not acceptable for anaerobic cultures. Anaerobes may be present in deep wounds with exudate.
2. Aspiration technique: a. Assess wound to be cultured. Most anaerobic cultures should be obtained by aspirating tissue with a sterile needle and syringe.	To limit contact with oxygen which destroys anaerobic pathogens.
b. Consult with physician, infection control practitioner, CNS, or ET nurse to obtain specmen.	

Table 9.4 Wound Culture: Aerobic and Anaerobic *(continued)*

TITLE: WOUND CULTURE: AEROBIC AND ANAEROBIC	PROCEDURE NO.___165___

PROCEDURE	RATIONALE/EMPHASIS
c. Cap the needle after the specimen is obtained or deposit aspirate into anaerobic specimen collector.	
d. Attach a stamped label to specimen container. Transport specimen to the lab immediately.	To prevent oxygen from destroying the pathogen.

DOCUMENTATION:
Nursing Shift Assessment, Specimen Section: Type of culture, source, time and initials.

REFERENCES:
Bergstrom N, Bennett MA, Carlson CE, et al. *Treatment of Pressure Ulcers.* Clinical Practice Guideline, No.15 Rockville, MD: U.S. Department of Health and Human Services. Public Health Service, Agency for Health Care Policy and Research. AHCPR Publication No. 95-0652. December 1994.
Depart of Path/Lab Informat manual (1984). E.1-E 13.3. Available from author.
Infection Control Manual (1985) Grace Hospital Detroit.
Eherlich M, & Hayes M (1985) *Guidelines For the Prevention and Management of Pressure Ulcers* The University of Michigan Hospitals 40-42 Ann Arbor MI: Author
Garner JS. CDC guidelines: for prevention of surgical wound infections. *Infection Control* 1985 7(3):193-200
Guevich I. Infected decubiti: patient placement and care. *Topics in clinical nursing.* 1983 5(7):55-62
Guevich I. Appropriate collection of specimens for culture and sensitivity. *Am J Infect Cont* 1980 8(4):113-119.
Rousseau P. Pressure ulcers in an aging society. *Wounds* 1989 1(2) August: 135-141.
Sapico FL, Witte JI, Canavati HN, et al. The infected foot of the diabetic patient: quantitative microbiology and analysis of clinical features. *Reviews of Infectious Disease* 1984 6(51) March-April:5171-5176.
Sapico FL, Quinumas, VJ, Thornhill-Joynes M, Canawati HN, Capen DA, Klein NE, Khawam S, Montgomerie JZ. Quantitative of pressure sores in different stages of healing. *DiagnMicrobiol Infect Dis* 1986 5(1) May:31-8.

RESOURCES:
Bartley, J., MPH. Director, Infection Control Department, Harper, March 1986.
Maklebust, J., MSN, RN, CS. Clinical Nurse Specialist, Harper, March 1986.

Table 9.5 Wound Irrigation

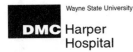 Wayne State University

DMC Harper
Hospital

PROCEDURE NO.___120___

NURSING PATIENT SERVICES

TITLE: WOUND IRRIGATION

POLICY:
1. Sterile technique is required for all wound irrigations.
2. A physician order is required for postoperative surgical wound irrigation.
3. A physician order is not required for pressure ulcer treatment.

PERSONNEL: RN, LPN, Nurse Technician, SNT

EQUIPMENT:
Clean gloves (2 pair)
Sterile Normal Saline 250 ml #101854 or sterile irrigant as ordered
Sterile gauze sponges
4x4 gauze sponges and/or abdominal pads
Skin sealant (optional)
Irrigation cap #105001
Paper tape
Impervious bag

PROCEDURE

RATIONALE/EMPHASIS

A. PREPARATION
1. Label bottle of saline with date and time.
2. Wash hands.
3. Apply non-sterile gloves and remove old dressings and place in impervious bag.
4. Remove gloves and wash hands.

Table 9.5 Wound Irrigation *(continued)*

TITLE: WOUND IRRIGATION   PROCEDURE NO.___120

PROCEDURE	RATIONALE/EMPHASIS
5. Measure wound and assess wound bed for presence of granulation tissue, necrosis, odor, amount and color of drainage.	Wound assessment aids in selection of appropriate irrigation technique.
6. Open irrigation cap package. Save the bubble package to cover cap after procedure.	
7. Tightly secure irrigation cap to a 250 ml bottle of saline.	
8. Open sterile gauze dressing supplies maintaining a sterile field.	

B. IRRIGATION

PROCEDURE	RATIONALE/EMPHASIS
1. Flush wound with prescribed irrigant. Hold tip 1-2 inches from wound:	Wound irrigation may dilute the bacterial count.
a. Gently irrigate clean granulating wounds.	Forceful irrigation may damage clean granulating wounds.
b. Forcefully irrigate necrotic wounds using full force to plunger of 30 ml syringe.	Forceful irrigation mechanically debrides loose necrotic tissue. Bacteria multiply and necrotic tissue easily accumulates in undermined areas of a wound or sinus tracts.
c. Flush away any wound drainage or residue from previous dressing.	
2. Apply non-sterile gloves.	
3. Dry surrounding skin with 4x4.	
4. Apply prescribed dressing.	
5. Consult Case Manager, ET Nurse, or wound care specialist for alternative types of dressings that may be used in clean and necrotic wounds.	

(continued)

Table 9.5 Wound Irrigation *(continued)*

TITLE: WOUND IRRIGATION   PROCEDURE NO.___120___

PROCEDURE	RATIONALE/EMPHASIS
6. Wash hands and discard impervious bag containing old dressings in soiled utility room. 7. Replace the bubble package on top of the irrigation cap to protect it from dust and contamination. After a 24 hour period, discard bottle.	

DOCUMENTATION:
Non-Critical Care:
Nursing Care Plan: As intervention for appropriate nursing diagnosis or clinical problem.
Nursing Treatments/Procedures Sheet: Chart treatment and signature.
Progress Notes: Date and assessment of wound.

ICU/CCU:
Critical Care 24 Hour Flow Sheet: Treatment and assessment of wound.

REFERENCES:
Brown, L., MD, Shelton, H., MD, Barnside, G., PhD. & Cohn, I., Jr. MD. (1978). Evaluation of wound irrigation by pulsatile jet and conventional methods. *Annals of Surgery.* 187(2), 170-173.
Cooper, D.M., Watt, R.C., & Alterescu, V. (1983). *Guide to wound care,* USA: Hollister Incorporated.
Diekmann, C.M., Smith, J.M., & Wilk, J.R. (1985). A double life for a dental irrigation device. *American Journal of Nursing,* 85(10). 1157.
Green, V.A., Carlson, H.C., Briggs, R.L., Stewart, J.L. (Eng.) (1971). A comparison of the efficacy of pulsed mechanical lavage with that of rubber bulb syringe irrigation in removal of debris from avulsive wounds. *Oral Surgical Oral Medical Pathology.* Jul; 32(1): 158-164.
Hamer, M.L., Robson, M.C., Krizek, T.J., (1975). Quantitative bacterial analysis of comparative wound irrigations. 181(6), 819-822. *Annals of Surgery.*
Lehmann S.L., Konstantindes N.N. (1989). Wound healing and management, *Critical CareNurse Curr* 7(3):9-12.
Longmire, A.W., & Broon, L.A. (1987). Wound infection following high-pressure syringe and needle irrigation. *Americal Journal Emergency Medicine.* March 5(2):179-181.
Maklebust, J., & Sieggreen, M. (1991). *Pressure Ulcers: Guidelines for prevention and nursing management.* S-N Publications, West Dundee, IL, pp. 118-119.
Parkinson, R.W., & Hirst, P. (Eng.) (1990). A simple needle guard for low-volume high-pressure irrigation. *Injury.* 21(2): 128.
Rodeheaver, G.T., Pettry, D., Thacker, J.G., Edgerton, M.T., & Edlich, R.F. (1975). Wound cleansing by high pressure irrigation. *Surgical Gynecological Obstetrics.* Sep; 141(3):357-362. 76013726.

Table 9.5 Wound Irrigation (continued)

TITLE: WOUND IRRIGATION   PROCEDURE NO.___120

Rogness, H. (1985). High-pressure wound irrigation. *Journal of Enterostomal Therapy.* (12), 27-28.

Stots, N.A. (1983). The most effective method of wound irrigation. *Focus Critical Care.* 10(5): 45-48.

Weller, K. (1991). In search of efficacy and efficiency. An alternative to conventional wound cleansing modalities. *Ostomy/Wound Management,* Nov-Dec; 37:23-28.

RESOURCES:

Flanagan, E., RN, BSN, CIC, Coordinator, Hospital Epidemiology, August, 1991.
Mott, M., RN, BSN, Wayne State University Graduate Student, 1993.

AUTHORS:

Maklebust, J., RN, MSN, CS, Case Manager, Surgical Patient Services, July, 1993.
Seiggreen, M., RN, MSN, CS, Case Manager, Surgical Patient Services, July, 1993.

APPROVAL:

Shirley L Green 5/2/95

Shirley L. Green   Date
Vice President Patient Services

Table 9.6 Dressings: Continuously Moist Saline

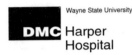

Wayne State University

Harper
Hospital

PROCEDURE NO.___121___

NURSING PATIENT SERVICES

TITLE: DRESSINGS: CONTINUOUSLY MOIST SALINE

GENERAL INFORMATION: Continuously moist saline gauze dressing: technique in which gauze moistened with normal saline is applied to the wound and remoistened with normal saline frequently enough so it will remain moist. The goal is to maintain a continuously moist environment.

POLICY:
1. Physician order is not required.
2. When an order is written for pressure ulcer care or wound care, the nurse will decide when to use a moist dressing. Consult a Case Manager, Wound Care Specialist, or Enterostomal Therapy Nurse for complex cases.

EQUIPMENT:
Sterile normal saline
Clean gloves
Impervious bag
Tape
4x4 gauze sponge and/or abdominal pads
Skin sealant (optional)

PROCEDURE	RATIONALE/EMPHASIS
A. PREPARATION	
1. Wash hands.	
2. Apply clean gloves.	To prevent introduction of additional bacteria into wound and to comply with universal precautions.
3. Remove moist dressing and dispose of in impervious bag. If dressing is dry, soak with normal saline before removal.	Removal of dried dressing may damage granulating tissue. Granulating tissue is a genatinous film that can easily be wiped or flushed away.

Table 9.6 Dressings: Continuously Moist Saline *(continued)*

TITLE: DRESSINGS: CONTINUOUSLY   PROCEDURE NO. <u>121</u>
         MOIST SALINE

PROCEDURE	RATIONALE/EMPHASIS
4. Remove soiled gloves and wash hands.	
5. Open dressings and normal saline.	
6. Use normal saline to moisten enough gauze to fill the wound.	
7. Apply non-sterile gloves.	
8. Irrigate wound using a 250 ml bottle of NS and Baxter Irrigating Tip.	Irrigation dilutes the bacteria. Irrigation assists in debriding by washing loose necrotic tissue from wound. See wound irrigation Procedure 120.

9. Apply moist gauze dressing:
  a. Squeeze excess saline from gauze sponges.
  b. Place layer of moist gauze against ulcer base. Tuck loosely into under-mined areas or sinus tracts. Be sure there is a moist dressing next to all the tissue in the wound.	

c. Fluff remaining gauze sponges and gently place into remainder of wound to fill dead space. Avoid overpacking the wound.	Overpacking increases pressure on tissue in wound bed causing additional tissue damage.
d. Keep intact skin dry.	Moisture will macerate intact skin.
e. May apply skin sealant to skin surrounding wound. Air dry.	To prevent tissue maceration from damp dressing and skin stripping when tape is removed.
10. Cover with a dry dressing and secure in place. Date, time and initial.	

(continued)

Table 9.6 Dressings: Continuously Moist Saline *(continued)*

TITLE: DRESSINGS: CONTINUOUSLY   PROCEDURE NO. _121_
        MOIST SALINE

PROCEDURE	RATIONALE/EMPHASIS
11. Maintain moist dressing by remoistening with saline.	
12. Change dressing a minimum of every 8 hours. If the dressing is dry when changed, the frequency of change must be increased.	
13. Remove gloves, wash hands and dispose of refuse in soiled utility room.	

DOCUMENTATION:
Non-ICU/CCU:
Nursing Care Plan: As intervention for appropriate nursing diagnosis or clinical problem.
Nursing Procedure/Treatments Sheet: Dressing change
Progress Notes: Chart assessment

ICU/CCU:
24 Hour Flow Sheet

REFERENCES:
Alm, A., Hornmark, A.M., Fall, P.A., Linder, L., Bergstrand, B., Ehrnabo, M., Madsen, S.M., & Setterberg, G. (1989). Care of pressure sores: A controlled study of the use of a hydrocolloid dressing compared with wet saline gauze compresses. *Acta Derm Venereal Suppl* (Stockh) 149, 1-10.
Bergstrom, N, Bennett, MA, Carlson, CE, et al. *Treatment of Pressure Ulcers*. Clinical Practice Guideline, No. 15. Rockville, MD: U.S. Department of Health and Human Services. Public Health Service, Agency for Health Care Policy and Research. AHCPR Publication No. 95-0652. December 1994.
Colwell, J.C., Foreman, M.D., & Trotter, J.P. (1992). *A comparison of the efficacy and cost-effectiveness of two methods of managing pressure ulcers.* Washington, D.C.: AHCPR.
Garner, J.S., Javier Emori, et al. (1988). CDEC Guidelines for prevention of surgical wound infections, 1985, *Infection Control*, 7(3), 193-200.
Maklebust, J., & Sieggreen, M. (1991). *Pressure ulcers: Guidelines for prevention and nursing management*. West Dundee, IL: S-N Publications.
Panel for the Prediction and Prevention of Pressure Ulcers in Adults. (1992). *Pressure ulcers in adults: Prediction and prevention clinical practices guideline. Number 3.* AHCPR Publication No. 92-0047. Rockville, MD: Agency for Health Care Policy and Research, Public Health Service, U.S. Department of Health and Human Services.

Table 9.6 Dressings: Continuously Moist Saline *(continued)*

TITLE: DRESSINGS: CONTINUOUSLY MOIST SALINE	PROCEDURE NO. <u>121</u>

Sieggreen, M. (1987). The healing of physical wounds. *Nursing Clinics of North America*, 22(2).

Xakellis, G.C., & Chrischilles, E.A. (1992). Hydrocolloid versus saline gauze dressings in treating pressure ulcers: A cost effectiveness analysis. *Archives Physical Medicine Rehabilitation*, 73, 463-9.

AUTHORS:
Maklebust, J., RN, MSN, CS, Case Manager, 1994.
Seiggreen, M., RN, MSN, CS, Case Manager, 1994.

APPROVAL:

Shirley L Green   5/2/95

Shirley L. Green   Date
Vice President Patient Services

Table 9.7 Dressings: Wet-to-dry for Debridement

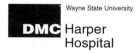 Wayne State University

DMC Harper
Hospital

PROCEDURE NO. __122__

NURSING PATIENT SERVICES

TITLE: DRESSINGS: WET-TO-DRY FOR DEBRIDEMENT

GENERAL INFORMATION: Wet-to-Dry saline gauze: a dressing technique in which gauze moistened with normal saline is applied wet to the wound and removed once the gauze becomes dry and adheres to the wound bed. The goal is to debride the wound as the dressing is removed.

POLICY:
1. A physician order is not required.
2. When an order is written for pressure ulcer care or wound care, the nurse will decide when to use a "Wet-to-Dry" dressing. Consult a Case Manager, Enterostomal Therapy Nurse or Wound Care Specialist for complex cases.

EQUIPMENT:
Sterile normal saline
Clean gloves (2 pairs)
Impervious Bag
Sterile 4x4 gauze sponges
Tape
Irrigation tray
Abdominal pad (optional)
Skin Sealant (optional)

PROCEDURE	RATIONALE/EMPHASIS
1. Wash hands.	
2. Apply non-sterile gloves.	
3. Remove dry dressing from wound pulling away necrotic debris with dressing. Discard in impervious bag.	More frequent dressing changes may be necessary to facilitate a more rapid debridement when there is excess wound drainage.
4. Remove gloves and wash hands.	

Table 9.7 Dressings: Wet-to-dry for Debridement *(continued)*

TITLE: DRESSINGS: WET-TO-DRY   PROCEDURE NO.___122_
          FOR DEBRIDEMENT

PROCEDURE	RATIONALE/EMPHASIS
5. Open normal saline and dressings.	
6. Moisten sterile gauze with normal saline.	
7. Apply non-sterile gloves.	
8. Irrigate wound using a 250 ml bottle of NS and Baxter Irrigation Tip.	Irrigation dilutes the bacteria. Irrigation assists in debriding by washing loose necrotic tissue from wound. See wound irrigation procedure #120 for technique.
9. Apply moist dressing: a. Unfold moist gauze. b. Spread it in a single layer over open wound. c. Tuck moist gauze loosely into undermined areas or sinus tracts.	Gauze should be just moist enough to allow it to dry between dressing changes.
d. Keep intact skin dry.	Moisture will macerate intact skin.
10. Gently place fluffed gauze into remainder of wound.	The additional dressing assists with drying. Absorption of exudate into the gauze will aid in debriding the wound. May cover gauze with abdominal pad.
11. May apply skin sealant to skin surrounding wound. Air dry. Secure dressing. Write date, time and initial.	To prevent tissue maceration from damp dressing.
12. Remove gloves, wash hands and discard impervious bag in soiled utility room.	
13. Change dressing as needed. Dressing should be dry when removed.	

(continued)

Table 9.7 Dressings: Wet-to-dry for Debridement *(continued)*

| TITLE: DRESSINGS: WET-TO-DRY FOR DEBRIDEMENT | PROCEDURE NO. __122__ |

DOCUMENTATION:

Non-ICU//CCU: Nursing Care Plan: As intervention for appropriate nursing diagnosis or problem.
Nursing Procedures/Treatments Sheet: "Dressing changed per care plan".
Progress Notes: Chart progress towards expected outcomes.
ICU/CCU: Critical Care 24 Hour Flow Sheet: Chart treatment and assessment of wound.

REFERENCES:

Alvarez, O.M., Mertz, P.M., & Eaglestein, W.H. (1983). The effect of occlusive dressings on collagen synthesis and re-epithelialization in superficial wounds. *Journal Surgical Research*, 35(2), 142-148.

Bergstrom, N, Bennett, MA, Carlson, CE, et al. *Treatment of Pressure Ulcers.* Clinical Practice Guideline, No. 15. Rockville, MD: U.S. Department of Health and Human Services. Public Health Service, Agency for Health Care Policy and Research. AHCPR Publication No. 95-0652. December 1994.

Fowler, E., & Goupil, D.L. (184). Comparison of the wet-to-dry dressing and a copolymer starch in the management of debrided pressure sores. *Journal of Enterostomal Therapy*, 11(1), 22-25.

Maklebust, J., & Sieggreen, M. (1991). *Pressure ulcers: Guidelines for prevention and nursing management.* West Dundee, IL: S-N Publications.

Panel for the Prediction and Prevention of Pressure Ulcers in Adults. (1992). *Pressure ulcers in adults: Prediction and prevention. Clinical practice guidelines, Number 3.* AHCPR Publication No. 92-0047. Rockville, MD: Agency for Health Care Policy and Research, Public Health Service, U.S. Department of Health and Human Services.

Sieggreen, M. (1987). The healing of physical wounds. *Nursing Clinics of North America.* 22(2).

Xakellis, G.C., & Chrischilles, E.A. (1992). Hydrocolloid versus saline gauze dressings in treating pressure ulcers: A cost-effectiveness analysis. *Archives Physical Medicine Rehabilitation*, 73, 463-469.

RESOURCE:

Flanagan, E., BSN, RN, CIC. Coordinator, Hospital Epidemiology, August, 1994.

AUTHORS:

Maklebust, J., RN, MSN, CS, Case Manager, Surgical Patient Services, July, 1994.
Sieggreen, M., RN, MSN, CS, Case Manager, Critical Care/Cardiology Services, July, 1994.

APPROVAL:

Shirley L Green 5/2/95
Shirley L. Green   Date
Vice President Patient Services

Table 9.8 Dressings: Foam Dressing to Maintain a Moist Wound Environment

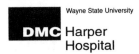 Wayne State University

**Harper
Hospital**

PROCEDURE NO.___111___

NURSING PATIENT SERVICES

TITLE: DRESSINGS: FOAM DRESSING TO MAINTAIN A MOIST
        WOUND ENVIRONMENT

POLICY: Physician order for skin/wound care required.

EQUIPMENT:
  Clean gloves - 2 pair
  250 cc bottle sterile normal saline
  Baxter irrigation cap
  Foam dressing
  Paper tape
  Impervious disposal bag

PROCEDURE	RATIONALE/EMPHASIS
A. PREPARATION	
1. Wash hands and put on clean gloves.	
2. Remove old dressing and discard in impervious bag.	
3. Remove soiled gloves and discard.	
4. Wash hands, apply second pair of clean gloves and use 250 cc normal saline with Baxter irrigation tip to forcefully irrigate wound.	Thorough cleansing and/or irrigation is needed to flush out cellular debris or loose necrotic tissue and reduce the bacterial count. Normal saline does not damage granulation tissue.
5. Dry skin surrounding the wound with a 4x4 sponge.	To keep periulcer skin clean and dry.
6. Assess wound bed and surrounding tissue for necrosis, erythema, odor, drainage, and size.	Foam dressings can absorb exudate and facilitate removal of superficial necrotic tissue by autolysis in pressure ulcers or partial- and full-thickness wounds.

(continued)

Table 9.8 Dressings: Foam Dressing to Maintain a Moist Wound Environment *(continued)*

TITLE: DRESSINGS: FOAM DRESSING TO MAINTAIN A MOIST WOUND ENVIRONMENT

PROCEDURE NO. __111__

PROCEDURE	RATIONALE/EMPHASIS
7. Select dressing size large enough to extend 1 inch beyond the wound margins on all sides.	Absorbs wound exudate and maintains moist wound bed.

B. APPLICATION
Foam dressing:

PROCEDURE	RATIONALE/EMPHASIS
a. Assess wound depth to determine necessity of filling wound bed prior to application of foam covering.	To avoid dead space in the wound.
b. If wound is superficial, cover wound with foam dressing positioning the dressing directly over the wound with the dressing extending one inch beyond wound bed on all sides.	To maintain moist wound environment.
c. If wound is not flush with skin, select moist dressing material to fill wound crater prior to covering with foam.	To avoid dead space in wound.
d. Do not cover the foam dressing with occlusive films or tapes.	Covering the foam can interfere with water vapor transmission and reduce dressing effectiveness.
e. Adhere dressing with tape, roll gauze or netting depending on periulcer skin condition.	

Table 9.8 Dressings: Foam Dressing to Maintain a Moist Wound Environment *(continued)*

TITLE: DRESSINGS: FOAM DRESSING TO MAINTAIN A MOIST WOUND ENVIRONMENT

PROCEDURE NO. __111__

PROCEDURE

f. Change dressing frequently enough to absorb exudate and keep wound bed moist.
g. Discontinue foam dressing if wound bed is sufficiently moist, wound exudate exceeds absorption capability, or frequency of dressing change needs to be decreased.
h. Remove gloves, wash hands and discard impervious bag containing old dressings in soiled utility room.

RATIONALE/EMPHASIS

Large necrotic or heavily draining wounds may require more frequent dressing changes due to exudate leakage. Wounds with a necrotic base may increase in size and depth during the initial phase of management as the necrotic debris is cleaned away.

DOCUMENTATION:

Nursing Care Plan: As intervention for nursing diagnosis or collaborative problem.
Shift Assessment Sheet; Treatment Section: Chart date, treatment, time and signature in shift column.
Progress Notes: Date, problem, assessment of wound and/or dressing.

REFERENCES:

Bergstrom, N, Bennett, MA, Carlson, CE, et al. *Treatment of Pressure Ulcers*. Clinical Practice Guideline, No. 15. Rockville, MD: U.S. Department of Health and Human Services, Agency for Health Care Policy and Research. AHCPR Publication No. 95-0652. December 1994.
Lyofoam dressing package insert, Acme United Corporation, 1995.
Wiseman, DM, Rovee, ST & Alvarz, OM (1992). Wound dressings: design and use. In Cohen, IK, Diegelmann, RF & Lindbald, WJ (eds). *Wound Healing: Biochemical and Clinical Aspects*. Philadelphia: WB Saunders.

AUTHORS:

Maklebust, J, MSN, RN, CS, Clinical Nurse Specialist/Case Manager, 1995.
Sieggggreen, M, MSN, RN, CS, Clinical Nurse Specialist/Case Manager, 1995.

APPROVAL:

Shirley L Green   5/2/95

Shirley L. Green   Date
Vice President Patient Services

Table 9.9 Dressings: Hydrogel Impregnated Gauze Dressing to Maintain a Moist Wound Environment

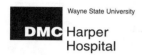

Wayne State University

Harper
Hospital

PROCEDURE NO. 118

NURSING PATIENT SERVICES

TITLE: DRESSINGS: HYDROGEL IMPREGNATED
GAUZE DRESSING TO MAINTAIN A MOIST
WOUND ENVIRONMENT

POLICY: Physician order for skin/wound care required.

EQUIPMENT:
Clean gloves - 2 pair
250 cc bottle sterile normal saline
Baxter irrigation cap
Hydrogel impregnated gauze dressing materials
Gauze sponges or rolls
Paper tape
Impervious disposal bag

PROCEDURE	RATIONALE/EMPHASIS
A. PREPARATION	
1. Wash hands and put on clean gloves.	
2. Remove old dressing and discard in impervious bag.	
3. Remove soiled gloves and discard.	
4. Wash hands, apply second pair of clean gloves and use 250 cc normal saline with Baxter irrigation tip to forcefully irrigate wound.	Thorough cleansing and/or irrigation is needed to flush out cellular debris or loose necrotic tissue and reduce the bacterial count. Normal saline does not damage granulation tissue.
5. Dry the area surrounding wound with a 4x4 sponge.	To keep periulcer skin clean and dry.

Table 9.9 Dressings: Hydrogel Impregnated Gauze Dressing to Maintain a Moist Wound Environment *(continued)*

TITLE: DRESSINGS: HYDROGEL IMPREG-   PROCEDURE NO. 118
NATED GAUZE DRESSING TO MAIN-
TAIN A MOIST WOUND ENVIRONMENT

PROCEDURE

6. Assess wound bed and surrounding tissue for necrosis, erythema, odor, drainage, and size.

7. Select dressing size that will cover the wound bed.

B. APPLICATION
Hydrogel impregnated dressing:
a. Assess wound depth to determine amount of hydrogel gauze dressing necessary to cover wound.
b. Place hydrogel dressing into wound covering all exposed wound surface.
c. Cover with secondary dressing.
d. Adhere dressing with tape or roll gauze depending on periulcer skin condition.
e. Change dressing every day and prn to keep wound bed moist.

RATIONALE/EMPHASIS

Hydrogel dressings can facilitate removal of superficial necrotic tissue by autolysis in pressure ulcers or partial-and full-thickness wounds.

Maintains moist wound bed.

Large necrotic or heavily draining wounds may require more frequent dressing changes due to exudate leakage. Wounds with a necrotic base may increase in size and depth during the initial phase of management as the necrotic debris is cleaned away.

(continued)

Table 9.9 Dressings: Hydrogel Impregnated Gauze Dressing to Maintain a Moist Wound Environment (continued)

TITLE: DRESSINGS: HYDROGEL IMPREG-   PROCEDURE NO. 118
NATED GAUZE DRESSING TO MAIN-
TAIN A MOIST WOUND ENVIRONMENT

PROCEDURE	RATIONALE/EMPHASIS
f. Discontinue hydrogel dressing if wound bed is sufficiently moist or frequency of dressing change needs to be decreased.	
g. Wash hands and discard impervious bag containing old dressings in soiled utility room.	

DOCUMENTATION:
Nursing Care Plan: As intervention for nursing diagnosis or collaborative problem.
Shift Assessment Sheet; Treatment Section: Chart date, treatment, time and signature in shift column.
Progress Notes: Date, problem, assessment of wound and/or dressing.

REFERENCES:
Bergstrom, N, Bennett, MA, Carlson, CE, et al. *Treatment of Pressure Ulcers*. Clinical Practice Guideline, No. 15. Rockville, MD: U.S. Department of Health and Human Services, Agency for Health Care Policy and Research. AHCPR Publication No. 95-0652. December 1994.
Carrington Laboratories product insert, 1995.
Panel for the Prediction and Prevention of Pressure Ulcers in Adults. (1992). *Pressure ulcers in adults: Prediction and prevention. Clinical practice guidelines, Number 3*. AHCPR Publication No. 92-0047. Rockville, MD: Agency for Health Care Policy and Research, Public Health Service, U.S. Department of Health and Human Services.
Wiseman, DM, Rovee, DT & Alvarez, OM (1992). Wound dressings: design and use. In Cohen, IK, Dieglemann, RF, & Lindbald, WJ (eds). *Wound Healing: Biochemical and Clinical Aspects*. Philadelphia: WB Saunders.

AUTHORS:
Maklebust, J, MSN, RN, CS Clinical Nurse Specialist/Case Manager, 1995.
Sieggreen, M, MSN, RN, CS Clinical Nurse Specialist/Case Manager, 1995.

APPROVAL:

Shirley L Green   5/2/95

Shirley L. Green   Date
Vice President Patient Services

Table 9.10 Dressings: Hydrocolloid

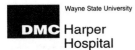 Wayne State University
Harper
Hospital

PROCEDURE NO. __123__

NURSING PATIENT SERVICES

TITLE: DRESSINGS: HYDROCOLLOID

POLICY: Physician order for skin/wound care is required.

EQUIPMENT:
 Clean gloves - 2 pair
 250 cc bottle sterile normal saline
 Baxter irrigation tip
 Hydrocolloid dressing, 4x4 or 8x8
 Skin sealant (optional)
 Paper tape
 Impervious disposal bag

PROCEDURE	RATIONALE/EMPHASIS
A. PREPARATION	
1. Wash hands and put on clean gloves.	
2. Remove old dressing by pressing down on the skin with one hand and lifting dressing edge toward the wound with the other hand.	Liquefied wound drainage may appear purulent and odiferous. Both are normal reactions to the hydrocolloid dressing.
3. Discard dressing and soiled gloves in impervious bag.	
4. Set up normal saline irrigation bottle and tip.	
5. Wash hands, apply second pair of clean gloves, and use 250 cc normal saline with Baxter irrigation tip to forcefully irrigate wound.	Thorough cleansing and/or irrigation is needed to flush out cellular debris or loose necrotic tissue and reduce the bacterial count. Normal saline does not damage granulation tissue.

(continued)

Table 9.10 Dressings: Hydrocolloid *(continued)*

TITLE: DRESSINGS: HYDROCOLLOID   PROCEDURE NO. 123

PROCEDURE	RATIONALE/EMPHASIS
6. Dry the skin surrounding wound with a 4x4 sponge.	Promotes adhesion and wear time of dressing.
7. Assess wound bed and surrounding tissue for necrosis, erythema, odor, drainage, and size.	Hydrocolloid dressings can absorb exudate and facilitate removal of superficial necrotic tissue by autolysis in pressure ulcers or partial-and full-thickness wounds.
8. Select dressing size large enough to extend 1 1/2 inch beyond the wound margins on all sides.	Facilitates adhesion of the wafer and dressing wear time.

B. APPLICATION

1. Remove backing from hydrocolloid wafer. Do not stretch wafer.
2. Apply wafer directly over wound surface in a rolling motion. The dressing may be cut if necessary to conform to different areas of the body.
3. Smooth the wafer firmly into place especially at the wound margins.
4. Picture frame or tape edge of dressings especially in sacral or perianal regions.

   Dressings on irregular surfaces are difficult to keep intact.

5. Leave dressing in place for 3-5 days. Change dressing frequently enough to avoid leakage.

   Wounds with a necrotic base may increase in size and depth during the initial phase of management as the necrotic debris is cleaned away.

6. Discontinue hydrocolloid dressings if wound exudate exceeds absorption capability or frequency of dressing change needs to be increased.

Table 9.10 Dressings: Hydrocolloid *(continued)*

TITLE: DRESSINGS: HYDROCOLLOID   PROCEDURE NO.___123_

PROCEDURE	RATIONALE/EMPHASIS
7. Remove gloves, wash hands and discard impervious bag containing old dressings in soiled utility room.	

DOCUMENTATION:
Nursing Care Plan: As intervention for nursing diagnosis or collaborative problem.
Shift Assessment Sheet; Treatment Section: Chart date, treatment, time and signature in shift column.
Progress Notes: Date, problem, assessment of wound and/or dressing.

REFERENCES:
Alm, A., Hornmark, A.M., Fall, P.A., Linder, L., Bergstrand, B., Ehrnabo, M., Madsen, S.M., & Setterberg, G. (1989). Care of pressure sores: A controlled study of the use of a hydrocolloid dressing compared with wet saline gauze compresses. *Acta Derm Venereal Suppl* (Stockh) 149, 1-10.
Bergstrom, N, Bennett, MA, Carlson, CE, et al. *Treatment of Pressure Ulcers*. Clinical Practice Guideline, No. 15. Rockville, MD: U.S. Department of Health and Human Services. Public Health Service, Agency for Health Care Policy and Research. AHCPR Publication No. 95-0652. December 1994.
Colwell, J.C., Foreman, M.D., & Trotter, J.P. (1992). *A comparison of the efficacy and cost effectiveness of two methods of managing pressure ulcers*. Washington, D.C.: AHCPR.
Maklebust, J., & Sieggreen, M. (1991). *Pressure ulcers: Guidelines for prevention and nursing management*. West Dundee, IL: S-N Publications.
Neill, K.M., Conforti, C., Kedas, A. & Burris, J.F. (1989). Pressure sore response to a new hydrocolloid dressing. *Wounds*. 1(3), 173-185.
Oleske, D.M., Smith X.P., White, P., Pottage, J., & Donavan, M.L. (1986). A randomized clinical trial of two dressing methods for the treatment of low-grade pressure ulcers. *Journal Enterostomal Therapy*, 13(3), 90-98.
Panel for the Prediction and Prevention of Pressure Ulcers in Adults. (1992). *Pressure ulcers in adults: Prediction and prevention. Clinical practice guidelines, Number 3*. AHCPR Publication No. 92-0047. Rockville, MD: Agency for Health Care Policy and Research, Public Health Service, U.S. Department of Health and Human Services.
Shannon, M.L., & Miller, B. (1988). Evaluation of hydrocolloid dressings on healing of pressure ulcers in spinal cord injury patients. *Decubitus*, 1(1), 42-46.

Table 9.10 Dressings: Hydrocolloid *(continued)*

TITLE: DRESSINGS: HYDROCOLLOID   PROCEDURE NO.___123_

Tudhope, M. (1984). Management of pressure ulcers with hydrocolloid occlusive dressing: Results in twenty-three patients. *Journal Enterostomal Therapy*.

Wiseman, DM, Rovee, DT & Alvarez, OM (1992). Wound dressings: design and use. In Cohen, IK, Dieglemann, RF, & Lindbald, WJ (eds). *Wound Healing: Biochemical and Clinical Aspects*. Philadelphia: WB Saunders.

Xakellis, G.C., & Chrischilles, E.A. (1992). Hydrocolloid versus saline gauze dressings in treating pressure ulcers: A cost effectiveness analysis. *Archives Physical Medicine Rehabilitation*, 73, 463-9.

AUTHORS:
Maklebust, J., RN, MSN, CS, Clinical Nurse Specialist/Case Manager, 1995.
Sieggreen, M., RN, MSN, CS, Clinical Nurse Specialist/Case Manager, 1995.

APPROVAL:

_____*Shirley L Green*_____ 5/2/95____

Shirley L. Green   Date
Vice President Patient Services

Table 9.11 Dressings: Polyurethane Film

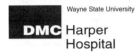 Wayne State University

DMC Harper
Hospital

PROCEDURE NO. ___124___

NURSING PATIENT SERVICES

TITLE: DRESSINGS: POLYURETHANE FILM

POLICY:
1. A physician's order is not required.
2. Polyurethane film is contraindicated for infected wounds and/or wounds that extend to fascia, muscle, or bone.

EQUIPMENT:
Polyurethane Film Dressing
    Small - 10 CM x 12 CM
    Large - 15 CM x 20 CM
Skin sealant
Clean gloves
250 ml sterile Normal Saline
Baxter irrigation tip
4x4 gauze sponge
Tape
Impervious bag
Syringe and 25g needle

PROCEDURE	RATIONALE/EMPHASIS
A. PREPARATION	
1. Wash hands.	
2. Apply non-sterile gloves and remove old dressing.	
3. Discard dressing and gloves in impervious bag.	
4. If skin is broken, apply sterile gloves and cleanse wound and surrounding skin gently with normal saline.	Normal saline will not damage tissue.
5. Dry intact surrounding skin with gauze. Clip hair if necessary.	Transparent film dressings will not stick to hair or a wet surface.

(continued)

Table 9.11 Dressings: Polyurethane Film *(continued)*

TITLE: POLYURETHANE FILM   PROCEDURE NO.___124_

PROCEDURE	RATIONALE/EMPHASIS
B. APPLICATION	
1. Select a dressing size that will cover at least two inches beyond the wound margin.	Dressing border on skin facilitates adhesion and wearing time of the dressing. Large wounds may be covered with overlapping pieces of film dressing.
2. Apply a skin sealant to the surrounding skin as needed. Air dry.	Protects skin from maceration from wound drainage and prolongs seal or dressing.
3. Remove and discard center cutout window.	
4. Peel printed paper backing from the paper frame of dressing exposing adhesive surface.	
5. View the wound site through the window and center dressing over the site.	
6. Press in place, firmly smoothing from center to edges of dressing.	Pulling or stretching the film dressing across wound area causes excessive tension on skin, tissue shearing, and patient discomfort.
7. Slowly remove the paper frame from the dressing and firmly smooth the dressing edges. Smooth entire dressing using firm pressure.	
8. Wipe edges of film dressing with skin sealant.	
9. Put a piece of tape on the dressing, if needed, and record date and initials on tape.	

Table 9.11 Dressings: Polyurethane Film *(continued)*

TITLE: POLYURETHANE FILM   PROCEDURE NO.___124_

PROCEDURE	RATIONALE/EMPHASIS
10. Inspect wound and integrity of film dressing every day and prn.	
11. If excessive exudate forms under the dressing compromising the seal, use sterile technique to aspirate exudate with a 25 gauge needle. Patch the puncture site with a small piece of film dressing.	It is normal for the wound to form a layer of fluid under the dressing.
12. Dispose of needle in sharps container.	
13. Change dressing if:	Film dressings may be left on for 2-3 days.
a. Leakage occurs.	
b. Edges roll up or dressing naturally sloughs off.	
c. Excessive granulation tissue forms in the wound bed.	Excess tissue may extend above and beyond wound margins.
14. Remove film dressings by stretching and releasing edges slowly in direction of hair growth. For fragile skin, use warm water soaks to release dressing from skin.	
15. Discontinue use of dressings if clinical signs of wound infection are present.	Drainage under film dressing will appear purulent and have a foul odor. This is a result of bacteria and white blood cell interaction. Wound culture and/or tissue biopsy may be indicated if there are clinical signs of infection (erythema, increased size of wound, pain, swelling, fever, and excessive purulent drainage).

(continued)

Table 9.11 Dressings: Polyurethane Film *(continued)*

TITLE: POLYURETHANE FILM   PROCEDURE NO.   124

DOCUMENTATION:
NON ICU/CCU:
Nursing Care Plan: As intervention for appropriate nursing diagnosis or clinical problem.
Nursing Procedures/Treatments Sheet: name of dressing.
Progress Notes: assessment of wound and/or dressing; progress towards expected outcome of nursing diagnosis/collaborative problem.

ICU/CCU:
24 Hour Flow Sheet: assessment of wound and/or dressing.
Nursing Care Plan: As intervention for appropriate nursing diagnosis or clinical problem.
Progress Notes: assessment of wound and/or dressing; progress towards expected outcome of nursing diagnosis/collaborative problem.

REFERENCES:
Ahmed, M. (1982). Op-Site for decubitus care. *American Journal of Nursing*, 82(1), 61-64.
Alvarez, O., Rozent, J., & Wiseman, D. (1989). Moist environment for healing: Matching the dressing to the wound. *Wounds*, 1(1), 35-51.
Bergstrom, N, Bennett, MA, Carlson, CE, et al. *Treatment of Pressure Ulcers*. Clinical Practice Guideline, No. 15. Rockville, MD: U.S. Department of Health and Human Services, Agency for Health Care Policy and Research. AHCPR Publication No. 95-0652. December 1994.
Brady, S.M. (1987). Management of pressure sores with OCC/SIU dressings in a select population. *Nursing Management*, 18, 41.
Ligner, C., & Rolstad, S., et al. (1984). Clinical trial of a moistrue vapor-permeable dressing on superficial pressure ulcers. *Journal of Enterostomal Therapy*, 11(4), 147-149.
Maklebust, J., & Sieggreen, M., (1991). *Pressure ulcers: Guidelines for prevention and nursing management*. West Dundee, IL: S-N Publications.
Sebern, M.D. (1986). Pressure ulcer management in home health care: Efficiency and cost effectiveness of moisture vapor permeable dressings. *Archives of Medicine Rehabilitation*, 67(10), 729.

RESOURCE:
Flanagan, E., BSN,CIC, Coordinator, Hospital Epidemiology, 1994.

AUTHORS:
Maklebust, J., RN, MSN, CS, Case Manager, Surgical Services, 1994.
Sieggreen, M., RN, MSN, CS, Case Manager, Critical Care/Cardiology, 1994.

APPROVAL:

Shirley L Green   _5/2/95_

Shirley L. Green   Date
Vice President Patient Services

Table 9.12 Dressings: Alginate

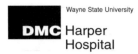 Wayne State University
DMC Harper
Hospital

PROCEDURE NO.___138___

NURSING PATIENT SERVICES

TITLE: DRESSINGS: ALGINATE

POLICY: A physician order is required for skin/wound care.

EQUIPMENT:
Clean gloves
Sterile normal saline
4x4 gauze sponge and/or abdominal pads
Impervious bag
Paper tape
Barrier agent
Gauze wrap (optional)
Normal saline 250 ml bottle
Irrigation cap #105001

PROCEDURE	RATIONALE/EMPHASIS
A. PREPARATION	
1. Wash hands. Apply clean gloves and remove old dressing.	Alginate is used for moderately to heavily draining wounds. It turns into a gel as it absorbs drainage.
2. Discard soiled dressing and gloves in impervious bag.	
3. Throughout the procedure, assess wound and surrounding tissue for erythema, degree of necrotic tissue, odor, amount of drainage, and size.	Alginate dressings are not effective for ulcers with dry eschar or clean granulation wound beds. Alginate dressings are not debriding agents; as much necrotic tissue as possible should be debrided prior to applica-
4. Wash hands. Apply clean gloves. Use "no touch" technique to irrigate wound with normal saline. See irrigation procedure #120 for technique.	tion.

(continued)

Table 9.12 Dressings: Alginate *(continued)*

TITLE: DRESSINGS: ALGINATE   PROCEDURE NO.___138___

PROCEDURE	**RATIONALE/EMPHASIS**
5. Leave wound bed moist. Dry intact skin with 4x4.	
6. Apply a barrier agent to intact skin around the wound and allow to dry.	To keep absorbent dressing off healthy skin.
B. APPLICATION	Hydrophilic absorptive dressings must have room for expansion in the wound bed, as they absorb drainage and odor.
1. Apply alginate to the moist wound surface.	Absorption dressings should be applied to a moist wound surface. Do not overfill or pack the wound bed.
2. Pat down to conform to the wound surface.	Do not use alginate in deep fistulae, sinus tracts or body cavities, where complete removal is not assured.
3. Cover alginate: a. For a moderately draining wound, use a secondary absorbent dressing or semi-occlusive film dressing. b. For a heavliy draining wound, use a thick absorbent dressing such as layers of gauze or an ABD pad.	
4. Secure alginate and cover dressing over bony promi-nence with stretch gauze wrap. Where stretch gauze would not be indicated, such as over a hip wound, secure in place with tape along the edges.	

Table 9.12 Dressings: Alginate *(continued)*

TITLE: DRESSINGS: ALGINATE   PROCEDURE NO. __138__

PROCEDURE	RATIONALE/EMPHASIS
C. DRESSING CHANGE	
1. Wash hands, apply clean gloves.	
2. Gently remove outer dressings down to the gel.	The frequency of dressing changes will depend upon the volume of exudate. The dressing should be changed when the secondary dressing becomes moist. A heavily draining wound may require one or two changes daily for the first 3 to 5 days.
3. Remove non-gelled alginate and discard.	As the wound begins to heal and drainage decreases, dressing changes may be made less frequently; every 2 to 4 days, or as directed by nurse specialist.
4. Irrigate the wound with normal saline to rinse away the remaining gel. Should the gel be too thick to rinse, the bulk of the gel should be wiped from the wound. Any remaining gell should then be rinsed away.	Retained foreign bodies have been associated with impaired wound healing.
5. Remove gloves, wash hands, and apply clean gloves.	
6. Redress the wound.	
7. Discontinue treatment when the wound has a healthy granulation base and is no longer draining.	

(continued)

Table 9.12 Dressings: Alginate *(continued)*

TITLE: DRESSINGS: ALGINATE   PROCEDURE NO.___138__

PROCEDURE	RATIONALE/EMPHASIS
8. Collaborate with physician or wound specialist to select another primary dressing that will continue to maintain a moist wound environment.	

DOCUMENTATION:
Non ICU/CCU:
Nursing Care Plan: As intervention for appropriate nursing diagnosis or collaborative problem.
Treatment/Procedure Sheet: date, type of "dressing changed per nursing care plan", time, and initials.
Progress Notes: Date, time, nursing diagnosis or collaborative problem and progress toward identified outcomes.

ICU/CCU:
24 Hour Flow Sheet
Progress Notes
Nursing Care Plan

REFERENCES:
Attwood, A.I. (1989). Calcium alginate dressing accelerates spit skin graft donor site healing. *British Journal of Plastic Surgery*, 42(4), 373-379.
Maklebust, J., Sieggreen, M. (1991). *Pressure ulcers: Guidelines for prevention and nursing management*. West Dundee, IL: S-N Publications.
Motta, G.J. (1991). Calcium alginate topical wound dressings, a new dimension in the cost-effective treatment for exudating dermal wounds and pressure sores. *Ostomy/Wound Management*, 25, 52-56.
Thomas, S. (1989). Sorbsan in the management of leg ulcers. *Pharmacology Journal*, 243, 706-709.
Tintle, T.E., & Jeter, K. (1991). Early experience with a calcium alginate. *Ostomy/Wound Management*, 28, 74-81.

AUTHORS:
Maklebust, J, MSN, RN, CS Clinical Nurse Specialist/Case Manager, March, 1995.
Sieggreen, M, MSN, RN, CS Clinical Nurse Specialist/Case Manager, March, 1995.

APPROVAL:

_____Shirley L Green____ 5/2/95__
Shirley L. Green   Date
Vice President Patient Services

Table 9.13: Enzymatic Agent to Debride Necrotic Tissue

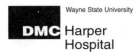 Wayne State University

DMC Harper
Hospital

PROCEDURE NO. ___126___

NURSING PATIENT SERVICES

TITLE: ENZYMATIC AGENT TO DEBRIDE
   NECROTIC TISSUE

POLICY: A physician's order is required for collagenase and polysporin powder.

EQUIPMENT:
 Clean gloves
 Sterile tongue blade
 4x4 gauze sponge and/or abdominal pads
 250 ml bottle sterile Normal Saline
 Collagenase (Santyl)
 Baxter irrigation tip
 Tape
 Impervious bag
 Skin sealant (optional)
 Polysporin powder

PROCEDURE	RATIONALE/EMPHASIS
A. PREPARATION	
1. Wash hands.	
2. Apply clean gloves.	To protect against nosocomial infec-
3. Remove old dressing.	tions.
4. Discard gloves and dressing in impervious bag.	
5. Wash hands.	
6. Open tongue blade or sponge and squeeze enzymatic debriding ointment on tongue blade or sponge.	Amount of ointment used depends upon size of necrotic area.
7. Open normal saline, apply Baxter Irrigation Tip. Set bubble cap aside.	

(continued)

Table 9.13: Enzymatic Agent to Debride Necrotic Tissue *(continued)*

TITLE: ENZYMATIC AGENT TO DEBRIDE
NECROTIC TISSUE

PROCEDURE NO.___126_

PROCEDURE	RATIONALE/EMPHASIS
8. Apply clean gloves.	
9. Irrigate wound by squeezing bottle of saline with full force.	See Procedure #120, Wound Irrigation. Forceful irrigation mechanically debrides loose necrotic tissue. The wound must be cleansed of antiseptics or heavy metal antibacterials which may denature the enzyme.
10. Dry intact surrounding skin.	To prevent maceration of skin.
11. Measure wound. Assess wound and surrounding tissue for erythema, degree of necrotic tissue, odor and drainage.	Surgical debridement and/or crosshatching of dry hard, necrotic tissue may be necessary. Debriding agents cannot penetrate dry, hard necrotic tissue (eschar). Crosshatching refers to using a scalpel to cut through the depth of the eschar allowing the enzymatic agent to penetrate.
12. Apply skin sealant to skin surrounding wound. Air dry.	To prevent tissue maceration and skin stripping when tape is removed.
B. APPLICATION	
1. Apply polysporin powder to surface of wound. This may be applied by sprinkling into the wound directly or onto a 4x4 and touching to the wound surface.	A topical antibiotic is applied to the wound prior to application of enzymatic agent to decrease the risk of bacteria entering healthy tissue as the enzymes debride.
2. Apply Santyl to necrotic tissue staying within the lesion area.	To prevent a transient erythema in surrounding intact skin areas.
3. Cover wound with dry 4x4 and/or ABD dressing.	

Table 9.13: Enzymatic Agent to Debride Necrotic Tissue *(continued)*

TITLE: ENZYMATIC AGENT TO DEBRIDE NECROTIC TISSUE	PROCEDURE NO.___126_

PROCEDURE	RATIONALE/EMPHASIS
4. Change dressing at least once a day. 5. Remove gloves and discard in impervious bag. 6. Secure dressing. Date and initial.	More frequent dressing changes may be necessary due to excessive drainage.

DOCUMENTATION:
NON ICU/CCU:
Nursing Care Plan: Intervention for appropriate nursing diagnosis or problem.
Progress Notes: Assessment of wound.
Nursing Procedure/Treatments Sheet: Type of dressing or "dressing changed per nursing care plan", time, and initial.
Scheduled and non-scheduled Medication Administration Record.

ICU/CCU:
Critical Care 24 Hour Flow Sheet: Dressing change.
Progress Notes: Progress toward expected outcome.

REFERENCES:
Alterescu, V. (1984). Debriding enzymes, *Journal of Enterostomal Therapy*, 11(3), 122-124.
Bergstrom, N, Bennett, MA, Carlson, CE, et al. *Treatment of Pressure Ulcers*. Clinical Practice Guideline, No. 15. Rockville, MD: U.S. Department of Health and Human Services, Agency for Health Care Policy and Research. AHCPR Publication No. 95-0652. December 1994.
Boxer, A.M., Gottesman, N., Bernstein, H., & Mandl, I. (1969). Debridement of dermal ulcers and decubiti with collagenase. *Geriatrics*, 24(7), 75-86.
Cuzzeli, J.Z.(1985). Wound care forum: Artful solutions to chronic problems. *American Journal of Nursing*, 85(2), 162-166.
Lee, L.K., & Ambrus, J.L.(1975). Collagenase therapy for decubitus ulcers. *Geriatrics*, 30(5), 91-3, 97-8.
Maklebust, J., & Sieggreen, M. (1991). *Pressure Ulcers: Guidelines for prevention and nursing management*, 134-36, West Dundee, IL: S-N Publications.
Rao, D.B., Sane, P.G., & Georgiev, E.L. (1975). Collagenase in the treatment of dermal and decubitus ulcers. *Journal of American Geriatrics Society*, 23(1), 22-30.
Varma, A.O., Bugatch, E., & German, F.M. (1973). Debridement of dermal ulcers with collagenase. *Surgery Gynecology Obstetrics*, 136(2), 281-282.

Table 9.13: Enzymatic Agent to Debride Necrotic Tissue *(continued)*

TITLE: ENZYMATIC AGENT TO DEBRIDE   PROCEDURE NO.   126
        NECROTIC TISSUE

RESOURCES:
Flanagan, E., BSN, CIC, Coordinator, Hospital Epidemiology, 1995.
Pressure Ulcer Committee, Harper Hospital, 1995.

AUTHORS:
Maklebust, J., RN, MSN, CS, Case Manager, Surgical Services, March, 1995.
Sieggreen, M., RN, MSN, CS, Case Manager, Critical Care/Cardiology, March, 1995.

APPROVAL:

Shirley L Green   5/2/95

Shirley L. Green   Date
Vice President Patient Services

Continuum of Care

An increasingly important part of health care delivery is planning for care across service settings. Careful planning is necessary to ensure continuity and to match resources to the level of services needed. The plan may require that patients receive
care from different people in various settings along a continuum as medical or social conditions change. A continuum of care has been described as an "integrated,
client-oriented system of care composed of both services and integrating mechanisms that guides and tracks clients over time through a comprehensive array of
health, mental health, and social services spanning all levels of intensity of care."[1]
The Joint Commission for Accreditation of Healthcare Organizations (JCAHO) recognizes the need for continuity as it states that each health care organization must
view the care it provides as part of a continuum that enables patients to have access
to an integrated system of settings, services, and care levels as the need occurs.
Within this continuum of care, each organization defines, shapes, and sequences
over time the following processes and activities to maximize coordination of care:
appropriate level of care based on patient's needs; coordination among health professionals; referral, transfer, or discharge to another level of care, health professional,
or setting; and exchange of patient care and clinical information.[2]

Essential components of an effective continuum of care are suggested by Vladeck:
- *Integration of payment sources.* Providing integrated services requires integration
of payment sources. Currently, patients may have insurance for a service only if that
service is provided in an acute-care setting, such as a hospital. The service may be
more appropriately provided in a less expensive setting, but no one person is addressing the comprehensive services needed by the patient and determining the best
way to meet those needs in a cost-effective way. As payment sources are integrated,
finances will be more wisely managed.
- *Shared data.* Establishing a communication system across settings may include
sharing procedures and forms. A shared data base should reduce the time needed
for data collection. Use of a common language across services improves communication and facilitates continuity of care.
- *Management.* Determining how the patient and system converge must be done by
an individual who recognizes the patient's needs and preferences and knows the
available services. Which discipline is best suited to provide this service has not yet
been determined, but one person or discipline should manage the care continuum.
The patient and system must somehow interface in a way that is beneficial to both.

- *Multidisciplinary team.* Providing effective, comprehensive, integrated, ongoing services requires effective multidisciplinary teamwork. It is essential to develop mechanisms that ensure continuation of teamwork.[3]

A continuum of health services can be classified from wellness to illness and return to wellness. It also can be seen as a type of service, such as preventive care, primary outpatient care, inpatient care, restorative care, or supportive care. Preventive care for those at risk for pressure ulcers includes education of patient and caregivers, referrals to community resources, and provision of equipment and supplies for prevention. Primary care of patients with a pressure ulcer problem requires a knowledgeable provider who periodically performs comprehensive assessments of health status and pressure ulcer risk factors. Individuals with severe conditions that cannot be managed without the service intensity of a hospital receive inpatient care. Examples of conditions requiring hospital services are sepsis and reconstructive operations to repair deep pressure ulcers. Restorative care can be received in a long-term care facility, a rehabilitative agency, or at home. Restorative care may include physical therapy, occupational therapy, or wound management. Supportive care may occur in multiple settings. Supportive care includes sitters for caregiver respite, day care, assisted living arrangements, and hospice.

Individuals requiring long-term or chronic care may use all the services in a system at one time or another. By addressing the chronic care needs of people with pressure ulcers, anticipatory management can be initiated at the preventive end of the continuum where care is financially, socially, and personally more economical.

For many years, ill or injured people were cared for in acute care hospitals. They were not sent home until wounds and diseases were under control or cured. Historically, a hospitalized patient was discharged by order of the physician when medically stable. Today patients are discharged in the midst of workups, sometimes before a definitive diagnosis is made and well before they can safely care for themselves.

The physician is only one of a number of people who plan and determine readiness for discharge. Several factors influence the discharge date:

- Availability of appropriate living arrangements
- Appropriate community resources
- Adequate financial resources
- Patient's ability to direct the activities of caregivers/assistants.[4]

Discharge planning, a logical concept but never so important as it is in today's world, emerged as a result of new reimbursement mechanisms, high-tech medical care, and regulations in the health care delivery system. In 1982, the prospective payment system for Medicare was enacted. The goals of this payment system clearly forced hospitals to reduce cost and length of stay in the acute care setting. Hence, planning for early discharge became a hospital priority. Length of stay in the acute care setting dropped, and the utilization of services was shifted to the community. Continuity of care became even more imperative in an era when earlier discharge from the hospital was the norm rather than the exception.[4,5]

Realizing that emphasis on controlling hospital costs might impinge on the quality of patient care, legislative action amended the Social Security Act to require hospitals to have a discharge planning program. The Joint Commission on Accreditation of Healthcare Organizations issued special guidelines to its member hospitals to recognize discharge planning as part of high-quality services.[6]

The American Hospital Association's General Council published guidelines on discharge planning that contain the definition, purpose, principles, essential elements, and need for quality assurance. The elements of a discharge planning program are:

- Early identification of patients likely to need complex posthospital care
- Patient and family education
- Patient and family assessment and counseling
- Discharge plan development
- Discharge plan coordination and implementation
- Postdischarge follow-up to determine outcomes.[5]

Because of its complexity, the discharge planning process has taken on a multidisciplinary focus. To increase the chance of successful outcomes, patients and families are expected to participate. Participation of patient and family members in planning ensures that their strengths and limitations are addressed as they will influence the effectiveness of implementation.

Hospital care

Planning for hospital discharge begins at the time the physician and patient or family agree on the need for hospitalization. Admitting nurses begin planning for discharge on their initial interview with the patient.[7] At Harper Hospital a new form was added to the admission data base for discharge planning documentation. Formerly, information about anticipated discharge needs was recorded in a section on the general admission data base. The intent was to initiate discharge planning on admission. However, information on the old form was static. Ongoing information regarding discharge plans, equipment ordered, or intended patient disposition was found everywhere in the record.

The new form allows discharge information to be located easily. Discharge information collected on admission is recorded on the discharge planning assessment form (see Figure 10.1). The form is kept in the discharge information section of the patient's record. On one side of the form the anticipated discharge disposition is recorded as well as consults requested, current living arrangements, support systems, barriers to self care, and other significant discharge data. The form also has a place for new consults and for additions to or changes in the plan. It is a reference for more detailed discharge information found elsewhere in the record.

As the patient's condition or needs change, information such as wound care treatment and supplies is updated in the progress notes. A simple statement on the discharge form (such as "see progress notes 9/15 for mattress ordered for home delivery") will ensure that discharge information elsewhere in the record is easily available to all caregivers. Many agencies have developed discharge planning tools to assist nurses in obtaining important information for home care.[8] To facilitate nursing doc-

(Text continued on page 216)

Wayne State University

DMC Harper
Hospital

DISCHARGE PLANNING ASSESSMENT

Patient lives with _____ ☐ Alone

Legal Guardian: ☐ No ☐ Yes   Name/Phone #: _____

Emergency Contact (name/phone#) : _____

Responsible for the care of someone else: ☐ No ☐ Yes Relation(s): _____

Services pre-hospitalization: ☐ None ☐ Home Care   Reason _____

   If yes, Agency _____   Last visit _____

   Equipment in home_____   Name of Company _____

   ☐ Meal Service   ☐ Chore Service/Housekeeper

Mobility: ☐ No problems ☐ Need assistance _____ ☐ Assistive devices/type_____

Self Care: ☐ No problems ☐ Need assistance/type_____

(Feed self, bathe, take own meds , energy for required activities, home maintenance, shopping)

Environment: ☐ No problems ☐ Architectural barriers in home ☐ Bathroom not on 1st level
☐ Bed not on 1st level ☐ Stairs in home ☐ Stairs to enter home ☐ Other_____

Transportation needs: ☐ No problems ☐ Transport to appointments ☐ Clinic/MD appointments
☐ ROC ☐ Van Service   ☐ Other _____

Financial: ☐ No problems ☐ Unable to obtain medications ☐ Assist with insurance ☐ Other: _____

Caregivers (name/relation): _____

Discharge plan at time of admission	(complete this section on admission) Disposition:	Referral made to:
☐ ☐	Home - Independently or with adequate support / Dependent on response to treatment	☐ None at this time / ☐ None at this time
☐ ☐ ☐	Home - With skilled Home Care / Home with Medical Equipment / Home - Hospice Care	☐ Home Care Coordinator / Name _____ / Reason for referral: _____ See HCC notes for detailed plan.
☐ ☐ ☐ ☐ ☐ ☐ ☐ ☐ ☐ ☐	Home with other community support / Nursing Home / Hospice - Inpatient / Hospice - Nursing Home / Ventilator Hospital / Adult Foster Care / Shelter / Psych Hospital / Rehabilitation Facility / Other Hospital	☐ Social Worker / Name _____ / Reason for referral: _____ / See SW notes for detailed plan.

Additional Self-Care Assessment

_____
_____
_____
_____
_____
_____
_____
_____
_____
_____
_____
_____
_____
_____
_____
_____

Date/Signature: _____

Figure 10.1 Discharge Planning Assessment Form

Discharge Planning Assessment Form *(continued)*

DISCHARGE PLAN REVISIONS

Additional discharge related consults placed to:
(Check all that apply)

Date/Signature   Date/Signature

Complex Nursing Issues
❑ Case Manager _____

Special teaching needs _____   ❑ Physical therapy _____
❑ Diabetes Educator _____   ❑ Occupational therapy _____
❑ Enterostomal Therapist _____   ❑ Speech therapy _____
❑ Pharmacist _____   ❑ Pulmonary Rehab/Home O$_2$ _____
❑ IVDT_____   ❑ Home Care Coordinator _____
❑ TPN Team _____   ❑ Social Worker _____
❑ Other _____   ❑ Dietitian _____
❑ Other _____   ❑ Other _____

Ongoing Revisions to Discharge/Disposition

Date	Disposition Plan	Signature

umentation, some agencies have developed a discharge criteria checklist for patients with pressure ulcers. Areas of instruction for patients with pressure ulcers include wound care, insurance coverage, pressure ulcer prevention techniques, and where to obtain specific durable medical equipment and supplies. Development of a discharge criteria checklist may facilitate communication of vital information to the receiving health care agency.[9] Much of the essential information for discharge planning can be obtained at group conferences or multidisciplinary rounds. Communication between nursing and other disciplines enhances the patient discharge planning process.[10]

The nurse's ability to identify the functional status of the patient is instrumental in determining the discharge plan. The acute care nurse is able to evaluate exactly what the patient is able to do and what support staff can contribute to meeting the patient's activities of daily living in the home setting. The acute care nurse tries to foresee problems that the patient may encounter in different levels of care. In order to ease the transition from one health care setting to another, the acute care nurse completes a continuing patient care form for home care or an interagency transfer summary for transfer to another health care facility (see Figure 10.2), including as much information as possible for the professional caregiver in the new setting. To implement the medical and nursing plans of care, the community health nurse assesses the patient's home for safety and comfort and makes appropriate requests for assistive devices as necessary.[5]

Many health care agencies have developed criteria for screening patients who are at risk for postdischarge problems.[7] Patients at risk for pressure ulcers generally fall into this category. With the advent of prospective payment, patients are discharged from the hospital sicker and more dependent than ever before, increasing their risk for developing pressure ulcers. Patients who are discharged from the hospital with pressure ulcers require intense observation and treatment at home because they are at risk for further tissue breakdown.

One way to monitor patients as they move from a controlled inpatient setting into the home is to contact them after discharge. Investigators found geriatric patients with newly diagnosed incontinence, pressure ulcers, and cognitive impairment to be at risk for functional decline or death during or following hospitalization.[11,12] Another study examined the feasibility of a postdischarge home assessment and follow-up intervention for geriatric patients. Elderly patients were selected 1 to 2 days before expected discharge. A geriatric nurse practitioner performed a screening history and physical examination on eligible patients. Within 24 to 72 hours after discharge, the nurse practitioner visited the intervention group of patients at home and conducted a second assessment. Immediately following the visit, all previously unrecognized and worsening problems related to medical status, nursing needs, patient function, medication use, and social circumstances were recorded. New or worsening problems were found in 99% of 150 patients. This study demonstrated the feasibility of a geriatric assessment and follow-up program that could be modified for hospitalized patients at risk for pressure ulceration.[13]

(Text continued on page 219)

Harper Hospital
Detroit, Michigan 48201

INTER-AGENCY
TRANSFER SUMMARY

1. PATIENT'S LAST NAME	2. FIRST NAME	3. MIDDLE	4. SEX M F	5. DATE OF TRANSFER	6. RELIGION

7. ADDRESS (street number, city, state, zip)	8. DATE OF BIRTH

9. TRANSFER TO: NAME	10. TRANSFER FROM:
ADDRESS:	

11. CONTACT PERSON

NAME	ADDRESS:	PHONE NUMBER:	RELATIONSHIP

12. PATIENT LIVES

Alone ☐   with spouse ☐   with Family ☐   Other ☐   Please specify:

13. INSURANCE INFORMATION:	14. PHYSICIAN AT TIME OF TRANSFER
	NAME: PHONE NUMBER:

15. ALLERGIES:	16. Previous hospitalizations and / or extended care facilities:

PHYSICIAN INFORMATION

17. DIAGNOSIS (ES) AT TIME OF TRANSFER
Primary:
Other Conditions:

18. SURGICAL PROCEDURES AND DATES

19. PHYSICIAN ORDERS ON TRANSFER:
a. DIET:
b. MEDICATIONS - NAME   DOSE / ROUTE / FREQUENCY

c. THERAPIES:

d. OTHER:

e. WEIGHT BEARING:
FULL _____ PARTIAL _____ NONE _____ ON _____ LEG

20. LABS:

CBC	date _____ result _____	Mode of Transport:
URINALYSIS	date _____ result _____	
SEROLOGY	date _____ result _____	Ambulance _____
OTHER	date _____ result _____	
CHEST X-RAY*	date _____ result _____	Car _____
	(* Report to be sent with patient)	

21. PATIENT*FAMILY AWARE OF DISEASE PROCESS   Yes ☐   No ☐

PHYSICIAN SIGNATURE   Date:

FORM NO. 300145 (10/91)

Figure 10.2 Interagency Transfer Summary

Inter-Agency Transfer Summary *(continued)*

Harper Hospital
Detroit, Michigan 48201

INTER-AGENCY TRANSFER SUMMARY

N U R S I N G	22. VITAL SIGNS: BLOOD PRESSURE _____ PULSE_____ TEMPERATURE _____ HEIGHT _____ WEIGHT _____			
	23. SPEECH: normal ☐	impaired ☐	unable to speak ☐	speaks no English ☐ understands no English ☐
	24. HEARING: normal ☐	impaired ☐	deaf ☐	hearing aid ☐
	25. SIGHT normal ☐	impaired ☐	blind ☐	glasses ☐
	26. MENTAL STATUS: oriented ☐	confused ☐	agitated ☐	other ☐
	27. FEEDING: independent ☐	needs help ☐	cannot feed self ☐	dentures ☐ tube ☐
	28. DRESSING independent ☐	needshelp ☐	cannot dress self ☐	
	29. BATHING: independent ☐	needs help ☐	bedbath with help ☐	bedbath ☐
	30. ELIMINATION independent ☐ incontinent:	help to bathroom ☐ urine ☐ stool ☐	bedpan or urinal ☐ foley ☐ ostomy ☐	last bowel movement _____
	31. AMBULATORY STATUS: independent ☐ assistance: equipment	chair ☐ one ☐	help with ambulation ☐ bedbound ☐ two ☐	three ☐
E V A L U A T I O N	32. DRESSING AND BANDAGES OR, CHECK NONE ☐			
	33. SKIN INTEGRITY: normal ☐ other ☐ Special skin Products: _____	pressure sore ☐	Stage I ☐ Stage II ☐ Stage III ☐ Stage IV ☐	
	34. UNRESOLVED NURSING DIAGNOSIS (ES) AND PLAN:			
	35. SPECIAL NEEDS:			
	SIGNATURE AND TITLE		DATE:	
	36. SPECIAL HOSPITAL SERVICES: SOCIAL WORK, DIETARY, PHYSICAL THERAPY, PHARMACY & PATIENT EDUCATION.			

Patients with pressure ulcerations may be discharged to any one of a variety of alternative care settings. Posthospital placement may be in a subacute, long-term care, or rehabilitation facility or in the patient's home with community support resources. Patients who are terminally ill may be discharged home with hospice services. It is essential that health care staff in every agency be educated regarding pressure ulcer prevention. Registered nurses, licensed practical nurses, home health aides, and other caregivers must be included in the education process.

Subacute care

Subacute care facilities evolved from the need for health care that is more intensive than that provided by nursing homes or home care. These agencies provide posthospital care at a less expensive cost than hospital care. Patients qualify for subacute care if they are stable but require either 24-hour nursing care or an intensity of service that cannot be provided in a long-term agency. The duration of stay is expected to be short.[14] Many patients with open pressure ulcers requiring complex dressing changes and patients who are in a lengthy postoperative phase after pressure ulcer reconstruction will spend part of their recovery in a subacute care facility. Patients admitted to subacute care facilities without pressure ulcers but requiring high-technology care and equipment are at risk for pressure ulcers while they are in the facility. Policies and procedures must be in place in the facility for pressure ulcer prevention and treatment.

Long-term care

Residents of long-term care facilities and nursing homes frequently are at high risk for pressure ulceration. The Omnibus Budget Reconciliation Act (OBRA) of 1991 established that all residents of long-term care facilities must be assessed with a standardized assessment tool, the Minimum Data Set (MDS). This tool contains "triggers" that are components of the assessment considered to be potential problems and may require development of a care plan. Triggers in the MDS associated with pressure ulcers and risk for pressure ulcers include presence of a pressure ulcer and the following 12 pressure ulcer risk factors: impaired transfer or bed mobility; bedfast, hemiplegia, quadriplegia; urinary or bowel incontinence; peripheral vascular disease; diabetes mellitus; hip fracture; weight loss; history of pressure ulcers; impaired tactile sensory perception; medications, such as antipsychotics and tranquilizers; restraints used daily; and no adequate skin care program.

Admitting patients with existing pressure ulcers generates tremendous anxiety among caregivers in long-term care facilities. Patients with pressure ulcers often are denied admission or readmission to skilled or long-term care facilities because their wound cultures show growth of multiple organisms. Some nursing homes require two "negative" wound cultures as criteria for admission. There is an erroneous concern that pressure ulcers with positive cultures are infected. The problem stems from lack of knowledge about colonization versus infection in chronic wounds. All chronic wounds will grow organisms when cultured, just as organisms will grow from a skin surface culture. It is inappropriate to use wound cultures as a criterion for denial for admission to a health care agency. If discharge planners are informed that a negative wound culture is required for placement in a given institution, the hospital epidemiologist should be consulted to assist the agency in interpreting the regulations.[15]

Home care

Home care agencies have registered nurses, licensed practical nurses, physical therapists, and home health aides who participate in the care of patients with pressure ulcers. Each of these providers must be educated about pressure ulcer prevention and treatment. As patients move through the system, periodic assessments are performed by professionals to update patient information and to determine the continued accuracy of the treatment plan. A home care agency admission assessment form can be a useful tool. Because this tool includes a body diagram, information about pressure ulcer location and characteristics can be communicated easily to caregivers. Specific instructions for pressure ulcer care are written on the Home Health Aide Care Plan. This includes required procedures, the duration and frequency of treatments, activity allowed, and body positioning to avoid pressure (see Figure 10.3). Routine pressure ulcer documentation by home care providers includes weekly wound measurements, ulcer stage, location, appearance, and drainage.

Providing home care for a patient with a pressure ulcer often is complicated and overwhelming for the caregiver. The professional nurse's time in the home is intermittent, and the family caregiver's skills are limited. For the lay person, most medication regimens, treatments, diet, and wound care management plans are complex. Even treatments that professionals think of as "easy" can be frightening for patients at home without professional supervision. Family members who usually are adept at routine care may be overwhelmed by the task of preventing and treating pressure ulcers on their own. The age and physical condition of the caregiver plays an important role in determining whether or not a specific treatment protocol will work.[16] During the patient's first few days at home, it is not unusual for the patient or caregiver to perform wound care once or twice a day with a nurse visiting daily to participate in a third dressing change. When the nurse believes that the caregiver is comfortable with the technique, the number of visits to the home can be reduced. Sebern[16] suggests that home care of pressure ulcers be broken down into three steps:
- Explain the cause of pressure ulcers.
- Assess each pressure ulcer and select the appropriate treatment plan.
- Explain the treatment plan to the family member.

See Chapter 11 for more detailed patient and family education regarding home care of the patient with pressure ulcers.

(Text continued on page 222)

RENAISSANCE HOME HEALTH CARE

HOME HEALTH AIDE CARE PLAN

Patient				Age	Sex	Pt. No.	Today's Date		Times Weekly (Range)
Patient Address			Apt. #	Team	Insurance ☐ BC ☐ Care ☐ HMO ☐ Caid ☐ Other		Therapy Only ☐	Diagnosis	
City		Zip		Phone		Directions (cross streets)			

P E R S O N A L C A R E	Encourage Participation ADL/bathing	**V I T A L S I G N S**	X TEMPERATURE NOTIFY:
	Assist Bath		X PULSE NOTIFY:
	Complete bed bath		X RESPIRATIONS NOTIFY:
	Progress to:		X DATE OF LAST BM Report if no BM x days
	Assist bath as tolerated		X Maintain Clean, Safe Environment
	Tub/shower as tolerated		DIET ☐ Regular ☐ _____
	Skin Care	**L I M I T A T I O N S**	**PLEASE NOTE:** ☐ Speech Impaired ☐ Disoriented ☐ Blind
	Shave Client		☐ Hard of Hearing ☐ Unconscious ☐ Incontinence ☐ Amputation
	Shampoo ___ Weekly and PRN		☐ Contractures ☐ Hemiplegia ☐ Quadriplegia ☐ Paraplegia
	___ Bi-Monthly and PRN		
	Comb Hair	**P R E C A U T I O N S**	Safe Disposal of contaminated materials
	Oral Hygiene		No smoking with oxygen in use
	Nail Care		Seizures
	Linen Change ___ Weekly and PRN		Lock wheelchair with transfers
	___ Other (specify) _____		Side rails up
A C T I V I T Y	Ambulation with Assistance of _____		Total hip precautions
	Transfer Bed/Chair with Assistance of _____		Other (specify) _____
	Complete Bed Rest		**REPORT TO RN:**
	ROM to _____		Dizziness, Headache, Blurred Vision, Fainting
O T H E R D U T I E S	Catheter Care: Dsg change/cleanse with _____	**S I G N S A N D S Y M P T O M S**	Report foley plugged, leaking, blood in urine, cloudy, burning
			or strong odor to urine.
	Irrigate with _____ Every _____		Report redness, warmth, change in wound drainage or foul odor
	Change Bag Every _____		Change in LOC/Change in Gait
			Excessive Thirst, Urination, and Hunger
	Wound/Decubitus Care (specify) _____		Abrupt onset of excessive sweating, faintness, trembling and
	_____		confusion
			Severe SOB, Unrelieved Chest Pain, Swelling Lower Extrem.
	Frequency for HHA: q. _____ .		Weight gain/loss greater than _____ #'s
	Oxygen at _____ Liters/min Per _____		OTHER:_____
	Weigh: q. _____ .		
	Other (specify)_____		

RN SIGNATURE:	PRIMARY YES ☐ NO ☐	REVISION YES ☐ NO ☐	AIDE ASSIGNED:	FIRST HHA VISIT:	SUPERVISORY VISIT DUE:

FORM # 2502 (12/93)

Figure 10.3 Home Health Aide Care Plan

Hospice care

The occurrence of pressure ulcers in hospice patients greatly complicates care, increases cost, and seriously threatens quality of life. In an article on pressure ulcer prevention for hospice patients, recommended nursing strategies include care to increase comfort. Needless pain and suffering associated with pressure ulceration can be avoided by implementing a pressure ulcer prevention program for hospice personnel.[17]

Pressure ulcer cost considerations

Home health care is growing rapidly, primarily because of the pressures on hospitals to discharge patients early. Recuperation with home-based nursing care is an essential link between the hospital and a return to daily living. A recent study focused on the health care characteristics and the nursing needs of a sample of elderly patients following discharge from the hospital. The patient's medical diagnoses fell into the categories of orthopedic, cardiovascular, pulmonary, and diabetes-related diagnoses. However, nursing diagnoses formed the framework for the home health care data base. The four most frequent nursing diagnoses—knowledge deficit, impaired physical mobility, impaired skin integrity, and altered comfort—accounted for 74% of the total nursing diagnoses. If self-care deficit was added to the list, these top five nursing diagnoses accounted for 83% of the total number used by home care nurses.[18] The authors emphasized that home care nurses used a limited number of nursing diagnostic categories that did not reflect all of the nursing care delivered. If this lack of documentation reflects the reimbursement atmosphere that only direct physical care is reimbursable, then nurses need to pursue changes in reimbursement mechanisms for home health care.[18]

Nurses employed in a Pennsylvania visiting nurse association tracked the cost of home care in a sample of 541 patients who were discharged from home nursing services. The resulting charges were highest for the nursing diagnosis of potential for impaired skin integrity. The patients in this category were chronically ill or had end-stage disease and were at high risk for developing pressure ulcers. The fifth most costly nursing diagnosis was actual impairment of skin integrity. Most of the patients with actual skin breakdown had acute, nonchronic, episodic type diseases, such as fractured hip or pneumonia. They were expected to return to pre-illness levels of functioning and required less care.[19]

Immobile patients are at high risk for pressure ulcers and require a pressure-relieving sleep surface at home. Often the choice of a pressure-relieving device will be determined by the family's financial situation and not by what is best for the patient. If a pressure-relieving surface is not sent home from the acute care setting, the patient who is at risk for pressure ulcers may not be able to obtain one after discharge. Currently, Medicare selectively reimburses for prevention and treatment of pressure sores under the Part B home care benefit.[18] The patient may not be eligible to receive reimbursement for a pressure-relief device obtained for home use. This is despite the fact that it is much less expensive to treat a patient in the home setting than in the hospital. Nurses need to continue to track such cases and submit the findings to fiscal intermediaries. Home care nursing agencies are lobbying for legislative changes to ensure quality nursing care. All nurses need to support changes in Medicare reimbursement for interventions that affect pressure ulcer management.

Summary

Health care cost containment policies have been the major impetus for the increasing importance of discharge planning. Volland points out that health care cost containment will remain a major concern for the foreseeable future because of the following:

- The aging of America
- Medical technology that is prolonging life without cure
- The shift of care from inpatient to outpatient
- Recognition that there are limited resources
- Uneven distribution of health care professionals
- Ensuring access to care while also trying to guarantee quality of life.[6]

It is anticipated that discharge planning will increase in importance as prospective payment is adopted by more third-party payers. Nurses must begin to shift their thinking from caring for the patient on an episodic acute incident to thinking of their encounters with the patient as a part of a large health care continuum. Responsibility for discharge planning takes on an expanded dimension as patients become part of a system that offers lifetime health and illness care and insurance companies assume responsibility for "covered lives." This is no less the situation for patients who have or are at risk for pressure ulcers, because these are chronic problems that demand lifetime surveillance as part of a management program. Discharge planning takes on a global dimension as it shifts from discharge planning to ongoing planning. Discharge from one agency to another or from an agency to the home is not a discharge of the patient from the system. It is merely a transition along the continuum of care.

References

1. Evashwick, C. "Definition of the Continuum of Care," in Evashwick, C., and Weiss, L.J., eds. *Managing the Continuum of Care.* Gaithersburg, Md.: Aspen Publishers, Inc., 1987.
2. Joint Commission for Accreditation of Healthcare Organizations. *1995 Comprehensive Accreditation Manual for Hospitals.* Oakbrook Terrace, JCAHO, 1994.
3. Vladeck, B.C. "The Continuum of Care: Principles and Metaphors," in Evashwick, C., and Weiss, L.J., eds. *Managing the Continuum of Care.* Gaithersburg, Md.: Aspen Publishers, Inc., 1987.
4. Volland, P.J. *Discharge Planning: An Interdisciplinary Approach to Continuity of Care.* Owings Mills, Md.: National Health Publishing, 1988.
5. Fitzig, C. "Discharge Planning: Nursing Focus," in Volland, P.J., ed. *Discharge Planning: An Interdisciplinary Approach to Continuity of Care.* Owings Mills, Md.: National Health Publishing, 1988.
6. O'Leary, D. "Joint Commission Sets Agenda for Change," *JCAH Perspectives,* 6-8, November/December 1986.
7. Siegel, H. "Nurses Improve Hospital Efficiency Through a Risk Assessment Model at Admission," *Nursing Management* 19(10): 38-47, 1989.

8. Ridley, M.A. "Discharge Planning Considerations for the Pressure Ulcer Patient," *Ostomy/Wound Management* 19: 70-77, Summer 1988.

9. Oot-Giromini, B., et al. "Pressure Ulcer Prevention and Management: Developing Discharge Criteria," *Continuing Care* 9(6): 20-27, 1990.

10. Esper, P.S. "Discharge Planning—A Quality Assurance Approach," *Nursing Management* 19(10): 66-68, 1988.

11. Kosekoff, J., et al. "Prospective Payment System and Impairment at Discharge: The Quicker and Sicker Story Revisited *JAMA* 264:1980-1983, 1990.

12. Inouye, S.K., et al. "A Predictive Index for Functional Decline in Hospitalized Elderly Medical Patients," *J Gen Intern Med* 8: 645-652, 1993.

13. Krafitz, R.L., et al. "Geriatric Home Assessment after Hospital Discharge," *J Amer Geriat Soc* 42(12):1229-1234, 1994.

14. Micheletti, J.A., and Shlala, T.J. "Understanding and Operationalizing Subacute Services," *Nursing Management* (Continuing Care Edition) 26(6): 49-56, June 1995.

15. Gurevich, I. "Infected Decubiti: The Problem of Patient Placement and Care," *Topics in Cl Nurs* 15: 55-63, July 1983.

16. Seburn, M. "Home-Team Strategies for Treating Pressure Sores," *Nursing* (4): 50-53, April 1987.

17. Colburn, L. "Pressure Ulcer Prevention for the Hospice Patient: Strategies for Care to Increase Comfort," *AM J Hospice Care* 2: 22-26, March/April 1987.

18. Motta, G. "Quality Review and Assurance Strategies of the Medicare Program," *Journal of Enterostomal Therapy* 16(1):1-3, 1989.

19. Harris, M.D., et al. "Tracking the Cost of Home Care," *American Journal of Nursing* 11: 1500-1502, November 1987.

Education

Education is one of the most important elements of providing care for patients in any situation or environment. As patients move from inpatient settings of hospitals and long-term-care facilities into their homes, more responsibility for care is assumed by family members and patients themselves. With this shift from professional care, the need for patients and caregivers to obtain health care knowledge and skills increases dramatically. Research has demonstrated that patient education results in positive outcomes for risk-related behaviors, decreased postoperative pain, less patient distress, fewer hospital readmissions, and decreased length of stay.[1,2,3]

Identifying educational needs of family members or caregivers for patients with pressure ulcers is a difficult process. There are no statistics available on the number of people with pressure ulcers who are being cared for at home. Baharestani[4] studied the experiences of wives caring for their homebound, frail, elderly husbands with pressure ulcers. The wives had no idea how to obtain knowledge about pressure ulcers and no awareness that they needed information. Five themes were identified among these elderly wife-caregivers: 1) difficulty with providing care (physical, emotional, safety, and financial), 2) frailty of the caregiver, 3) limited socialization, 4) limited social support systems, and 5) limited caregiving knowledge. The wives reported increasing and progressive fatigue related to the physical work of moving and repositioning their spouses. The emotional difficulty stemmed from each wife's need to "be there" for her husband. The wives allowed their own health to suffer in order to provide the care they believed was needed by their husbands. Since Medicare reimbursement did not cover the bulk of supplies, the cost of dressings, equipment, and nutritional supplements created a financial burden for these families. Because of their extensive caregiving activities, the wives had little time or energy left for socialization. In addition, they had little social support. Home care services were not covered by insurance, and none of the wife-caregivers felt they were able to pay for 24-hour assistance with care.

The caregivers in this study reported that they learned to care for their husbands through experience. They did not have the opportunity to interact early with health care professionals and, therefore, solicited advice from neighbors. When their husbands developed pressure ulcers, the wives contacted "Doctors-on-Call" or dermatologists. They were given prescriptions for various topical applications. They did not receive education and community referrals until their husbands were hospitalized for sepsis or other medical diagnoses. Many wives had never heard of pressure ulcers and had no information on risk factors or preventive measures. Yet, when their husbands were hospitalized, the wives reported that they were blamed by professionals for providing poor care. This study clearly indicates the need to identify and to educate family caregivers. The author suggests that creative strategies are needed to reach the public, such as: 1) using educational television programming, 2) attaching a toll-free number to social security checks for information, assistance, counseling, and literature, 3) providing free hotlines to answer caregivers' questions, 4) marketing home nursing services and 5) placing literature in places where people regularly go, such as grocery stores and physician's offices.[4]

Patients and caregivers are empowered through education. Health care professionals have a responsibility to educate patients and families about risk factors and pressure ulcer prevention measures while they are in hospitals, long-term-care facilities, outpatient clinics, and offices. The optimal time for teaching each person is determined on an individual basis. One study found that patient education is more effective when given in more than one session with a follow-up. Presenting large amounts of new educational content at once has a detrimental effect on the patient's abilities to process information. Information is more likely to be retained if given over time.[5] Patient education should focus on promoting the acquisition of knowledge and skills and on supporting decision making.[6]

Guidelines for adult learning

Patients and families enter the health care environment with a variety of beliefs and a wide range of educational experiences and abilities. They approach learning new tasks with their unique value systems and views of life. Their interpretations of current situations reflect their own past experiences. When educating adults, consideration should be given to these factors. The educator may believe that the learner should know how to perform a procedure or modify risk factors, but the patient must value this knowledge in order to learn. If the patient is not interested in learning, no learning will take place. Adult learning principles should be used to provide health education for adult patients and families. Knowles[7] identified the following concepts regarding adult learning:

- Adults have a need to know why they should learn something.
- Adults have a deep need to be self-directed.
- Adults have a greater volume and different quality of experiences than youth.
- Adults become ready to learn when they experience a need to know or do something to perform more effectively and satisfyingly.
- Adults enter into a learning experience with a task-centered, problem-centered, or life-centered orientation to learning.
- Adults are stimulated to learn by extrinsic and intrinsic motivators.[7]

These principles should be applied as formal or informal education is developed.

Assessment of learning needs

Nurses collect comprehensive data to determine a patient's current and past health status, functional status, and coping patterns.[8] This database must include assessment of patient and family learning needs and identification of available resources for patient/caregiver education. Assessment of patients with pressure ulcers includes identification of caregivers and patient and family characteristics that may inhibit or enhance learning. Interpersonal and intrapersonal patient and caregiver characteristics may influence both the teaching-learning process and the outcome. Pressure ulcer prevention information should be directed toward the principal learner.[9] In some cases, the patient is able to obtain information and either carry out the functions or direct someone else to perform the skills. In other situations, the patient may be cognitively impaired, unable to retain information, or physically unable to perform the tasks necessary for self-care. For any number of reasons, a capable patient may wish to have someone else assume the primary provider role. The patient's chosen primary caregiver is taught skills to perform the care required.

Familiarity with people of different cultures and their expectations of the health care system is essential. Cultural values of the patient and caregiver must be considered. Patients may have "healing remedies" that are detrimental to a healing wound. The patient may be uncomfortable having another person perform skin inspection, particularly in the pelvic girdle, an area that often is vulnerable to pressure ulceration. Health care professionals must develop culturally sensitive strategies to teach pressure ulcer prevention and treatment.[9]

A comprehensive pressure ulcer history and risk assessment must be obtained before learning needs are identified. Health professionals then will be able to identify current practices that increase the risk for pressure ulcers. Risk factors and health practices provide the basis for determining what educational content should be stressed.[9]

Establishing goals and objectives

Goals and objectives for health care are mutually determined by the patient/caregiver and provider.[10] These goals guide the teaching-learning process. They identify what needs to be accomplished. Objectives are the behaviors expected at completion of the process. They are stated in behavioral terms so that they can be measured. For example, one goal may be to have the patient's pressure ulcer heal. Objectives related to this goal may include a patient demonstration of a dressing change or preparation of a menu with a balanced nutrition plan for wound healing.

Combining the expertise of clinicians with the patient's and caregiver's desires ensures more realistic goal setting. Individuals may have many reasons for being at risk for pressure ulcers. Multiple goals may be necessary to reduce these risks or to promote pressure ulcer healing. Often risks are embedded in lifestyles or routines, or the patient may have priorities that are in conflict with risk factor management. For example, young insensate wheelchair-bound individuals may need a reminder to perform wheelchair pushups or shifts in body weight while attending long school lectures. One mother found a watch with an alarm that she could set to remind her wheelchair-bound daughter to shift her weight on a predetermined schedule. Because the alarm brought attention to her handicap, the young girl chose not to use it. A watch with a vibrating alarm turned out to be a more acceptable alternative.

A more manageable plan might be developed by dividing long-term goals into short-term goals. Facing a large number of goals may be an overwhelming experience for both patients and caregivers. Whenever possible, additional family members should be encouraged to participate in goal setting and caregiving. If there is more than one person in the household to assist, sharing the care relieves the burden and reduces caregiver strain.[11,12] Matching tasks to individual family member skills creates a sense of teamwork and mutual responsibility. If it is acceptable to the patient and family, children can participate in care by moisturizing skin and providing oral fluids.[9] Adolescents may assume responsibility for running errands. Participation in the team helps all members of the family understand frustrations when they occur. When the number of goals seems overwhelming, consideration should be given to the importance of subjective goal setting. In some instances, a subjective goal may be more important to the caregiver than an objective goal. For example, the objective goal of decreasing the pressure ulcer size provides the patient or caregiver with the subjective goal of experiencing a sense of relief as the frequency of dressing changes decreases.[9] Health care providers should continuously assess the patient situation in relation to goals or expected outcomes. The goals may be adjusted or completely revised as patient risk factors change. Patients and caregivers should consider plan revision as a sign of caregiver attentiveness. Revision is an ongoing part of the goal-setting process. As new information is obtained and patient characteristics change, the goals must be modified to fit the situation. Revisions indicate that caregivers are responding to the needs of the patient and not just working with a routine plan that has no benefit.

Teaching strategies and methods of instruction

An effective educator uses a variety of teaching strategies to reach the desired educational outcome. Matching the health care provider's teaching style with the patient's preferred learning style increases the chance that learning will take place. The majority of learners require multisensory stimulation in order to learn.[13] Selection of a particular strategy is based on the specific learner or on the type of outcome expected. When there is a need for caregivers to master a necessary task, they may not be given a choice of learning strategies. Health care professionals may request a return demonstration if the essential component of a lesson is mastering a required skill. Other teaching strategies include written instruction and diagrams. One family videotaped the physical therapist as she taught the patient safe transfer techniques. The patient could view the video to reinforce learning after the physical therapy visits concluded.

The demonstration-practice method of instruction is effective for teaching pressure ulcer prevention and care skills. Positioning, use of equipment, and dressing change procedures are best taught by demonstration and practice. Procedure teaching is accompanied by written patient outcome criteria, often in the form of a checklist. The patient is told how to do the procedure, a demonstration is performed by the nurse, and the patient is asked to repeat the demonstration, including all the items on the written checklist. The checklist can serve as a reminder to the patient when a procedure is performed at home without supervision. Procedure instructions should accompany the checklist. All instructions should be written in clear, simple terminology so that family members may refer to them whenever they feel the need.[14] When referring a hospitalized patient for continuing care, the discharging nurse should document patient education covered during the hospital stay and the patient's/family's level of understanding and ability for care at the time of discharge.

A patient outcome checklist is a method that provides an organized system of nursing documentation. The purpose of the checklist is to determine when the patient has reached a desired outcome for specific tasks or for a series of related tasks. Health care providers develop teaching outcome checklists based on their experience in caring for many patients with the same type of health care problem. Checklists may be modified to fit the desired objectives, goals, and needs of each patient (see Table 11.1).

Reading levels

The reading level of printed educational material should match the reading ability of the learner. If the reading level is too high, the written information will not be understood by less educated patients. If the level is too low, more educated patients will lose interest. Formulas are available to assess the reading level of written educational material. For example, the SMOG Readability Formula[15] is used to determine if the written material is appropriate for a specific patient or caregiver. See Table 11.2 for how to use the SMOG formula and conversion table.

What patients need to know

All patients with pressure ulcers and those who are at risk for pressure ulcers need to know basic information about pressure ulcer prevention and treatment. The AHCPR Consumer Guides *Preventing Pressure Ulcers: A Patient's Guide* and *Treating Pressure Sores* are available from the U.S. Department of Health and Human Services for patient and caregiver education.[16,17] These guides describe how pressure ulcers form, how to identify risk factors, steps to prevent pressure ulcers, and how to treat them if they do occur. The guides also include skin care, pressure reduction, nutrition, mobility and activity, positioning, ulcer treatment, complications, and what to report to a health care provider. Pharmaceutical companies, durable medical equipment manufacturers, and wound care companies also have commercial educational

Table 11.1 Dressing Changes and Wound Care: Teaching Outcome Checklist

Initial and date each criteria.

DMC Harper
Hospital

Performance Criteria: Dressing Change/Wound Care		Initiated by Nurse	Verbalized or Demonstrated by Patient
1. Patient verbalizes need/rationale and frequency for dressing changes.	1.	_____	_____
2. Selects the correct amount and type of dressing supplies.	2.	_____	_____
3. Discusses technique of dressing changes (e.g., clean, sterile)	3.	_____	_____
4. Demonstrates steps of dressing change/wound care:			
a. Washes hands and prepares new dressings	4a.	_____	_____
b. Removes old dressing	b.	_____	_____
c. Rewashes hands	c.	_____	_____
d. Changes dressing per correct procedure	d.	_____	_____

☐ dry   ☐ soaks

☐ wet and dry   ☐ other (specify)

☐ packing   _____

☐ other (specify)

e. Disposes of old dressing properly	e.	_____	_____
5. Verbalizes confidence in changing dressing	5.	_____	_____
6. States intended method of changing dressing at home:			
a. Sitting	6a.	_____	_____
b. Standing	b.	_____	_____
c. Use of Mirror	c.	_____	_____
7. States where to obtain dressing supplies/ needed resources.	7.	_____	_____
8. States signs and symptoms to report to physician:			
a. Color of tissue in wound	8a.	_____	_____
b. Color of drainage from wound	b.	_____	_____
c. Color of tissue surrounding wound	c.	_____	_____
d. Chills, fever, pain, swelling, tenderness of wound	d.	_____	_____
9. States date of and intention to keep follow-up appointment with physician.	9.	_____	_____

COMMENTS _____

_____

Initials	Signature/Title	Initials	Signature/Title	Initials	Signature/Title

Table 11.2 SMOG Readability Formula and Conversion Table

1. Count off 10 consecutive sentences near the beginning, in the middle, and near the end of the text. If the text has fewer than 30 sentences, use as many as are provided.
2. Count the number of words containing three or more syllables, including repetitions of the same words.
3. Look up the approximate grade level on the SMOG Conversion Table.

Total polysyllabic word count	Approximate grade level (+1.5 grades)
0-2	4
3-6	5
7-12	6
13-20	7
21-30	8
31-42	9
43-56	10
57-72	11
73-90	12
91-110	13
111-132	14
133-156	15
157-182	16
183-210	17
211-240	18

From the United States Department of Health and Human Services. *Pretesting in Health Communications.* NIH Pub No 84-1493. Washington, DC, 1984, US Government Printing Office. Table developed by Harold C. McGraw, Office of Education Research, Baltimore County Schools, Towson, Maryland.

material that can be adapted for individual use. The AHCPR pressure ulcer consumer guidelines provide a foundation for teaching patients and caregivers about pressure ulcers.

Prevention and treatment

A program for pressure ulcer education should address both prevention and treatment (see Chapters 6 and 7). Patients and caregivers are taught that unrelieved pressure is the main cause of pressure ulcers. Simple explanations should be given about compression of blood vessels and the need for tissue oxygenation and nutrition. The effect of pressure against soft tissue can be demonstrated by pressing the fingers tightly around a clear drinking glass. With enough pressure, the finger pads become pale from compression of the blood vessels. Patients can see the effect of pressure through the clear glass. Reactive hyperemia is demonstrated on the finger pads when the pressure is relieved. A description of the consequence of prolonged pressure is more easily understood with these visual signs.

Skin care

Inspection and care of the skin should be done at least twice daily. In addition, areas over bony prominences should be inspected after each position change. Pressure points may vary when joints become contracted, after flap operations for repair of pressure ulcers, and with redistribution of soft tissue after weight changes. Pressure points unique to each individual should be identified. It is helpful to create a diagram of the patient's body with identified pressure points to be used as a check sheet for inspection. Inspection of the entire skin surface is essential. A hand mirror can be useful for self-inspection when checking hard-to-see areas.[18] Reddened areas that remain after position changes should receive special attention. Reddened areas should be completely free from pressure when repositioned. Pillows, rolled towels, or foam wedges should be used to position the body to completely relieve pressure for reddened areas of skin. Massage over bony prominences or reddened areas is contraindicated. Massage may disrupt capillaries and damage the tissue under the skin.

Skin should be cleaned when it is soiled. Warm water is safer than hot water for bathing or showering, particularly over skin areas that are insensate. If daily bathing is preferred, measures may be needed to prevent dry skin. Creams or oils can be used for moisturizing.

Urine, stool, and perspiration remaining on skin are irritants that increase pressure ulcer risk. A program for incontinence management should be in place to reduce the risk for skin breakdown. The cause of incontinence should be investigated and treated. *Managing Urinary Incontinence: A Patient's Guide*[19] can be ordered from AHCPR Publications. Fecal incontinence is especially detrimental to skin. Use of a skin barrier will help protect the skin. Incontinence pads that wick moisture away from the skin should be used to help keep the skin dry. Peri pads are easily available and can be used if there is minimal urinary or fecal incontinence. Patients and caregivers should be encouraged to use these products and to cleanse and dry the peri-anal and pelvic area after each soiling. For more information about continence products and services,[20] contact Help for Incontinent People, P.O. Box 544, Union, SC 29397.

Friction against the skin can be avoided during repositioning by lifting, rather than dragging, the body across a bed or chair surface. Friction can rub away the skin surface. Use of an overbed trapeze allows the patient to help lift the body during repositioning. Use of lift sheets prevents friction when caregivers are repositioning. Wearing clothing, such as long-sleeved pajamas and socks, or using a thin film of cornstarch on the skin will also reduce friction.

How to perform a skin check

Caregivers should take the following steps when performing a skin check:
1. Remove the patient's clothing. Position the patient so that areas to be checked are accessible. The patient's position will depend on the previous activity or position and the current nursing care plan.

2. Identify the areas to be inspected. All surface areas are checked at least twice daily. Convenient times may be on waking and at bedtime. Pressure points are checked with every change in position. Previously reddened areas may be checked every 15 minutes to 1 hour as indicated by the care plan.

3. Examine the skin for signs of pressure (redness, loss of skin, changes in color or temperature), moisture or dryness, and presence of rashes. Temperature changes can best be checked by placing the back of the hand against the skin surface. Compare findings with the temperature of other skin surface areas. Using this method will detect even a 5-degree difference in temperature. If there are reddened areas, reassess them in 15 minutes. If there is no change in the reddened area, do not position the patient on this area. Continue to monitor until the condition resolves. Report the finding to the professional health care provider.

4. If signs of rash are present, cleanse the area with plain water and pat dry. Report findings to the professional health care provider. Apply topical lotions, powders, or ointments only under the direction of the health care provider.

Pressure reduction

Removing pressure is the most important part of prevention and treatment of pressure ulcers. Individuals who are confined to bed need a special mattress or mattress overlay made of foam, air, gel, or water. Selection of the best product must be made with the patient's health care provider. Insurance companies with case management services may identify preferred products.

Positioning, repositioning, and the use of special devices and surfaces to support the body must be included in the teaching plan. Good body positioning while in bed begins with good body alignment. Pillows and wedges should be used for positioning (see Chapter 6 for more information on pressure-reduction devices and proper positioning). While the patient is on bedrest, the head of the bed should be raised as little as necessary and for as short a time as possible. Maintaining the head with less than 30 degrees elevation will avoid a shearing effect of the bony skeleton sliding inside the soft tissue of the pelvis. Use of a knee gatch or a foot board on a hospital bed will help prevent the patient from slipping while in a sitting position. The 30-degree lateral sidelying position avoids direct pressure on the greater trochanter of the femur and places the weight of the pelvis on the soft tissue of the buttocks. Use of a diagram may be necessary to explain to caregivers how to use this position for patients. A support surface can be assessed for effectiveness in reducing pressure by a "hand check" procedure (see Chapter 6). The caregiver places a hand under the support surface beneath the pressure point. The palm is up and the fingers are flat. If there is less than 1 inch of support surface between the pressure point and the caregiver's hand, there is not enough support. A different support surface may be recommended.

Heels require extra protection. Devices that suspend the heels are preferred. Pillows placed under the ankle and calf are an inexpensive method to protect the heels.

Effectiveness can be assessed by sliding a piece of paper between the heel and the surface of the bed. Avoid placing pillows or other support devices behind the knee, as this may cause undue pressure to the popliteal area. Pillows and foam wedges should be used to maintain correct body alignment and support the patient's position.

Patients who use wheelchairs should be taught to avoid sitting directly on a pressure ulcer. Special chair cushions can be used to reduce pressure areas while sitting. Correct posture for chair sitting is shown in Chapter 6. Instruct the patient to keep the thighs horizontal to the chair seat. The feet should rest comfortably on the foot rest and the arms horizontal on the arm rests. A pressure-reducing chair cushion is needed for wheelchair-bound individuals. Cushions are available in foam, gel, or air. Selection of appropriate products is made with the health care provider. Donut-type cushions should not be used because they cause pressure and reduce blood flow to the tissue surrounding the ulcer. Use of a chair cushion does not eliminate the need for frequent moving and repositioning or shifting body weight. If an individual is confined to a chair, the position should be changed at least every hour with small shifts in body weight at 15-minute intervals. Persons with sufficient upper body strength should be taught wheelchair pushups.

Teaching pressure-reduction activities

The purpose of these activities is to provide regular relief of pressure over bony prominences. Develop an individualized schedule for pressure relief activities that is compatible with the patient's daily routine. Be sure to consider the following:

Frequency of activity. Determine the capacity of the patient to tolerate position changes, shifts in body weight, and the individual's tissue tolerance. Skin inspection should be done every 15 minutes initially. Evaluation time can be extended by 15-minute intervals until the maximum time is established. There should be no evidence of redness at the pressure points.

Length of pressure relief. Relieve the pressure for at least 10 seconds every 15 minutes when the patient is in the sitting position.

Assistance. When the patient is unable or unwilling to carry out the recommended measures for pressure ulcer prevention, a caregiver must perform the activities. Use of assistive devices may increase the patient's independence. Suggestions for devices can be made by the physical therapist and occupational therapist. Whenever possible, the patient should direct the care that others provide.

Effectiveness. Absence of tissue breakdown and skin redness is the goal of pressure relief. If there is no redness and the skin is intact, the pressure-relief activities are effective. The first sign of tissue injury—redness—requires a revision in the plan. Complete pressure relief is needed until the tissue is healed. A shorter time interval between pressure-relief activities is instituted. Determine whether the patient is following the plan as established. Does the patient have any problems in carrying out the activity? Are the risks and benefits of the activity clear to the patient? Can the procedure be simplified in any way to improve compliance? Are there any incentives that can be used for this patient to encourage desired behavior?

Wheelchair pressure relief

The goal for sitting tolerance should be established with the patient. For most patients, tolerance of several hours is required to resume life activities.

- Inform the patient of frequency for pressure relief. Teach pushups or leans if the patient has the upper body strength and coordination to perform these activities.
- Gradually increase sitting time by 30 minutes.
- Maintain increased time for 2 days before increasing sitting time again.
- Examine skin over ischia, posterior trochanters, and sacral-coccygeal bony prominences for hyperemia whenever the patient returns to bed.
- Remind the patient to perform pressure-relief activities every 30 minutes.[18]

Nutrition

Malnutrition may be present because of an underlying disease process or because of social or economic reasons. Sometimes individuals are just not aware of what constitutes a balanced diet. Patients need to be taught that skin breaks down easier and wounds will not heal with inadequate nutrition. Protein is needed for growth of new tissue. Nutritional deficiencies predispose patients to wound infections, wound dehiscence, sepsis, and other complications. Nutrition is integral for healing wounds, preventing infections, and maintaining a general sense of well-being. Nutritional assessments should be done periodically by health care providers in order to recognize early signs of malnutrition, to correct problems, and to minimize the loss of patient strength. Individualization of nutrition intervention is as important as any other part of goal setting. Patients are instructed to report weight loss, poor appetite, or gastrointestinal disturbances that interfere with eating.[21,22,23]

An elderly person is at high risk for dehydration with a decrease in oral fluid intake. Without water, nutrients can't reach the wound. Fluid also helps cushion the cells and organs. The National Research Council recommends 1 ml of water per calorie intake or 30 ml per kilogram of body weight per day.[24] For a 110-pound person, this would be approximately six to eight cups of fluid per day. (See Table 11.3 for suggestions on how to increase fluid intake.)

Diet education for patients and their families should include information about types of foods that contain nutrients necessary for wound healing. Protein, vitamins, and minerals are needed for tissue growth and calories are needed for energy. High-protein, high-calorie supplements may be necessary. Families should be encouraged to bring in any favorite foods that might stimulate the patient's appetite. They also should be taught to read labels on food products. Often there are less expensive supplements available in grocery stores with the same nutritional value as brand-name products. Enteral feedings should be considered for those patients who cannot or will not consume adequate oral intake. The National Center for Nutrition and Di-

Table 11.3 Suggestions for Increasing Fluid Intake

1. Offer large amounts of fluids with medications.
2. Add flavoring such as a lemon or lime slice to water.
3. Mix ginger ale or other carbonated soft drinks with fruit juice.
4. Offer popsicles, soup and jello between meals.
5. Provide ice cream or frozen yogurt cones.
6. Serve hot or cold cereal with extra milk.
7. Remind all visitors to offer fluids at periodic intervals.

Adapted from Kobriger, A. (1995). The healing power of water. *Contemporary Long Term Care,* 18(6): 68-69.

etetics of the American Dietetic Association and its Foundation recommends using The Food Guide Pyramid as a guide to nutritional well-being (see Figure 11.4). Teaching patients and their caregivers to perform their own nutritional assessments is part of comprehensive self-care education. The nutritional checklist developed by the Nutrition Screening Initiative can be used for this purpose[22] (see Table 11.4). The checklist is based on the warning signs of nutritional deficiencies listed in Table 11.5.[22] Problems identified by patients and caregivers need to be reported to a health care provider. Consultation with a dietitian may be indicated for assistance with menu selection, food substitution, and dietary instruction.

Treatment

A treatment plan is developed by a team that includes the patient, the patient's caregiver(s), physicians, nurses, dietitians, physical and occupational therapists, social workers, and pharmacists. Case managers working for insurance companies may participate as part of the team. According to the AHCPR Consumer Guide for Pressure Ulcer Treatment, the patient and caregiver need to:

- Know their roles in the treatment program.
- Learn how to perform care.
- Know what to report to the doctor or nurse.
- Know how to tell if the treatment works.
- Help change the treatment plan when needed.
- Know what questions to ask.
- Get understandable answers.[17]

Patients are able to participate in their care more effectively if they understand the reason for the plan. They should be informed that the health care provider will ask about general health, other illnesses, medications, and available support of family and friends. The plan is developed based on information obtained from the history and physical examination and the goals of the patient. It will include pressure reduction, pressure ulcer care, and promotion of healing.

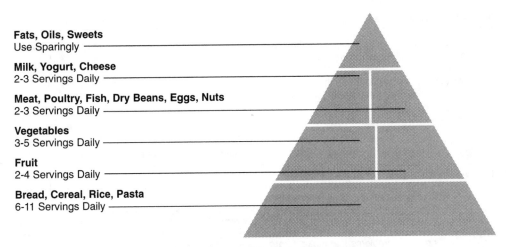

Fats, Oils, Sweets
Use Sparingly

Milk, Yogurt, Cheese
2-3 Servings Daily

Meat, Poultry, Fish, Dry Beans, Eggs, Nuts
2-3 Servings Daily

Vegetables
3-5 Servings Daily

Fruit
2-4 Servings Daily

Bread, Cereal, Rice, Pasta
6-11 Servings Daily

Source: U.S. Department of Agriculture/U.S. Department of Health and Human Services.

What Counts as a Serving?

Bread, Cereal, Rice, Pasta
- 1 slice of bread, ½ bagel or hamburger bun
- 1 ounce of ready-to-eat cereal
- ½ cup of cooked cereal, rice, or pasta

Vegetable
- 1 cup of raw leafy vegetables
- ½ cup of other vegetables, cooked or chopped raw
- ¾ cup of vegetable juice

Fruits
- 1 medium apple, banana, orange
- ½ cup of chopped cooked or canned fruit
- ¾ cup fruit juice

Milk, Yogurt and Cheese
- 1 cup of milk or yogurt
- 1 ½ ounces of natural cheese
- 2 ounces of processed cheese

Meat, Poultry, Fish, Dry Beans, Eggs, and Nuts
- 2-3 ounces of cooked lean meat, poultry, or fish
- ½ cup of cooked dry beans, 1 egg, or 2 tablespoons of peanut butter counts as 1 ounce of lean meat

Source: *Nutrition and Your Health: Dietary Guidelines for Americans,* 3rd ed. U.S. Department of Agriculture/
U.S. Department of Health and Human Services, 1990.

Figure 11.1 The Food Guide Pyramid

Table 11.4 Self-Assessment of Nutritional Health

The Warning Signs of poor nutritional health are often overlooked. Use this checklist to find out if you or someone you know is at nutritional risk.

Read the statements below. Circle the number in the yes column for those that apply to you or someone you know. For each yes answer, score the number in the box. Total your nutritional score.

	YES
I have an illness or condition that made me change the kind and/or amount of food I eat.	2
I eat fewer than 2 meals per day.	3
I eat few fruits or vegetables, or milk products.	2
I have 3 or more drinks of beer, liquor or wine almost every day.	2
I have tooth or mouth problems that make it hard for me to eat.	2
I don't always have enough money to buy the food I need.	4
I eat alone most of the time.	1
I take 3 or more different prescribed or over-the-counter drugs a day.	1
Without wanting to, I have lost or gained 10 pounds in the last 6 months.	2
I am not always physically able to shop, cook and/or feed myself.	2
TOTAL	

Total Your Nutritional Score. If it's—

0-2....................Good! Recheck your nutritional score in 6 months.

3-5....................You are at moderate nutritional risk. See what can be done to improve your eating habits and lifestyle. Your office on aging, senior nutrition program, senior citizens center or health department can help. Recheck your nutritional score in 3 months.

6 or more ....You are at high nutritional risk. Bring this checklist the next time you see your doctor, dietitian or other qualified health or social service professional. Talk with them about any problems you may have. Ask for help to improve your nutritional health.

Remember that warning signs suggest risk but do not represent diagnosis of any condition.

Used with permission. Nutrition Screening Initiative, a project of the American Academy of Family Physicians, the American Dietetic Association, and the National Council On the Aging, Inc., funded in part by Ross Products, a division of Abbott Laboratories.

Table 11.5 Warning Signs of Nutritional Deficiencies

The Self-Assessment of Nutritional Health is based on the warning signs described below. If your patient exhibits one or more warning signs, he or she may be at risk for nutritional deficiency.

Disease

Any disease, illness or chronic condition which causes you to change the way you eat, or makes it hard for you to eat, puts your nutritional health at risk. Four out of five adults have chronic diseases that are affected by diet. Confusion or memory loss that keeps getting worse is estimated to affect one out of five older adults. This can make it hard to remember what, when or if you've eaten. Feeling sad or depressed, which happens to about one in eight older adults, can cause big changes in appetite, digestion, energy level, weight and well-being.

Eating Poorly

Eating too little and eating too much both lead to poor health. Eating the same foods day after day or not eating fruit, vegetables, and milk products daily will also cause poor nutritional health. One in five adults skip meals daily. Only 13% of adults eat the minimum amount of fruit and vegetables needed. One in four older adults drink too much alcohol. Many health problems become worse if you drink more than one or two alcoholic beverages per day.

Tooth Loss/Mouth Pain

A healthy mouth, teeth and gums are needed to eat. Missing, loose or rotten teeth or dentures which don't fit well or cause mouth sores make it hard to eat.

Economic Hardship

As many as 40% of older Americans have incomes of less than $6,000 per year. Having less— or choosing to spend less—than $25-30 per week for food makes it very hard to get the foods you need to stay healthy.

Reduced Social Contact

One-third of all older people live alone. Being with people daily has a positive effect on morale, well-being and eating.

Multiple Medicines

Many older Americans must take medicines for health problems. Almost half of older Americans take multiple medicines daily. Growing old may change the way we respond to drugs. The more medicines you take, the greater the chance for side effects such as increased or decreased appetite, change in taste, constipation, weakness, drowsiness, diarrhea, nausea, and others. Vitamins or minerals, when taken in large doses, act like drugs and can cause harm. Alert your doctor to everything you take.

Involuntary Weight Loss/Gain

Losing or gaining a lot of weight when you are not trying to do so is an important warning sign that must not be ignored. Being overweight or underweight also increases your chance of poor health.

Needs Assistance in Self Care

Although most older people are able to eat, one of every five have trouble walking, shopping, buying and cooking food, especially as they get older.

Elder Years Above Age 80

Most older people lead full and productive lives. But as age increases, risk of frailty and health problems increase. Checking your nutritional health regularly makes good sense.

Used with permission. Nutrition Screening Initiative, a project of the American Academy of Family Physicians, the American Dietetic Association, and the National Council On the Aging, Inc., funded in part by Ross Products, a division of Abbott Laboratories.

Table 11.6 Recipe for Making Saline

1. Use 1 gallon of distilled water or boil 1 gallon of tap water for 5 minutes. *Do not use well water or sea water.*

2. Add 8 teaspoons of table salt to the distilled or boiled water.

3. Mix the solution well until the salt is completely dissolved. Be sure that the storage container and mixing utensil are clean (boiled).

Note: Cool to room temperature before using. This solution can be stored at room temperature in a tightly covered glass or plastic bottle for up to 1 week.

Pressure ulcer care

Three aspects of pressure ulcer care include cleansing, debridement, and dressing application. The purpose of cleansing the wound is to provide an optimum environment for wound healing to occur. Cleansing removes exudate, loose necrotic tissue, dressing residue, residual topical agents, and metabolic wastes. There are a variety of commercial wound cleansing agents available, but the safest agent to use is normal saline. Normal saline will not harm the new cells present in a healing wound. Normal saline can be purchased or made in the home (see Table 11.6 for directions on how to prepare normal saline solution at home). Professionals teaching patients about cleansing should assess the resources available in the home. If the water supply in the home is unsafe for drinking, it may be unsafe for use in the wound. Bottled water can be purchased to create the saline solution.

Pressure ulcers should be cleansed with each dressing change. The AHCPR Treatment Guideline recommends the use of irrigation pressures from 4 to 15 psi for safe and effective cleansing. A soft plastic 250-cc bottle of commercially prepared normal saline fitted with an irrigation cap provides approximately 4 to 5 psi when squeezed with full force (see Chapter 9 for use of this irrigation device). These containers can be used, cleaned, and refilled by patients and caregivers in the home environment. If the pressure ulcer contains necrotic tissue, debridement may be necessary. (See Tables 11.7 and 11.8 for charts that the patient and caregiver can use in pressure ulcer prevention and care.)

Patients or caregivers expected to perform dressing changes should be taught handwashing techniques, how to perform the dressing changes, how to store and care for the dressings, and how to dispose of the soiled dressings. In addition to local wound care,[23,24] the family needs to know how to relieve pressure in the home setting. They must be taught that a pressure-reducing device does not substitute for frequent repositioning. A pictorial illustration of the recommended positioning schedule can remind the caregiver to routinely turn the patient. Sole caregivers who cannot withstand an every-2-hour around-the-clock turning schedule should be taught to use the 30-degree laterally inclined position for nighttime hours (see Table 11.9). Because this position simultaneously relieves pressure on the trochanter and the sacrum, it is the position of choice if the patient must stay in the same position for an extended time.[25]

Table 11.7 Educating Your Patient on Pressure Ulcers, Prevention and Care

What are they? Pressure ulcers are red areas or sores on the skin. Pressure ulcers are also called bed sores, pressure sores and decubitus ulcers. The sores can occur over any bony part of the body such as heels, hips and back. There may be drainage or odor from these areas if they are deep.

What causes them? Pressure ulcers are caused from lying in one place "too long." The skin and body need blood to get oxygen and food. Pressure on the skin blocks the blood supply. If the blood supply is stopped for a long time, a red area may be seen over a bony part of the body. Pressure can cause ulcers in less than two hours. If the pressure is NOT removed, the red area will turn into a pressure ulcer or sore.

Who gets pressure ulcers? People who are sick or have been hurt may not be able to move. Because they are not able to move, they may get pressure ulcers.

What can be done to keep from getting pressure ulcers? Pressure ulcers are prevented by moving, turning or lifting in the bed or wheelchair.

DO ....move or turn every two hours.

DO ....make small turns in between turning every two hours.

DO ....use padding on the bed or chair.

DO ....use a trapeze to lift if possible.

DO ....look at the skin three times a day for any red areas or any skin change. A mirror may be used to look at the back of the legs. Ask someone to help if needed.

DO ....keep skin clean and dry.

DO ....keep bed sheets smooth.

DO ....use an extra sheet to help turn, lift or change position. This helps prevent sheet burns.

DO ....eat the right kind of food and drink a lot of fluids. Ask the nurse or doctor about special foods and vitamins.

DO ....ask the nurse or doctor about the use of lotions or medicines.

DO ....tell the nurse or doctor about changes or more drainage.

DO NOT..................sit on a rubber or plastic air ring.

DO NOT..................rub any sore areas.

DO NOT..................use heat on any pressure sore.

DO NOT..................sit in a chair more than two hours without shifting weight.

When to call the health care provider

Caregivers should notify a health care professional if any of the following problems occurs:

- bleeding that does not stop with pressure
- foul, odorous drainage
- increased redness or warmth of the skin surrounding the ulcer
- a fever over 101 degrees, especially if accompanied by chills
- generalized decrease in activity or alertness.[26]

Patients must be taught that healed pressure ulcers continue to be at risk for ulceration. The scar resulting from granulation and re-epithelialization of soft tissue

Table 11.8 Educating Your Patient on Ulcer Characteristics

Patients and caregivers should be taught to report characteristics of pressure ulcers systematically. Use of common terminology will facilitate communication between patient and professional and ensure that ulcer changes will be correctly identified.

Size
Identify the size of the ulcer by using these steps
1. Use a ruler or measuring tape to measure across the ulcer at the widest points. Take two measurements.
2. If there is no ruler available, a piece of paper or a string can be placed across the ulcer. A pencil mark on the paper or string identifies the width of the ulcer. These marks on the paper or string can be measured later.

Depth
Depth can be measured by gently inserting a gloved finger into the wound and rotating the finger to touch all the sides of the wound bed. Note on the gloved finger how far the finger can extend. When the finger is removed, a measurement is taken of the depth of insertion.

Color of wound bed
Red color usually means there is a good blood supply. When new tissue is growing to fill in the wound, new blood vessels are made to feed the new tissue. This is called "granulation" tissue. This tissue is said to have a "beefy red" appearance.
Yellow, cream, or light green color of stringy tissue in the ulcer usually is fibrous tissue that will need to be removed. If it is allowed to dry, it will become a dark black hard crust.
Black hard tissue is dead. It may need to be removed by the healthcare provider before healing can take place.

Location
Patients may have pressure ulcers in more than one area. The same characteristics should be assessed for each ulcer.

Drainage
Thickness, color, and odor of any drainage should be reported.

Swelling
The surrounding tissue should be felt with the back of the hand to check for increase in firmness or temperature. It should be examined for redness and swelling.

ulceration has only 80% of the tensile strength of normal body tissue. Lifelong surveillance of this tissue is necessary. Health care providers should discuss the rationale for treatment decisions with patients so that they will be able to make informed decisions about new treatment options.

Evaluation of learning

Evaluation of learning should reflect the achievement of goals and objectives.[12] Knowledge about pressure ulcer prevention and acquisition of necessary skills to use that knowledge should be evident by changes in behavior. Patients and caregivers should be able to verbalize the information and perform the procedures. Evaluation is ongoing. If the plan is underway and conditions change, the plan may have to be altered. For example, the type of dressing that was effective may no longer be avail-

Table 11.9 Teaching Caregivers the 30 Degree Laterally Inclined Position

1. Show the family/caregiver a picture of the 30-degree-angle side lying position. Point out that there is no pressure either on the hipbones (trochanter of the femur) or tailbone (sacrum).

2. Demonstrate the positioning technique by first moving the patient into the 30-degree-angle side lying position, then placing a pillow or wedge behind the patient to maintain the position.

3. Once the patient is properly positioned, have the caregiver slide a hand, palm upward under the patient's hip.

4. Tell the caregiver to feel how the weight of the body rests on the fleshy part of the buttocks, not on the hipbone.

5. Return the patient to a back lying position. Have the caregiver correctly position the patient while you provide verbal coaching. Once the patient is positioned, have the caregiver repeat the handcheck to validate the correct position.

able or affordable. The patient may develop a medical problem that necessitates changing the plan. The patient should be asked to evaluate the teaching methods. A modification or combination of methods may produce better results.

Summary

Recognizing the need for education in health care is the responsibility of the learner and the educator. Through experience, educators identify essential information and necessary skills for care of patients with pressure ulcers. Using a variety of educational techniques and methods increases the effectiveness of the learning experience. Setting realistic goals must be done with the patient and caregiver. The learner is responsible for incorporating newly acquired knowledge and skills into useful behavior. The AHCPR Pressure Ulcer Prevention and Treatment guides provide a basis for patients and professionals to build individualized educational programs. In addition to pressure relief, patients and families need to know how to reduce the pressure ulcer risk factors. Adequate nutrition, management of incontinence, good body hygiene, skin care maintenance, and relief of pressure are topics that need to be reviewed on every nursing visit.[27,28]

The purpose of education is to facilitate the patient's understanding of the pressure ulcer problem, encourage participation in decision making, maximize skills, and promote a healthful lifestyle. Educating patients about risk factors, pressure ulcer prevention, and pressure ulcer management gives them the power to manage their own care and to oversee the care others provide for them.

References

1. O'Connor, F.W., et al. "Enhancing Surgical Nurses' Patient Education: Development and Evaluation of an Intervention," *Patient Education & Counseling* 16: 21-28, 1990.

2. Cargill, J.M. "Medication Compliance in Elderly People: Influencing Variables and Interventions," *Journal of Advanced Nursing* 17: 422-426, 1992.

3. Goldstein, N.I. "Patient Learning Center Reduces Patient Readmissions," *Patient Education and Counseling* 17: 177-190, 1991.

4. Baharestani, M.M. "The Lived Experience of Wives Caring for Their Frail, Homebound, Elderly Husbands with Pressure Ulcers," *Advances in Wound Care* 7(3): 40-52, 1994.

5. Wikblad, K.F. "Patient Perspectives of Diabetes Care and Education," *Journal of Advanced Nursing* 16: 837-844, 1991.

6. Faller, N.A. "Patient Education: Patient Willingness vs. Nursing Skill," *Ostomy/Wound Management* 40(7): 32-40, 1994.

7. Knowles, M.S. "Adult Learning," in Craig, R.L. *Training and Development Handbook: A Guide to Human Resource Development,* 3rd ed. New York: McGraw-Hill, 1987.

8. Carpenito, L.J. *Nursing Diagnosis: Application to Clinical Practice,* 5th ed. Philadelphia: J.B. Lippincott, 1994.

9. Maklebust, J., and Magnan, M.A. "Approaches to Patient and Family Education for Pressure Ulcer Management," *Decubitus* 5(7): 18-28, 1992.

10. Redman, B.K. *The Process of Patient Education,* 6th ed. St. Louis: C.V. Mosby Company, 1988.

11. Ballie, V., et al. "Stress, Social Support and Psychological Distress of Family Caregivers of the Elderly," *Nursing Research* 37: 217-222, 1988.

12. Barnes, S.H. "Patient/Family Education for the Patient with a Pressure Necrosis," *Nursing Clinics of North America* 22(2): 463-474, 1987.

13. Gianella, A. "Effective Teaching and Learning Strategies for Adults," in Abruzzese, R.S., ed. *Nursing Staff Development: Strategies for Success.* St. Louis: C.V. Mosby, 1992.

14. Seburn, M. "Home-Team Strategies for Treating Pressure Sores," *Nursing* (4): 50-53, 1987.

15. "SMOG Readability Formula." United States Department of Health and Human Services: Pretesting in Health Communications NIH Pub No 84-1493, Washington, D.C.: U.S. Government Printing Office, 1984.

16. "Preventing Pressure Ulcers: A Patient's Guide." AHCPR Patient Care Guidelines. Publication No. 92-0048. Rockville, Md.: Agency for Health Care Policy and Research. Public Health Service, U.S. Department of Health and Human Services, 1992.

17. "Treating Pressure Sores." AHCPR Patient Care Guidelines. Publication No. 92-0047. Rockville, Md.: Agency for Health Care Policy and Research. Public Health Service, U.S. Department of Health and Human Services, 1994.

18. King, R.B. "Assessment and Management of Soft Tissue Pressure," in Martin, N., et al., eds. *Comprehensive Rehabilitation Nursing.* New York: McGraw-Hill, 1981.

19. "Managing Urinary Incontinence." AHCPR Publication No. Rockville, Md.: Agency for Health Care Policy and Research. Public Health Service. U.S. Department of Health and Human Services, 1993.

20. Verdell, L.L. *Resource Guide of Continence Products and Services,* 5th ed. Union, S.C.: Help for Incontinent People, 1992.

21. Breslow, R. "Nutritional Status and Dietary Intake of Patients with Pressure Ulcers: Review of Research Literature 1943 to 1989," *Decubitus* 4: 16-21, 1991.

22. Parsons, Y. "Healing More than Wounds," *Contemporary Long Term Care* 18(6): 57-76, 1995.

23. Weingarten, M.S. "Obstacles to Wound Healing," *Wounds* 5: 238-244, 1993.

24. National Research Council. *Recommended Dietary Allowances,* 10th ed. Washington, D.C.: National Academy Press, 1989.

25. *The Nutrition Checklist.* Washington, D.C.: The Nutrition Screening Initiative.

26. Watterworth, B., and Podrasky, D.L. "Meeting the Needs of the Person Discharged Home with an Open Wound," *Journal of Enterostomal Therapy* 16(1): 12-15, 1989.

27. Barr, J.E. "Standards of Care, Alteration in Skin Integrity: The Pressure Ulcer," *Journal of Enterostomal Therapy* 16(1): 16-20, 1989.

28. Seiler, W.O., et al. "Influence of the Thirty Degree Laterally Inclined Position and the "Super-Soft" Three Piece Mattress on Skin Oxygen Tension on Areas of Maximum Pressure: Implications for Pressure Sore Prevention," *Gerontology* 32: 158-166, 1986.

Continuous Quality Improvement

The 1990s have seen a transition from traditional quality assurance (QA) to continuous quality improvement (CQI). With CQI, there is a shift from the reactive approach of QA to a proactive approach. QA efforts began when a measured indicator fell below an established threshold. The 10% outliers of care were identified and corrective actions taken. With CQI, the entire performance curve is shifted upward. Surveillance of the 10% of care that falls below the accepted norm is continued, but the 90% of acceptable care also is monitored to make it even better. The transition from QA to CQI involves moving defect detection to defect prevention, while making continuous improvements in the processes concerned with the delivery of care. Continuous improvement can be made in two types of processes: operational and/or clinical.[1,2]

QA efforts traditionally focused on outcomes. CQI focuses on processes used to accomplish outcomes. CQI operates under a philosophy that when quality fails, the process is at fault.[3] When the process is improved, outcomes improve as a result. When selecting opportunities for continuous improvement, Mozena and Anderson[4] recommend that priority be given to high-volume, high-risk, problem-prone areas. Pressure ulcers fall into this category. The AHCPR Clinical Practice Guideline for Pressure Ulcer Treatment[5] directs clinicians to gain agency administrative support for pressure ulcer management as a major aspect of care.

Pressure ulcer quality improvement committee

Pressure ulcer management is most efficient if there is a Pressure Ulcer or Skin Care Committee of interested and knowledgeable people. Agency team members vary, depending on the patient setting. Nurses, physicians, dietitians, physical therapists, social workers, discharge planners, quality improvement specialists, and infection control practitioners compose many skin care committees. Staff nurses should be included in order to gain input and effect change among bedside caregivers. One person should serve as committee chairperson, and that person must have strong administrative support.

Pressure ulcer committee members should develop, implement, and evaluate pressure ulcer educational and quality improvement programs. Most pressure ulcer quality improvement programs have the following components:

• A measurement component that determines the size and severity of the problem, including agency pressure ulcer prevalence and incidence

• A risk assessment component that determines the population at risk for pressure ulcers

• A policy and procedure component that specifies agency pressure ulcer standards and treatment protocols

• A monitoring component to evaluate the clinical and operational processes associated with pressure ulcer management.

Operational processes are those that produce a service or a product for an internal or external customer. A CQI project might focus on improving operational processes to obtain supplies from pharmacy or central supply. Clinical processes focus on medical or therapeutic processes that improve a person's health, such as pressure ulcer management.[4] Specific aspects of clinical processes might be related to staff competence in care or value analysis of pressure ulcer dressing products or support surfaces. In order to improve processes associated with pressure ulcer management, support must be provided by clinical departments and nonclinical departments, such as data management, utilization management, purchasing, pharmacy, and central supply.[6]

Improving the pressure ulcer cost and quality equation

Pressure ulcers impact the cost of care, reimbursement, and quality of life. Assessment of agency prevalence rates, patient risk profile, standardization of therapy protocols, and increased staff awareness can positively impact the balance between cost and quality patient outcomes. A multidisciplinary team can positively impact this equation if given the authority to impact clinical and financial decisions.[7]

Measuring pressure ulcer prevalence and incidence rates

Pressure ulcer prevalence has been measured in acute, long-term, and home care settings. At Harper Hospital in the Detroit Medical Center, the Pressure Ulcer Quality Improvement Committee measures pressure ulcer prevalence twice yearly. All nursing units receive pressure ulcer audit instruction sheets (see Table 12.1), pressure ulcer data collection forms (see Table 12.2), and measuring grids to assess pressure ulcer dimensions. Every staff nurse caregiver inspects the skin of each assigned patient for that day. Every pressure ulcer found by the nurse caregiver is validated by another nurse. All pressure ulcers are recorded on the data collection forms. The depth, length, and width of each ulcer is determined and recorded. Relevant patient risk factors are identified by circling them on the data collection form. If nutritional consultation has been done or the patient is using pressure ulcer prevention products, this information also is recorded. Unit managers collect the completed data collection forms from their respective nursing units and take them to a central location in the nursing office for data analysis.

A second data collection form, the pressure ulcer medical record audit sheet, was designed to assess the medical record of patients with pressure ulcers in order to determine the accuracy of pressure ulcer documentation (see Table 12.3). Members of

(Text continued on page 252)

Table 12.1 Pressure Ulcer Audit Instruction Sheet

These steps should be followed for each patient on your unit. The data collection tool *must be completed by the staff nurse caring for the patient.*

1. STAMP PRESSURE ULCER DATA COLLECTION TOOL WITH ADDRESSOGRAPH PLATE.

2. CAREFULLY READ INSTRUCTIONS ON DATA COLLECTION FORM.

3. ASSESS EACH PATIENT'S ENTIRE BODY FOR PRESSURE ULCERS.
   (Do not include venous stasis ulcers, tape burns, skin lesions not caused by pressure, or skin irritation from incontinence)

4. IF PRESSURE ULCER IS PRESENT:

   a. Assess each ulcer for stage. (Redness that does not disappear when pressure is relieved is considered Stage I and should be recorded.)

   b. Measure each ulcer's length and width in centimeters (using Measuring Grid).

   c. Indicate where each ulcer was acquired (e.g., home, hospital).

   d. Complete Side 2 of audit form in its entirety.

   e. Date and sign the audit sheet.

5. If NO pressure ulcer is present, check the "No Pressure Ulcer" box.

   a. Complete Side 2 of the data collection form in its entirety.

   b. Date and sign the data collection.

6. Place the form in the designated area on your unit for Administrative Manager, CNS/Case Manager, or ET nurse to validate.

NOTE: DO assess ALL patients on your unit on the day shift.

    DO NOT include afternoon admissions.

    DO include patients being discharged.

    DO include patients going to the OR (assess them before they leave the unit).

Table 12.2 Pressure Ulcer Data Collection Form

1. <u>DO YOU THINK THE PATIENT IS AT RISK FOR PRESSURE ULCERS?</u>   YES ❑   NO ❑

2. <u>INSTRUCTIONS:</u>

   A. Read Pressure Ulcer Audit Instructions posted on unit.

   B. Inspect entire body from head to toe.

   C. Assess skin condition at each body site on numbered figure.

   D. Use stage key to determine stage of pressure ulcer and record after appropriate number at right.

   E. Measure and record the size of each pressure ulcer in cm.

   F. Indicate where each ulcer was acquired.

   G. Complete <u>BOTH SIDES</u> of audit sheet.

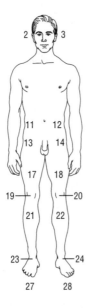 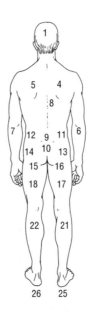

Stage Key

Stage 0	No redness or breakdown
Stage 1	Erythema only: redness that does not blanch
Stage 2	Break in skin such as blisters or abrasions
Stage 3	Break in skin exposing subcutaneous tissue
Stage 4	Break in skin tissue extending through tissue and subcutaneous layers, exposing muscle or bone
Stage 9	Non-stageable (Wound bed can't be observed)

(continued)

Table 12.2 Pressure Ulcer Data Collection Form *(continued)*

	Stage	Size (in cm)	Indicate Where Each Ulcer Was Acquired				
			Harper Hospital	Another Hospital	Nursing Home	Home	Unknown
1) Back of head	_____	_____	_____	_____	_____	_____	_____
2) Right ear	_____	_____	_____	_____	_____	_____	_____
3) Left ear	_____	_____	_____	_____	_____	_____	_____
4) Right scapula	_____	_____	_____	_____	_____	_____	_____
5) Left scapula	_____	_____	_____	_____	_____	_____	_____
6) Right elbow	_____	_____	_____	_____	_____	_____	_____
7) Left elbow	_____	_____	_____	_____	_____	_____	_____
8) Vertebrae (upper-mid)	_____	_____	_____	_____	_____	_____	_____
9) Sacrum	_____	_____	_____	_____	_____	_____	_____
10) Coccyx	_____	_____	_____	_____	_____	_____	_____
11) Right iliac crest	_____	_____	_____	_____	_____	_____	_____
12) Left iliac crest	_____	_____	_____	_____	_____	_____	_____
13) Right trochanter (hip)	_____	_____	_____	_____	_____	_____	_____
14) Left trochanter (hip)	_____	_____	_____	_____	_____	_____	_____
15) Right ischial tuberosity	_____	_____	_____	_____	_____	_____	_____
16) Left ischial tuberosity	_____	_____	_____	_____	_____	_____	_____
17) Right thigh (front/back)	_____	_____	_____	_____	_____	_____	_____
18) Left thigh (front/back)	_____	_____	_____	_____	_____	_____	_____
19) Right knee	_____	_____	_____	_____	_____	_____	_____
20) Left knee	_____	_____	_____	_____	_____	_____	_____
21) Right lower leg (front/back)	_____	_____	_____	_____	_____	_____	_____
22) Left lower leg (front/back)	_____	_____	_____	_____	_____	_____	_____
23) Right ankle (inner/outer)	_____	_____	_____	_____	_____	_____	_____
24) Left ankle (inner/outer)	_____	_____	_____	_____	_____	_____	_____
25) Right heel	_____	_____	_____	_____	_____	_____	_____
26) Left heel	_____	_____	_____	_____	_____	_____	_____
27) Right toe(s)	_____	_____	_____	_____	_____	_____	_____
28) Left toe(s)	_____	_____	_____	_____	_____	_____	_____
29) Other (specify)	_____	_____	_____	_____	_____	_____	_____

30) NO PRESSURE ULCER ☐

(continued)

Table 12.2 Pressure Ulcer Data Collection Form *(continued)*

31) Is the patient using a pressure-relieving device?   Yes ❑   No ❑
    If yes:
    A. Vascular Boot ❑
    B. Sof-Care bed cushion ❑
       On manual check, is the Sof-Care adequately inflated? Yes ❑   No ❑

    C. Special bed (specify type:) _____

    D. Other (specify:) _____

32) Is there a **completed pink nutrition assessment form**
    in the medical record?   Yes ❑   No ❑

33) The following list contains factors that increase the risk for developing pressure ulcers. Circle all
    that apply to your patient.
    1) Decreased mental status
    2) Impaired mobility
    3) Malnutrition
    4) Fecal incontinence
    5) Urinary incontinence
    6) Diabetes
    7) Vascular disease
    8) Spinal cord injury
    9) Multiple sclerosis
    10) Metastatic CA

Date: _____

Signature:_____

Title: _____

Validating Nurse: _____

Table 12.3 Pressure Ulcer Medical Record Audit Sheet

Date:_____

Time:_____ | Addressograph

	YES	NO	N/A	COMMENTS
IF ULCER WAS ACQUIRED OUTSIDE OF HOSPITAL:				
1. Is it documented on the Admission Data Base? (include date)				
2. Is there a Nursing Diagnosis and Plan of Care including pressure relief? (indicate date written)				
3. Is there evidence that interventions were carried out? (Shift Assessment, Nursing Notes, etc.)				
4. Was a pressure-relief device applied? (indicate date)				
IF ULCER WAS ACQUIRED AT HOSPITAL:				
1. Was there a High-Risk For Impaired Skin/Tissue Integrity Nursing Diagnosis and Plan of Care prior to the ulcer formation, including preventive measures?				
2. Was a pressure-relief device applied?				
3. Indicate date and nursing unit where pressure ulcer was first identified.				
4. Is there an Impaired Tissue Integrity Plan of Care including pressure relief and local wound care? (indicate date written)				
5. Is there evidence that the interventions were carried out? (Shift Assessment, Nursing Progress Notes, etc.)				

Signature of Validator: _____

the Pressure Ulcer Quality Improvement Committee reviewed the charts of those patients who had pressure ulcers within 24 hours of pressure ulcer measurement. The tool was used to determine whether or not nursing documentation supported onset of the ulcer (preadmission or unit-specific origin); description of the ulcer; treatment plan, including pressure relief and local wound care; and evidence that care was delivered according to the plan of care. Committee members tabulated and analyzed the data, which then were distributed to managers in tabular format (see Table 12.4).

Because pressure ulcer data can be interpreted in several ways, there is concern about the accuracy of some statistics.[8] When reporting data, it is important to include as much information as possible so that others will know exactly what the data mean. While it is important to report the number of ulcers within each stage, it is equally important to include the agency definitions for each pressure ulcer stage. Many pressure ulcer reports do not indicate whether or not nonblanchable reddened areas are counted as Stage I ulcers.

Prevalence

It is important to differentiate between pressure ulcer prevalence and incidence. Agency pressure ulcer prevalence reflects the total number of patients with pressure

Table 12.4 Pressure Ulcer Audit Report Form

SERVICE / CENSUS	NUMBER OF PATIENTS WITH ULCERS	TOTAL NUMBER OF PRESSURE ULCERS	STAGES					
			1	2	3	4	9	
Oncology /								
Medicine /								
Surgery /								
Cardiology / Critical Care/								
TOTALS /								

TOTAL = Prevalence Rate (ALL PRESSURE ULCER PATIENTS IN HOSPITAL ON DAY OF AUDIT)

Percentage of Ulcers Acquired at Harper Hospital =

ulcers on any given day. This includes all patients with pressure ulcers, regardless of where the ulcers were acquired.[8] Data are reported in percentage of patients with pressure ulcers per number of the patient population included in data collection. The formula for calculating a pressure ulcer prevalence rate is given below.

$$\text{PU Prevalence Rate} = \frac{\text{Number of patients with pressure ulcers on data collection day}}{\text{Number of patients in agency included in data collection}} \times 100$$

Incidence

Pressure ulcer incidence reflects the number of patients who acquire pressure ulcers while in the care of a given agency.[8] This can be determined only by assessing patients admitted without pressure ulcers and monitoring them over time to see if they develop pressure ulcers during their admission. Data are reported in percentages of patients developing pressure ulcers during a specified period per number of patient admissions for that period. Incidence can be calculated for an individual nursing

	HARPER HOSPITAL ACQUIRED ULCERS	OTHER HOSPITAL ACQUIRED ULCERS	NURSING HOME ACQUIRED ULCERS	HOME ACQUIRED ULCERS	SOURCE OF ULCERS UNKNOWN

NATIONAL ACUTE CARE PREVALENCE RATE = 5%-11%

NATIONAL ACUTE CARE INCIDENCE RATE = 1%-5%

unit or an entire agency. One formula for calculating a pressure ulcer incidence rate is given below.

$$\text{PU Incidence Rate} = \frac{\text{Total number of patients developing pressure ulcers per period}}{\text{Total number of patients admitted per period}} \times 100$$

Allman[9] believes a more accurate way to determine pressure ulcer incidence is to determine the number of patients at risk for pressure ulcers and then calculate the percentage of those patients who develop pressure ulcers within a specified time period. The formula to calculate pressure ulcer incidence using only at-risk patients is given below.

$$\text{PU Incidence Rate} = \frac{\text{Number of at-risk patients developing pressure ulcers per period}}{\text{Number of at-risk patients admitted per period}} \times 100$$

Once pressure ulcer prevalence and incidence rates are determined, it is important to compare data against national norms. Prevalence and/or incidence trends can be recorded on a graph for visual reinforcement (see Figure 12.1). In order to demonstrate a more complete picture, prevalence or incidence data can be shown in bar graphs or pie charts categorized by pressure ulcer stage (see Figure 12.2).

Each agency should determine intended improvements based on baseline data.[5] This means determining pre-established standards so that appropriateness of treatment can be evaluated and necessary changes can be made. Improvements may include changing policies and procedures, educating or redistributing staff, altering use of equipment and supplies, or correcting communication processes. If the incidence of pressure ulcers is lowered by instituting a pressure ulcer program, an agency usually can continue to improve outcomes by continuing to improve operational and clinical processes.

Various agencies have reported successes with continuous quality improvement. The entire resident population of one long-term care facility was followed for 4 years.[10] Protocols for quality improvement reduced the prevalence rate from 7% in 1988 to 4% in 1992. The average percentage of residents who developed pressure ulcers while in the long-term care facility was 3.4%, the majority of which were Stage I or Stage II ulcers. The 816-bed Jewish Home and Hospital for the Aged in the Bronx reports that a quality improvement approach to pressure ulcer management

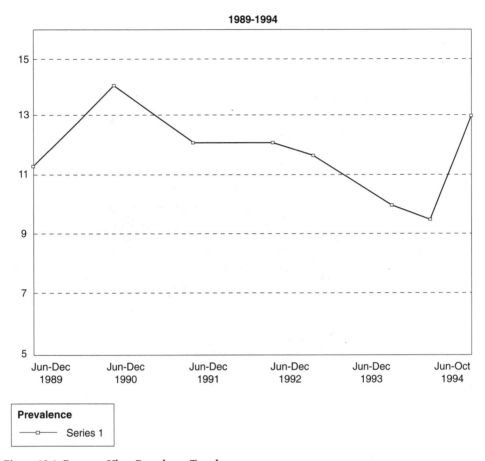

Figure 12.1 Pressure Ulcer Prevalence Trends

resulted in a nosocomial pressure ulcer prevalence rate of 3.1%. The authors believe that pressure ulcers are an ideal clinical entity for application of CQI principles.[11] A retrospective chart review of spinal cord-injured patients who developed pressure ulcers during an 18-month period revealed that 7.4% (35 of 468 patients) developed a total of 81 pressure ulcers. Newly injured patients, patients with longstanding spinal cord injury, and patients who used condom catheters appeared to have the most problems with pressure ulceration.[12] CQI processes were planned to address problems with these patients. In an acute-care example, a cluster of operating room-acquired pressure ulcers on cardiovascular patients led to a quality improvement project to search for the cause. It was determined that the severity of the problem warranted design of new pressure-reducing operating room table pads. No further incidences occurred after the new table pads were in place.[13]

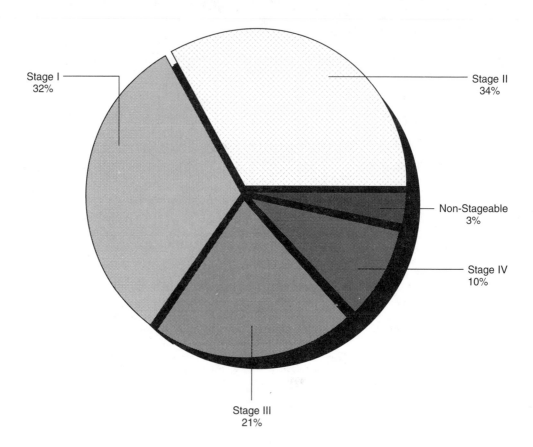

Figure 12.2 Pressure Ulcer Prevalence by Stage

Improving pressure ulcer outcomes with risk assessment

It is beneficial for an agency to determine the percentage of patients who are at risk for pressure ulceration. This allows for planning of human and material resources to lower the risk and improve outcomes. Incorporating risk assessment scales into a daily clinical flowsheet is an important way to detect changes in patient risk status. The pressure ulcer risk assessment scale must be simple to use to ensure that it will be completed. In today's climate of restructured health care delivery and patient-focused care, there will be fewer professional caregivers at the bedside. It is important for nurses to delegate collection of specific patient data and then have adequate time to interpret the clinical significance of data collected.

Analyzing pressure ulcer risk factors that impact an agency population can lead to natural improvements in care processes to compensate for risk. Gawron[14] reported risk factors for and prevalence of pressure ulcers among patients hospitalized in a university-based setting. A pressure ulcer prevalence rate was reported as 12%.

For patients who were determined to be at moderate risk on the Braden Scale, most were not placed on therapeutic support surfaces. As a quality improvement measure, pressure ulcer prevention practices will be closely monitored. At Harper Hospital in the Detroit Medical Center, the relationship between pressure ulcer risk factor and pressure ulceration was examined by secondarily analyzing pressure ulcer data collected from five hospital-wide prevalence measurements.[15] Pooled data showed a pressure ulcer prevalence rate of 12.3%. The most frequently occurring risk factor was immobility; however, immobility was not the risk factor associated with the greatest odds of acquiring a pressure ulcer. Because Harper nurses use pressure-reducing surfaces for immobile patients, it is suspected that the nursing staff may have compensated for the risk of impaired mobility. The risk factor with the greatest odds for causing a pressure ulcer was fecal incontinence. The odds of having a pressure ulcer were 22 times greater in patients who were fecally incontinent compared to patients who were not fecally incontinent. Patients with pressure ulcers who were fecally incontinent also had a greater number of pressure ulcers than patients who were not fecally incontinent. Based on analysis of these data, a new skin care program was developed to protect the skin from caustic fecal enzymes. Skin/wound care flowcharts were developed (see the Appendices), and the process was computerized so that nurses could independently order appropriate products from pharmacy or central supply while simultaneously printing an order on the patient kardex. A similar process could be used to reduce the risk for any relevant pressure ulcer risk factor.

Lyder et al[16] tested the efficacy of a structured skin care regimen to prevent perineal dermatitis in elderly incontinent patients. All subjects who had perineal dermatitis were incontinent of both urine and stool and were wearing adult diapers. While the results showed that nurses used their own preferred methods of skin care for incontinent patients, implications for nursing indicate that it is vitally important to keep moisture and feces away from patients' skin. After involving staff nurses in development and quality monitoring of a skin care protocol, Kravitz[17] noted a high level of compliance by both nurses and physicians. Frequently, staff at the bedside are best at developing patient-related protocols. Not only do they claim ownership of protocols that they design, but, if they believe it makes a difference, they also will make the process successful.

Pressure ulcer standards of care

The Pressure Ulcer Guidelines released by the Agency for Health Care Policy and Research (AHCPR) represent the best scientific information available for pressure ulcer prevention[18] and treatment.[5] The multidisciplinary pressure ulcer guideline panels wrote the guidelines after conducting extensive literature searches, hearing public testimony, and examining information provided by consultants. The guidelines are designed to enhance the quality, appropriateness, and effectiveness of care. Prior to the release of the AHCPR pressure ulcer guidelines, Harper Hospital was selected as a pilot site to test the national guidelines. As a result of the pilot project, the Pres-

sure Ulcer Quality Improvement Committee incorporated guideline recommendations into Harper Hospital Pressure Ulcer Standards of Care (see Table 12.5). The
standards are generic enough to allow individualization of patient care. Protocols,
policies, procedures, and patient documentation records elaborate more specific
clinical and operational processes of care. (See Chapter 9 for Harper protocols, policies, procedures, and documentation format.)

Implementing research-based findings can promote reduction in agency costs. A
study showed that 1-year treatment costs were $30,079 for 81 pressure ulcers in an
830-bed, long-term care facility following implementation of a research-based standard skin care protocol based on the AHCPR pressure ulcer prevention guideline.
Approximately 70% of these costs were attributable to nursing care. Mean cost of
the pressure ulcer treatment was $3.74/day after instituting the standard skin care
protocol, compared to $5.35/day prior to implementing the standard protocol.[19]

Improving processes associated with pressure ulcer management

Clinician education

The AHCPR Pressure Ulcer Guidelines[5,18] spell out the recommended content of
pressure ulcer education programs for health care providers involved with pressure
ulcer prevention and treatment. There is an extensive amount of information to re-
lay to caregivers. Educational content needs to be geared to various levels of learners. Agencies will need educational resources to assist in disseminating information
to personnel, patients, and families. The National Pressure Ulcer Advisory Panel
(NPUAP) developed slide sets to augment the AHCPR Pressure Ulcer Guidelines.
They are valuable for staff education. The slides contain clinical photographs of patients being cared for at agencies in various settings. To facilitate agency inservices,
each slide set is accompanied by a companion script. For information on how to obtain a set of slides, call NPUAP at 716-881-3358.

There are several ways in which the AHCPR Pressure Ulcer Prevention Guidelines
will impact nursing practice.[20] Some aspects of recommended care have been a part
of daily practice for many years. Other guideline recommendations will require
changes in usual nursing practice. For instance, massaging a patient's skin over bony
prominences to increase circulation has been a time-honored tradition in nursing.
Now, scientific evidence demonstrates that massaging skin over bony prominences
may be harmful to soft tissue.[21] Another example that may be unfamiliar to caregivers is the proper way to position and reposition patients. For many years, nurses
have been taught to turn bedbound patients from one side to another every 2 hours.
Now, there is research-based evidence that patients should not be placed on the
greater trochanter of the femur but instead in a 30-degree laterally inclined position
to avoid pressure over the bony prominence of the hip.[22] This 30-degree sidelying
position needs to be shown and demonstrated to bedside caregivers.

The Pressure Ulcer Treatment Guideline[5] specifies accurate wound assessment,

Table 12.5 Standards of Care for Prevention and Treatment of Pressure Ulcers

Standard for Pressure Ulcer Prevention

■ All patients with mobility or activity deficits will have a formal risk assessment tool administered to determine pressure ulcer risk.

■ All patients at risk will have a systematic skin assessment at least once daily.

■ Skin exposure to pressure, friction, shear, and moisture will be minimized.

■ At-risk patients will be repositioned according to their tissue tolerance.

■ At-risk patients will be placed on pressure-reducing surfaces.

■ At-risk patients' nutritional status will be assessed for adequacy.

■ At-risk patients and caregivers will be taught pressure ulcer prevention techniques.

■ Pressure ulcer prevention interventions and patient/family instruction will be documented.

Standard for Pressure Ulcer Treatment

■ Patients with pressure ulcers will have prevention standards instituted.

■ Pressure ulcers will be assessed for stage, size, condition, etiology, duration, and previous treatment.

■ Condition of skin surrounding pressure ulcers will be assessed.

■ Pressure ulcers with necrotic tissue will be assessed for need of debridement.

■ Pressure ulcers will be cleansed with physiologic solutions.

■ Pressure ulcers will be protected with appropriate dressings.

■ Pressure ulcers will be reassessed with each dressing change for improvement or deterioration.

■ Pressure ulcer treatment and patient outcomes will be documented.

■ Patients and families will be educated about pressure ulcer treatment.

appropriate wound irrigation pressure, and correct techniques for culturing wounds. It also differentiates colonization from infection and indicates toxicities of various topical treatments. Recommended infection control practices support use of clean, no-touch technique rather than sterile technique for pressure ulcer care. All of these recommendations need to be transferred to the caregiver level. It is a formidable task to educate all caregivers, but the guideline itself provides a good start by giving a rationale for each guideline recommendation.

Agencies can begin by inservicing nursing personnel taking direct care of patients, and nurses can be messengers for the other disciplines. Moody et al[23] demonstrated that education of caregivers alone was responsible for reducing the incidence and severity of pressure ulcers in hospitalized patients. Pre-testing and post-testing is a good way to determine if provider knowledge is gained from didactic or videotaped information. To determine the effectiveness of a teaching plan designed to increase a hospital staff's knowledge of pressure ulcer risk, assessment, and treatment, 102 RNs, LPNs, and nursing assistants were randomly selected and assigned to experimental or control groups. Both groups completed a 100-item pretest. The experimental group then was taught pressure ulcer risk, assessment, and treatment before completing a post-test. The control group viewed a videotape on general aspects of skin care for hospitalized patients before completing a post-test. There was no significant difference in pretest scores; however, post-test scores were significantly higher in the experimental group, both in total score and in subscores of risk, assessment, and treatment. The authors concluded that staff post-test knowledge improved when teaching was based on current pressure ulcer literature.[24]

It is helpful if bedside clinicians first are taught the relevant knowledge and then precepted clinically to determine competency in pressure ulcer prevention and management. Cardy[25] developed a clinical competency tool for preceptor documentation of pressure ulcer prevention and management (see Table 12.6). Studies of changes in nurses' behavior after continuing education showed that support from colleagues and superiors is the most important determinant of ongoing behavioral change in nursing practice.[26]

Value analysis of pressure ulcer products

Quality improvement includes measuring and analyzing the value of products used in a pressure ulcer management program.

Support surfaces

Understanding the principles of pressure relief assists in evaluating various support surfaces on the market. Pressure-reducing equipment options range from inexpensive, 1-inch, convoluted foam products to expensive, sophisticated specialty beds.[27,28] The effectiveness of a pressure-relieving device is not necessarily reflected by the cost of the product.[29,30]

The magnitude of pressure at the support surface/tissue interface must be considered when choosing products for pressure relief. Tissue interface pressures have

Table 12.6 Clinical Competency Tool

Clinician Signature: _____

Title/Department: _____

Intervention	Initial & Date—(Clinician)		Initial & Date—(Preceptor)
	Verbalized Knowledge	**Demonstrate Skill**	
1. Identifies clients at risk for loss of skin integrity.	_____	_____	_____
2. Completes risk assessment tool.	_____	_____	_____
3. Completes a thorough skin assessment.	_____	_____	_____
4. Develops and implements plan of care to maintain and improve skin integrity.			
- cleansing and remoisturizing	_____	_____	_____
- positioning (bed and chair)	_____	_____	_____
- support surface	_____	_____	_____
- nutritional support	_____	_____	_____
- management of incontinence	_____	_____	_____
- encourage mobility	_____	_____	_____
- minimize shear and friction	_____	_____	_____
- pain control	_____	_____	_____
- appropriate transfer	_____	_____	_____
5. Initiates appropriate referrals to consults.			
- nurse	_____	_____	_____
- physician	_____	_____	_____
- dietitian	_____	_____	_____
- pharmacy	_____	_____	_____
- physical therapy	_____	_____	_____
- enterostomal therapist	_____	_____	_____
- pharmacist	_____	_____	_____
- infection control	_____	_____	_____
6. Appropriately stages and identifies characteristics of a wound.			
- stage	_____	_____	_____
- size	_____	_____	_____
- undermining/tunneling	_____	_____	_____
- eschar	_____	_____	_____
- slough	_____	_____	_____
- drainage	_____	_____	_____
- hyperplasia	_____	_____	_____
- granulation	_____	_____	_____
- epithelialization	_____	_____	_____
- erythema	_____	_____	_____
- location	_____	_____	_____
- surrounding tissue	_____	_____	_____
- depth	_____	_____	_____
7. Identifies characteristics of wound healing physiology	_____	_____	_____
8. Differentiates clean, contaminated, and infected wounds.	_____	_____	_____
9. Demonstrates and discusses selective versus non-selective debridement.			
- surgical	_____	_____	_____
- autolytic	_____	_____	_____
- chemical	_____	_____	_____
- mechanical	_____	_____	_____

(continued)

Table 12.6 Clinical Competency Tool *(continued)*

Intervention	Initial & Date—(Clinician)		Initial & Date—(Preceptor)
	Verbalized Knowledge	Demonstrate Skill	
10. Identifies the goal of moist wound therapy in wounds that are:	_____	_____	_____
- granular, draining	_____	_____	_____
- granular, non-draining	_____	_____	_____
- necrotic, draining	_____	_____	_____
- necrotic, non-draining	_____	_____	_____
11. Selects and appropriately implements use of moist wound therapy dressings and cleansers.	_____	_____	_____
- surfactant	_____	_____	_____
- saline	_____	_____	_____
- transparent film	_____	_____	_____
- hydrocolloid	_____	_____	_____
- foam	_____	_____	_____
- skin protectant	_____	_____	_____
- hydrogel/gels	_____	_____	_____
- absorptive fillers	_____	_____	_____
- alginates	_____	_____	_____
12. Demonstrates the use of devices to control incontinence.	_____	_____	_____
- intermittent catheterization	_____	_____	_____
- indwelling catheterization	_____	_____	_____
- external catheter	_____	_____	_____
- external pouches	_____	_____	_____
13. Selects adjunctive topical treatments (antimicrobial, antibacterial).	_____	_____	_____
14. Appropriately obtains and interprets wound cultures.	_____	_____	_____
15. Demonstrates ability to assess the effectiveness of current wound therapy and initiates changed therapies as needed.	_____	_____	_____
16. Implements interventions that prevent recurrence of breakdown.	_____	_____	_____
17. Documents the prevention and management of pressure ulcers.	_____	_____	_____
18. Reports findings to the appropriate resource.	_____	_____	_____
- physician	_____	_____	_____
- supervisor	_____	_____	_____
- infection control	_____	_____	_____
- quality improvement	_____	_____	_____
- utilization review	_____	_____	_____
- social service	_____	_____	_____
- case management	_____	_____	_____
- PT/OT/ST	_____	_____	_____
- Enterostomal Therapist	_____	_____	_____
19. Participates in the development and evaluation of protocols.	_____	_____	_____

Preceptor's Signature: _____   Date of Completion:_____

Used with permission. ©Mary Cardy Weaver. "A tool to document the competence of clinicians to prevent and manage pressure ulcers," *Decubitus* 5(6): 47-48, Nov. 1992.

been measured with flexible inflatable transducers. Pressure in the electromagnetic sensor is indicated on a mercury manometer or aneroid gauge. Good agreement has been reported between interface pressures and internal compression.[31]

When tissue interface pressures quoted in the literature or advertising materials are used to screen devices for pressure relief, care must be taken to ensure that the data being compared are really comparable. Generally, one cannot compare data collected by different investigators using different tissue interface pressure measuring devices. If data from different studies are compared, it is likely that the data will be misrepresented.[32] It is recommended that interface pressure data be reported as both absolute values[33] and as percentages of the interface pressure generated on a control surface, such as a standard hospital mattress or unpadded chair.[32] The absolute value of an interface pressure measurement can be compared to average capillary closing pressure (32 mm Hg) in order to decide about the adequacy of pressure relief. The interface pressure measurement data expressed as a percentage of interface pressure obtained on a standard mattress would indicate the relative amount of pressure relief obtained. Biomedical engineers recommend that a standard format be developed for reporting research data on tissue interface pressure measurements. Kemp[34] offers valuable guidelines for critiquing clinical research on support surfaces.

Dressings

The choice of dressings and topical solutions for pressure ulcer treatment must be made with the same careful consideration as the choice of bed surfaces. Today's clinicians need a thorough knowledge of current research on wound healing and the effects of dressings and topical solutions on human tissue. Product selection depends on caregiver knowledge of wound healing principles. Measurement criteria for value analysis of dressings include several parameters (see Table 12.7). When evaluating marketing information on wound dressings, clinicians should ask company representatives for bonafide controlled clinical trials on dressings used for pressure ulcers. A template for pressure ulcer research (see Table 12.8) gives the information needed to make inferences from the results of pressure ulcer dressing studies.[35]

Medical exam gloves

The skin offers the body protection against infection. Medical exam gloves provide additional protection for both patients and caregivers. However, gloves alone do not offer total protection against infection. Good handwashing techniques and practices, along with the use of gloves, offers the best protection. Medical exam gloves may be made of latex, vinyl, or other substances. They are either sterile or nonsterile, powdered or powder free. Tests have shown that they can be an effective barrier against HIV and hepatitis. Latex gloves can be used for protection only if the person is not allergic to latex.[36]

There are many decisions to make when deciding on the type of medical exam gloves to use. Both latex and vinyl gloves can be used for protection against blood

Table 12.7 Measuring the Value of Dressings

Characteristics	WT.	Rating (Circle Score) Acceptable ⟶ Unacceptable					Subtotal
Wear time/Meltdown		5	4	3	2	1	
Skin protection		5	4	3	2	1	
Ease of application		5	4	3	2	1	
Ease of cutting		5	4	3	2	1	
Ease of molding		5	4	3	2	1	
Ease of removal		5	4	3	2	1	
Patient comfort		5	4	3	2	1	

and body fluids; however, vinyl gloves cannot be used when handling chemotherapeutic agents. Vinyl gloves do not stretch and fit as well as latex gloves. The decreased stretch of the vinyl gloves makes them less durable and more likely to leak.[36,37] A series of experiments tested the integrity of vinyl and latex procedure gloves. In simulations designed to approximate clinical use, the latex gloves were more watertight and less permeable to bacteria than vinyl gloves. The risk of bacterial transmission rate was not studied. The Centers for Disease Control recommends that gloves not be reused or washed between patients. Additionally, they recommend that gloves be changed after high-stress use in high-risk situations.[37]

Many gloves are lubricated with cornstarch to make it easier to put them on. When cornstarch powder is used on latex gloves, the cornstarch absorbs allergens from the latex, which may cause an allergic reaction in latex-sensitive individuals. Sterile gloves must be used for sterile procedures, and nonsterile or clean gloves may be worn when sterile technique is not necessary.[36]

Benchmarking

Benchmarking is a search for industry best practices.[38] A benchmark can be a source of best practice or a desired result or outcome. Many agencies do comparative benchmarking to identify improvement opportunities. Benchmarking data from one department to another or from one organization to another is useful only if data are collected and reported in such a way that data are comparable. The benchmarking process, like the nursing process, has sequential steps. With the nursing process, the phase that follows data analysis is diagnosis. With the benchmarking process, the phase that follows data analysis is discovery, which then leads to opportunities for continuous quality improvement.

With regard to pressure ulcers, the Sun Health Alliance of Hospitals is benchmarking the prevention and treatment of pressure ulcers.[38] Within their alliance, they are searching for hospitals with the best overall pressure ulcer program or with the best components of a pressure ulcer program. Examples of program components might be ease of use, content, staff education, patient education, policies and pro-

Table 12.8 Template for Pressure Ulcer Dressing Study Data

Category	Descriptions and Examples
Authors' Names, Places of Employment, Date	
Study Time Frame	
Research Design	Examples: Case series, randomized controlled trial
Setting	Examples: Hospital, long-term care, home
Inclusion/Exclusion Criteria	
Method of Pressure Ulcer Risk Assessment	Example: Pressure Ulcer Risk Assessment Scale
Study Protocol	Examples: randomization process; use of ulcers or patients as unit of analysis; how multiple ulcers on one patient were handled in study design; cleansing protocol, cleansing materials (e.g., saline, hydrogen peroxide); dressing protocol for experimental group, dressing protocol for control group, person changing dressing, frequency of dressing change, criteria for dressing change; use of adjunctive therapies, such as pressure reduction, turning regimens, or nutritional interventions.
Outcome Variables and Measurement	Primary outcome variables (usually a measure of healing):
	Examples: Time to healing; percentage healed within a specified period of time; change in ulcer surface area, depth, or volume; methods of healing measurement (e.g., tracings of ulcer perimeter and measurement length and width); frequency of measurement.
	Secondary outcome variables:
	Examples: Patient or caregiver subjective assessments; level of ulcer pain; occurrence of ulcer complications; time needed to change dressings; monetary costs associated with dressings (cost may be primary outcome variable in some studies); cost measurement methods and frequency of measurement.
Study Endpoints	
Identified End of Treatment for Individual Subjects Specified Apriori	Examples: All ulcers treated for 14 days; or, complete ulcer healing with pre-specified maximum length of treatment time for ulcers not healed.
Statistical Methods	Examples: Type of statistical tests; use of power analysis to detect whether sample size can show significant differences between or among treatments being studied.
Results	Subject's demographics: age, gender, pressure ulcer risk levels/score, etc.
	Medical diagnoses of subjects
	Baseline ulcer characteristics: etiology, size, stage, location, appearance (e.g., exudate, odor, necrosis, periulcer skin condition), ulcer duration, prior treatment.
	Outcome results: unit of analysis (subjects or pressure ulcers); number of subjects enrolled; number of subjects who reached study endpoint; number of subject dropouts; reason for dropped status (e.g., withdrew, died, discharged

(continued)

Table 12.8 Template for Pressure Ulcer Dressing Study Data *(continued)*

Category	Descriptions and Examples
Results *(continued)*	from care prior to study endpoint, had ulcer complications); number of subjects in data analysis; results of major outcome variables (e.g., time to healing, percentage healed) analyzed by appropriate statistical tests; operational definition of "improved" if used to describe major outcome variables; results of secondary outcome variables; presence or absence of complications; analysis of costs if appropriate.
Summary/Conclusion	Discussion of author's opinion and possible rationales for study findings; comparison of study results with findings from other published research on the topic; identified study weaknesses; implications for clinical practice or healthcare policy; suggestions for further research in the area.

Used with permission from Xakellis, G., and Maklebust, J. "Template for pressure ulcer research." *Advances in Wound Care* 8(1): 46-48, Jan/Feb 1995.

cedures, documentation, and so forth. Each of these components is rated by individuals from multiple disciplines of several other hospitals. All the best-rated components are combined into a new and better program for superior outcomes which, if all goes as planned, will represent industry's best practice.

Unit-based continuous quality improvement

Once a pressure ulcer program is established, the clinical staff needs a method to evaluate its effectiveness. Unit-based quality improvement programs can identify potential or actual practice-related strengths and problems. Administrative managers should include staff nurses and bedside caregivers in unit quality improvement activities to evaluate pressure ulcer policies, procedures, and patient outcomes.

Using skin care as an example, Leary[39] describes use of the nursing process to develop unit-specific quality improvement plans. Unit-based assessment of all patients can determine the prevalence and incidence of pressure ulcers. Tools for data collection may be found in the literature or developed by the nurses on the unit. Harper Hospital has a pressure ulcer quality assurance report form (see Figure 12.3). Nursing units keep the QA forms in a unit log so they can trend information on any patients with pressure ulcers. If problems surface on more than one unit, they can be discussed and solved in the hospital-wide pressure ulcer committee.

Other unit-based projects may be tackled by the nursing staff. Before data collection, unit committee members identify problem-prone areas and then aim for improving operational and clinical processes to improve outcomes. Data are collected by caregivers on the unit. This serves as both an educational process and a form of peer review. The findings are analyzed and summarized by unit committee members. The summary should include both feedback to the unit staff and an action plan to improve any problem clinical or operational processes. The results also will determine the next pressure ulcer project that the unit wishes to undertake. Staff

Initiate This Form for <u>ALL PRESSURE ULCERS</u>

Fill in the boxes below. Use the numbered figure and staging scale provided.

Ulcers on Admission		Ulcers Acquired at Harper		
Location by No.	Stage	Location by No.	Stage	Date Discovered
____	____	____	____	____
____	____	____	____	____
____	____	____	____	____
____	____	____	____	____
____	____	____	____	____
____	____	____	____	____

NONE _____

Circle all the patient's current pressure ulcer risk factors.

Decreased activity: Bedbound   Chairbound

Impaired mobility: Repositions self   Requires turning

Poor nutritional status

Incontinent of urine: Foley catheter   Condom catheter

Incontinent of stool: Fecal collector

Decreased mental status

Decreased sensation

Chronic Disease, Specify_____

Other _____

Circle all devices in use at this time.

None   Vascular boot

Sof-Care mattress   Sheepskin pad

Eggcrate mattress   Heel protectors

Acucair mattress   Chair cushion

Clinitron bed   Other _____

Has a "High-Risk for Impaired Skin Integrity" or "Impaired Tissue Integrity" problem been identified in the chart?

Yes ❑   No ❑

Name of person completing this form: _____

Nursing Unit: _____   Date: _____

PLEASE SUBMIT TO ADMINISTRATIVE MANAGER ON UNIT

Stage(s)

I) Non-blanchable erythema, intact skin

II) Skin loss through epidermis

III) Skin loss exposing subcutaneous fat

IV) Full thickness loss to muscle/bone.

E) Eschar—Not able to stage

Specify right or left when applicable

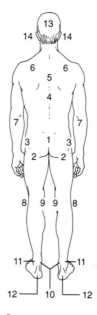

1. Sacrum
2. Ischial tuberosity
3. Trochanter
4. Lumbar vertebrae
5. Thoracic vertebrae
6. Scapula
7. Elbow (olecranon)
8. Lateral knee
9. Medial knee
10. Medial malleolus (inner ankle)
11. Lateral malleolus (outer ankle)
12. Heel
13. Occipital
14. Ear

Figure 12.3 Quality Assurance Report

nurses may suggest new procedure trials or new pressure ulcer products to improve outcomes of problem-prone areas. Some of the most beneficial outcomes of unit-based quality improvement occur when members of the unit staff rotate turns on the quality improvement committee. Participation in quality improvement assists clinicians to develop insight and perspective into standards of care for nursing. Involved staff nurses accept the professional responsibility for monitoring and evaluating their own practices.[39]

Clinical staff enjoy being involved in quality improvement efforts. When the AHCPR guidelines were first released, Harper staff on the pressure ulcer committee participated in an all-day pressure ulcer awareness day to disseminate the information hospital wide. Dietitians had posters and displays of nutrition information, physical therapists had positioning demonstrations and articles about hydrotherapy and debridement, and nurses had multiple tables representing pressure ulcer prevention and treatment strategies. The results of Harper-based research on pressure ulcers was highlighted on poster boards. Every nursing unit was given a set of the AHCPR Pressure Ulcer Guidelines[18] and educational material from the National Pressure Ulcer Advisory Panel.[40] A video monitor continuously played an educational tape on pressure ulcer care. To stimulate interest, attendees participated in a drawing for subscriptions to wound care journals. The "pressure ulcer day" was a big success, and many nurses asked that it be held twice yearly.[41]

As new scientific information is generated, AHCPR Guidelines will be revised and updated to reflect new research findings, emerging technologies, and innovative approaches. Pressure Ulcer Quality Improvement Committees can help keep pace by educating health care practitioners.

Summary

Ongoing systematic improvement of the quality of patient care will become increasingly important in today's health care market. Nurses in every health care facility need to be aware of the potential for pressure ulcer development. If information in the AHCPR guidelines is widely disseminated and incorporated into practice, the pressure ulcer incidence rate and associated pressure ulcer costs will come down. Nursing has both a responsibility and an opportunity to help decrease the number of individuals who suffer from pressure ulceration. Nurses can begin now to effect changes in practice by starting multidisciplinary skin care teams in their own agencies. By the year 2000, cost effectiveness and quality care will be more crucial than ever before.

References

1. Van Valkenburgh, D. "Continuous Quality Improvement (CQI) of Current Quality Assurance Programs," *Dialysis and Transplantation* 20(9): 530-567, 1991.
2. Peacock, E., et al. "The Transition from Traditional Quality Assurance to Continuous Quality Improvement," in Wick, G.S., and Peacock, E., eds. *Continuous Quality Improvement: From Concept to Reality.* Pitman, N.J.: ANNA, 1995.

3. Leebov, W., and Ersoz, C. *The Health Care Manager's Guide to Continuous Quality Improvement.* Chicago: American Hospital Publishing, Inc., 1991.

4. Mozena, J., and Anderson, D. *Quality Improvement Handbook for Health Care Professionals.* Madison, Wisc.: ASQC Press, 1993.

5. Bergstrom, N., et al. "Pressure Ulcer Treatment," Clinical Practice Guideline, No. 15. AHCPR Pub. No. 95-0652. Rockville, Md.: U.S. Department of Health and Human Services, Agency for Health Care Policy and Research, December 1994.

6. Baranoski, S. "Collaborative Roles Lead to Success in Wound Healing," *Decubitus* 5(3): 66-68, 1992.

7. Kuhn, B.A., and Coulter, S.J. "Balancing the Pressure Ulcer Cost and Quality Equation," *Nursing Economics* 10(5): 353-359, 1992.

8. National Pressure Ulcer Advisory Panel. "Pressure Ulcers: Incidence, Economics, Risk Assessment. Consensus Development Conference Statement," *Decubitus* 2(2) and (3), entire issues, 1989.

9. Allman, R.M. "On Calculating Incidence Rate," *Decubitus* 6(5): 12, 1993.

10. Lesham, O.A., and Skelskey, C. "Pressure Ulcers: Quality Management, Prevalence, and Severity in a Long-Term Care Setting," *Advances in Wound Care* 7(2): 50-54, 1994.

11. Levine, J., and Totolos, E. "A Quality-Oriented Approach to Pressure Ulcer Management in a Nursing Facility," *The Gerontologist* 34(3): 413-417, 1994.

12. Hammond, M.C., et al. "Pressure Ulcer Incidence on a Spinal Cord Injury Unit," *Advances in Wound Care* 7(6): 57-60, 1994.

13. Hoyman, K.H., and Gruber, N. "A Case Study of Interdepartmental Cooperation: Operating Room Acquired Pressure Ulcers," *Journal of Nursing Care Quality*, Special report: 12-17, 1992.

14. Gawron, C.L. "Risk Factors for and Prevalence of Pressure Ulcers Among Hospitalized Patients," *JWOCN* 21(6): 232-240, 1994.

15. Maklebust, J., and Magnan, M.A. "Risk Factors Associated with Having a Pressure Ulcer: A Secondary Data Analysis," *Advances in Wound Care* 7(6): 25-42, 1994.

16. Lyder, C.H., et al. "Structured Skin Care to Prevent Perineal Dermatitis in the Elderly," *Journal of ET Nursing* 19(1): 12-16, 1992.

17. Kravitz, R. "Development and Implementation of a Nursing Skin Care Protocol," *Journal of ET Nursing* 20(1): 4-8, 1993.

18. Panel for the Prediction and Prevention of Pressure Ulcers in Adults. "Pressure Ulcers in Adults: Prediction and Prevention," Clinical Practice Guideline, No. 3. AHCPR Publication No. 92-0047. Rockville, Md.: U.S. Department of Health and Human Services, Agency for Health Care Policy and Research, May 1992.

19. Frantz, R.A., et al. "The Cost of Treating Pressure Ulcers Following Implementation of a Research-Based Skin Care Protocol in a Long-Term Care Facility," *Advances in Wound Care* 8(1): 36-45, 1995.

20. Maklebust, J. "Impact of AHCPR Pressure Ulcer Guidelines on Nursing Practice," *Decubitus* 4(2): 46-50, 1991.

21. Ek, A.C., et al. "The Local Skin Blood Flow in Areas at Risk for Pressure Sores Treated with Massage," *Scandinavian Journal of Rehabilitation Medicine* 17(2): 81-86, 1985.

22. Seiler, W.O., et al. "Influence of the 30 Degrees Laterally Inclined Position and the Super Soft 3-Piece Mattress on Skin Oxygen Tension on Areas of Maximum Pressure: Implications for Pressure Sore Prevention," *Gerontology* 32(3): 158-166, 1986.

23. Moody, B.L., et al. "Impact of Staff Education on Pressure Sore Development in Elderly Hospitalized Patients," *Archives of Internal Medicine* 148(10): 2241-2243, 1988.

24. Hayes, P.A., et al. "Effect of a Teaching Plan on Nursing Staff's Knowledge of Pressure Ulcer Risk, Assessment, and Treatment," *Journal of Nursing Staff Development* 10(4): 207-213, 1994.

25. Cardy, M. "A Tool to Document the Competence of Clinicians to Prevent and Manage Pressure Ulcers," *Decubitus* 5(6): 46-49, 1992.

26. Francke, A.L., et al. "Determinants of Change in Nurses' Behaviour After Continuing Education: A Literature Review," *Journal of Advanced Nursing* 21(2): 371-377, 1992.

27. Andrews, J., and Balai, R. "The Prevention and Treatment of Pressure Sores by Use of Pressure-Distributing Mattresses," *Decubitus* 1(4): 14-21, 1988.

28. Jackson, B.S., et al. "The Effects of a Therapeutic Bed on Pressure Ulcers: An Experimental Study," *Journal of Enterostomal Therapy* 15(6): 220-226, 1988.

29. Greer, D.M., et al. "Cost-Effectiveness and Efficacy of Air-Fluidized Therapy in the Treatment of Pressure Ulcers," *Journal of Enterostomal Therapy* 15(6): 247-251, 1988.

30. Maklebust, J., et al. "Pressure-Relief Capabilities of the Sof-Care Bed Cushion and the Clinitron Bed," *Ostomy/Wound Management* 21: 32-41, 1988.

31. Clark, M. "Continuous Interface Pressure Measurement Using an Electropneumatic Sensor: the SCP Monitor," *Care: Science and Practice* 5: 5-8, June 1987.

32. Krouskop, T.A. "Interface Pressure Confusion," *Decubitus* 2(3): 8, 1988.

33. Stewart, T. "Another Option on Interface Pressure," *Decubitus* 2(3): 8-9, 1989.

34. Kemp, M. "Critiquing Clinical Research on Support Surfaces," *Ostomy/Wound Management* 40(2): 18-25, 1994.

35. Xakellis, G.C., and Maklebust, J. "Template for Pressure Ulcer Research," *Advances in Wound Care* 8(1): 46-48, 1995.

36. Henry Ford Health System Glove and Latex Task Force. *Gloves: What Every Health Care Worker Needs to Know.* Detroit, Mich.: Author, 1993.

37. Korniewicz, D.M., et al. "Integrity of Vinyl and Latex Procedure Gloves," *Nursing Research* 38: 144-146, 1989.

38. SunHealth Alliance. "Benchmarking the Prevention and Treatment of Pressure Ulcers," Charlotte, N.C., January 1995.

39. Leary, C.B. "Use of the Nursing Process to Develop Unit-Specific Quality Assurance Plans," *Journal of Nursing Quality Assurance* 4(2): 1-6, 1990.

40. The National Pressure Ulcer Advisory Panel. *Pressure Ulcer Prevention Points: A Summary of the AHCPR Clinical Practice Guidelines.* Buffalo: State University of New York at Buffalo, 1992.

41. Maklebust, J. "Using AHCPR Pressure Ulcer Guidelines to Improve Nursing Practice," *Michigan Nurse*, 1992.

CHAPTER 13

Meeting the Future Now

In today's evolving health care environment, there is search for the highest quality of care for the least cost. It is a challenge to find a model that is acceptable to patients, providers, and payors. We live in an age characterized by rapid technological advances and equally rapid change in health care. Healthcare delivery systems are being downsized and restructured. Health care businesses are both consolidating and purchasing one another. Methods of reimbursement are changing from prospective payment for DRGs to capitated payment rates for covered lives. The number of people enrolled in Health Maintenance Organizations (HMO) is increasing dramatically. Many of these changes in the health care system affect management of patients with pressure ulcers. Recently, medical policy for coverage and payment of surgical wound dressings and support surfaces changed significantly under Medicare part B.[1] This policy significantly impacts chronic wound care patients who reside at home or in long-term care facilities.

Managed care

It appears that America has a national passion for managed care. Originally, managed care was seen as a system that stressed continuity of care and a full range of services from prevention to complicated intervention in an inpatient setting. It was a system of organizing care, not just a mechanism of financing. Today managed care is seen as a method of cost containment. Managed care has become popular for limiting costs under Medicaid. Congressional reform of the Medicare program will include some form of managed care.[2] Fixed, negotiated rates, not charges, determine the mechanism of payment. Changes in funding rules are the norm rather than the exception.

Agencies that deliver health care are trying to find innovative ways to stay cost effective.[3] Many are contracting services, such as physical therapy and dietary services. Cost-effective care also is maintained through Materials Management Departments. Many health care agencies enter strategic planning and corporate buying agreements to help contain or neutralize costs. Other agencies outsource their central supply department and contract for "just in time services." Computerized systems can carefully track use of patient supplies for replenishment and utilization purposes.

New prospective payment systems bundle all healthcare services rather than provide separate reimbursement for wound care. Facilities that provide wound management under managed care contracts must know their costs. They must be able to deliver wound management for the agreed-upon price through apppropriate use of products and resources. These include surgical dressings, support surfaces, nutritional supplements, laboratory and diagnostic tests, nursing care, physical therapy, and other rehabilitative therapies. In long-term care, all of these wound care components will be reimbursed through an acuity-based system. The sicker the individual, the more money is reimbursed. It is up to the provider to calculate total costs for care of the patient. After calculating the cost, the agency must then monitor the actual cost of delivering the care. A postdischarge analysis can determine if resources could have been used more efficiently.[1]

Under managed care programs, wound care specialists need to develop and promote model wound programs that HMOs can use to incorporate management of chronic wounds. Wound care can become a product line with competitive bidding for the best managed chronic wound care program. Standard reporting measures can compare clinical outcomes, functional outcomes, patient satisfaction, and cost so that competing managed care plans can choose the most cost-effective wound management program. It will take a dedicated group of wound care specialists to design the most cost-effective pressure ulcer programs. Skilled clinicians from multiple disciplines are needed to embark on such an initiative.

Patient-focused care

Market forces, health care legislation, and managed care have combined to change the delivery of health care services. The prevailing operating philosophy changed from specialization and centralization to tightened cost controls and operational efficiency through restructuring. As a managed care survival strategy, many agencies are implementing new models of health care delivery called patient-focused care (PFC). The old health care delivery model focuses on care providers. The goal of PFC is to focus on the recipient of care in order to achieve improved continuity, quality, operational efficiency, and cost structure. Although PFC initiatives vary among facilities, the following common themes have emerged:
- grouping patients with similar resource needs
- decentralization or redeployment of ancillary services
- cross-training to produce multiskilled workers
- multidisciplinary team approach
- goverance restructuring and empowerment of employees
- clinical pathways (CareMaps[TM])
- charting by exception (CBE).[4]

In a PFC model, multiskilled workers are trained to perform a variety of tasks and responsibilities that previously were performed by health care professionals. They are given such titles as care partners or care associates and such duties as feeding and bathing patients, monitoring vital signs, changing wound care dressings, conducting phlebotomy procedures, and assisting patients to ambulate, transfer, and do range-of-motion exercises. Some multiskilled workers also apply traction, casts, and continuous passive motion machines. Other duties vary, depending on the patient mix of the work setting.[5,6,7] With PFC as a new entity, the hoped-for "increase in quality and quantity of time interacting with patients" has not yet materialized. As multiskilled workers assume a larger share of patient care, it will be interesting to evaluate outcome data on satisfaction among patients, physicians, nurses, and other licensed and unlicensed health care personnel. To evaluate outcomes from PFC, quality and cost data need to be collected prior to implementation in order to have a valid comparison from which cost-effective claims can be made.[8]

Case management

Under managed care, the cost of pressure ulcers takes on new meaning. Patients who develop pressure ulcers may require increased intensity of nursing services and increased length of stay. Yet, under managed care contracts, health care agencies do not receive additional money for pressure ulcer care. This represents a hidden cost to the agency. For health care agencies to afford delivery of needed care, it is important to have consistent protocols regarding pressure ulcer management. These protocols must emphasize primary care prevention to avoid unnecessary hospital care. Under managed care, a comprehensive skin integrity and pressure ulcer risk assessment should be done on all enrolled at-risk patients and pressure ulcer prevention should be started before risk becomes reality.[9,10]

As Medicare and Medicaid payment rates are reduced, establishing control over the cost of providing requisite care to patients with pressure ulcers is essential. Case management of these patients is a way to enhance quality improvement, meet internal and external documentation requirements, develop wound care pathways, improve patient and staff communication, streamline variance tracking, cut skyrocketing wound care costs, reduce length of stay, and boost agency revenues. The overall goal of case management is to provide a service delivery model that ensures cost-effective health care, offers alternatives to hospitalization, provides access to care, coordinates supportive services, and improves the patient's functional capacity. A specialized wound care program with an accountable case manager can streamline care and maintain standards across settings. Specialized nurse case managers can develop staff and patient education programs related to pressure ulcer management. Proper allocation of appropriate resources for patient care is accomplished with patient and family input. Wound care pathways can be developed and superimposed on pathways for other patient conditions or procedures.

Clinical pathways

Clinical pathways, or CareMaps[TM], are multidisciplinary plans of care that give direction to the health care team.[11] They can help providers give consistent, comprehensive, quality care for patients with pressure ulcers by describing the interventions that should be delivered to the patient each day. Patient outcomes are predefined, and progress toward these outcomes is documented. If expected patient outcomes are not achieved by the interventions of health care professionals, the plan of care must be reevaluated or the patient outcomes modified accordingly.

Reimbursement to an agency may be based on what is consistently documented in the medical record. Documentation plays a significant role in DRG assignment, and charts are reviewed by external peer review organization personnel.[12] The importance of documentation in proper coding and DRG assignment cannot be underestimated. Omissions in the medical record can be costly for any health care agency. A model pressure ulcer pathway can assist personnel to document required information in an efficient manner (see Chapter 7).

Omnibus Reconciliation Act

The 1986 Omnibus Budget Reconciliation Act (OBRA) mandated the development of a uniform needs assessment instrument by the Secretary of Health and Human Services. The purpose of the instrument was to collect consistent national data on Medicare patients in all health facilities. OBRA required the instrument to be developed for use by discharge planners, hospitals, nursing facilities, and fiscal intermediaries in evaluating a patient's needs for posthospital services. The needs assessment instrument was completed in 1989 by the Uniform Needs Assessment Advisory Panel. The assessment instrument includes pressure ulcer data. The date and process of implementation of the uniform needs assessment have not been determined. If this instrument is adopted, it will provide a rich data bank for tracking national pressure ulcer cost and prevalence data.

Recently, HCFA officials established new enforcement regulations for nursing homes. Operations manuals for HCFA surveyors have been drafted to enforce the regulations. Nursing homes will have to comply with complicated new rules regarding patients' rights. Expanded rights of nursing home residents include the right to refuse treatment, the right to give advance directives, and the right to avoid use of physical and chemical restraints.[13] Quality care of pressure ulcers also is the right of nursing home residents.

Caring for patients

Quality of life is becoming a crisis in America. Human suffering, financial cost of care, and legal and ethical problems created by life-or-death decisions are paramount to the issue. Health care professionals have acknowledged the ethical problems created by the tremendous improvement in life-sustaining techniques. As the number of elderly increases, health care administrators are increasingly concerned about the strain on our physical and financial capabilities. Patients and families are concerned about their right to control their own health care. The courts are concerned about mental competency and the right to refuse life-sustaining treatment. Agencies have appointed bioethics committees to help patients and professionals arrive at life decisions with peace of mind and some degree of certainty. Many states have advance directives guidelines that provide critical information about the patient's wishes concerning life-prolonging technology and who the patient delegates to make decisions in his behalf. A monumental study, *A Matter of Choice*, done for the Special Senate Committee on Aging, as well as the apparently overwhelming public consensus on individual rights, seem to be having an impact on changing society's attitude about what constitutes living and what constitutes dying.[14] The public is demanding that more attention be paid to their needs and desires.

Agency for Health Care Policy and Research

In 1989, Congress established the Agency for Health Care Policy and Research (AHCPR) to improve the quality, appropriateness, and effectiveness of health care and to improve access to health care services.[15] Several social and economic factors gave rise to the AHCPR, including delivery of inappropriate health care, lack of science-based health care, high cost of health care, and consumer demands for greater participation in health care decision making. Clinical practice guidelines for various health-related conditions have been released by the AHCPR. Designed to assist health care professionals and patients in making better choices about treatment options, the guidelines are developed by multidisciplinary panels of expert health care professionals and consumers. They result from a combination of scientific evidence and professional judgment.[16] Concern for patient preference is reflected in many ways, including a consumer version of each practice guideline. Each guideline has multiple algorithms indicating its organization and use. The guidelines are considered "living documents" that will be revised as new knowledge is generated from research. Much more scientific evidence is needed to support areas of the guidelines for which science is lacking, and many of the concepts in the guidelines need further testing. However, the AHCPR *Guideline on Prediction and Prevention of Pressure Ulcers*[17] and *Treatment of Pressure Ulcers*[18] represent the most sound comprehensive management of pressure ulcers to date.[19,20]

The AHCPR guidelines have become the standard of care and are used by many accrediting and regulating bodies. They are being converted to medical review criteria, which may affect payment mechanisms. Health care agencies should adopt the AHCPR guidelines for any clinical conditions relevant to their populations.[16,19,20]

National Pressure Ulcer Advisory Panel

The National Pressure Ulcer Advisory Panel (NPUAP) is a nonprofit multidisciplinary organization of health care professionals dedicated to the prevention of pressure ulcers. The mission of this group is to provide leadership, recommendations, guidance, and action toward pressure ulcer management. The panel acts as a steering committee for the country's efforts toward eradicating pressure ulcers. Through educational and legislative activities, the NPUAP stresses the responsibility of all health-related professionals in the management of pressure ulcers. In 1987, the group was instrumental in amending the Omnibus Reconciliation Act (OBRA) in order to strengthen the bill language that related to quality of care of patients in long-term care settings. An important aspect of the OBRA was to encourage the Secretary of Health and Human Services to list pressure ulcers as a parameter for evaluating the quality of care delivered by long-term care facilities.

The NPUAP was invited by the National Academy of Science to participate in formulating the Health Care Objectives of the Nation for the year 2000. As part of the alliance of organizations involved in Healthy People 2000, one of the NPUAP goals is to reduce pressure ulcer incidence by 50% by the year 2000. In another area, the NPUAP has been active in third-party reimbursement for prevention and treatment of pressure ulcers. Quality patient care and effective pressure ulcer interventions are difficult to provide when the required materials are not reimburseable. The NPUAP has been actively working with the Health Care Financing Administration on medical policy for durable medical equipment and supplies related to wound care. Meetings with the DMERC Medical Directors have been beneficial in establishing medical policy for surgical dressings and support surfaces.

In March of 1989, the NPUAP sponsored the first National Consensus Development Conference in Washington, D.C., to focus on the pressure ulcer problem. At this meeting, a panel of experts heard testimony concerning the incidence, cost, and risk for pressure ulcers. The final report was published as a monograph, and the entire proceedings were published in *Decubitus*.[21-22] The second and third national conferences sponsored by the NPUAP were formal multidisciplinary critiques of drafts of the AHCPR's *Guideline on Prediction and Prevention of Pressure Ulcers*[17] and *Guideline on Treatment of Pressure Ulcers*.[18] As an adjunct to the guidelines, leadership from the NPUAP is expected to set the standard for pressure ulcer education, research, and public policy. The NPUAP recently established a Pressure Ulcer Research Foundation, and NPUAP national conferences are held bi-annually to address the most critical issues related to pressure ulcers. Proceedings of a 1995 NPUAP conference on pressure ulcer assessment, measurement, and outcomes of care were published in *Advances in Wound Care*.[23]

Summary

The dynamic state of the health care system challenges both patients and health care providers. The crisis of care cuts across the boundaries of all health care professions. Patients in hospitals feel depersonalized, and they wonder if professionals really care about them. Caregivers seem to be rewarded for efficiency, technical skill, and measurable results while their concern and attentiveness go unnoticed within their institutions. Phillips and Benner[24] think the ethics of care and the sources from which caregivers draw inspiration must be restored to caregiving practices in the helping professions. In the future, as patient satisfaction becomes a marker of excellence, emphasis may swing from high technology to caring. As the health care system redefines itself, caring about patients must remain our overriding mission.

While continuously examining advances in pressure ulcer research, maintaining skin integrity must remain a conscious part of the complex management of the ill, disabled, and elderly. Primary emphasis should be placed on the prevention of pressure ulcers. Key management issues in this area should include: (a) education of the patient and family, focusing on early detection and intervention to decrease pressure ulcer risk factors, (b) an aggressive patient/team approach directed at pressure ulcer management when skin integrity is already compromised, and (c) implementation of a coordinated team approach that uses the expertise of all disciplines to manage the pressure ulcer problem.[20,25,26,27,28] It is hoped that these guidelines for pressure ulcer management will assist agencies and individuals to implement practices that will accomplish this goal.

References

1. Lusky, K. "Reimbursement under Managed Care," *Contemporary Long Term Care* 18(6): 58-66, 1995.
2. Schwartz, R.M. "Congress Advocates Medicare Managed Care," *Contemporary Long Term Care* 18(4): 21, 1995.
3. Sovie, M.D. "Tailoring Hospitals for Managed Care and Integrated Health Systems," *Nursing Economics* 13(2): 72-83, 1995.
4. Arthur, P.R. "Acute Orthopedic Services," *PT Magazine* 2(7): 35-47, 1994.
5. Strakal, M. "Patient-Focused Care in Private Practice," *PT Magazine* 3(4): 43-50, 1995.
6. Brumfield, J. "The Restructuring of America's Hospitals: Patient- Focused Care," *PT Magazine* 2(9): 76-89, 1994.
7. Bullock, K. "Patient-Focused Care," *PT Magazine* 2(11): 51-60, 1994.
8. "Hospitals of the Future: Can the Patient-Focused Model Really Work?" Chicago Health Executive Health Care Forum, September 19, 1991.
9. Levesque, L. "Making a Difference with the Right Kind of Case Management," *Subacute Care* (supplement), *Contemporary Long Term Care* 18(6S): 56, 1995.
10. Lyons, J.C. "Models of Nursing Care Delivery and Case Management: Clarification of Terms," *Nursing Economics* 11(3): 163-169, 1993.
11. Gartner, M.B. "Care Guidelines: Journey Through the Managed Care Maze," *JWOCN* 22(3): 118-121, 1995.
12. Hines, G.L. "DRGs: Nursing Documentation Contributes to the Bottom Line," *Nursing Clinics of North America* 23(3): 579-586, 1988.
13. Schwartz, R.M. "Inside Washington: Enforcement Manual, Schedule Raise Concerns," *Contemporary Long Term Care* 18(5): 25, 1995.
14. Hoopes, R. "Turning Out the Light," *Modern Maturity* June-July: 29-33, 88-93, 1988.
15. "AHCPR Fact Sheet." Rockville, Md.: Agency for Health Care Policy and Research, 1992.
16. Jacox, A. "Addressing Variances in Nursing Practice/Technology Through Clinical Practice Guidelines Methods," *Nursing Economics* 11(3): 170-72, 1993.
17. Panel for the Prediction and Prevention of Pressure Ulcers in Adults. *Pressure Ulcers in Adults: Prediction and Prevention.* Clinical Practice Guideline No. 3. AHCPR Publication No. 92-0047. Rockville, Md.: Agency for Health Care Policy and Research, Public Health Service, U.S. Department of Health and Human Services, May 1992.
18. Bergstrom, N., et al. *Treatment of Pressure Ulcers.* Clinical Practice Guideline No. 15. AHCPR Publication No. 95-0652. Rockville, Md: Agency for Health Care Policy and Research, Public Health Service, U.S. Department of Health and Human Services, December 1994.
19. Parsons, Y. "Healing More Than Wounds," *Contemporary Long Term Care* 18(6): 57-76, 1995.
20. Bergstrom, N. "The Big Picture: The Holistic Approach of the New Treatment Guidelines Can Help Providers Update Their Protocols," *Contemporary Long Term Care* 18(6): 58-60, 1995.
21. National Pressure Ulcer Advisory Panel. "Proceedings of the Consensus Development Conference on Pressure Ulcers: Prevalence and Incidence," *Decubitus* 2(2): 22-48, 1989.
22. National Pressure Ulcer Advisory Panel. "Proceedings of the Consensus Development Conference on Pressure Ulcers: Prevalence, Cost and Risk Assessment," *Decubitus* 2(3): 14-63, 1989.
23. National Pressure Ulcer Advisory Panel. "Proceedings of the Pressure Ulcer Conference: Controversy to Consensus: Assessment, Measurement and Outcomes," *Advances in Wound Care* 8(4): entire issue, 1995.
24. Phillips, S.S., and Benner, P. *The Crisis of Care: Affirming and Restoring Caring Practices in the Helping Professions.* Washington, D.C.: Georgetown University Press, 1994.
25. Breslow, R.A. "A Look at Nutritional Status: You May Be Doing the Right Thing but Your Patient Can't Heal Without Adequate Protein," *Contemporary Long Term Care* 18(6): 60-62, 1995.
26. Melton, E. "The Right Stuff: How a Facility That Wanted a Specialty in Wound Care Got a Lesson in Coordination," *Contemporary Long Term Care* 18(6): 62-66, 1995.
27. Kobriger, A. "The Healing Power of Water: Caregivers Should Be on Guard for Signs of Fluid Loss," *Contemporary Long Term Care* 18(6): 68-70, 1995.
28. Erwin-Toth, P. "The First Line of Care: Certified Nursing Assistants Are a Facility's Most Valuable Players in Terms of Wound Prevention," *Contemporary Long Term Care* 18(6): 75-76, 1995.

Appendix A: Norton Scale

PHYSICAL CONDITION		MENTAL CONDITION		ACTIVITY		MOBILITY		INCONTINENT		TOTAL SCORE
Good	4	Alert	4	Ambulatory	4	Full	4	Not	4	
Fair	3	Apathetic	3	Walk with help	3	Slightly limited	3	Occasional	3	
Poor	2	Confused	2	Chairbound	2	Very limited	2	Usually/ Urine	2	
Very bad	1	Stupor	1	Bed	1	Immobile	1	Doubly	1	

Appendix B: Gosnell Scale

I.D. _____   Medical Diagnosis _____

Age _____ Sex _____   Primary _____

Height _____ Weight _____   Secondary _____

Date of Admission _____   Nursing Diagnosis _____

Date of Discharge _____   _____

                                                                _____

Instructions: Complete all categories within 24 hours of admission and every other day thereafter. Refer to the accompanying guidelines for specific rating details.

DATE	Mental Status:	Continence:	Mobility:	Activity:	Nutrition:	TOTAL SCORE
	1. Alert	1. Fully Controlled	1. Full	1. Ambulatory	1. Good	
	2. Apathetic	2. Usually Controlled	2. Slightly Limited	2. Walks with Assistance	2. Fair	
	3. Confused	3. Minimally Controlled	3. Very Limited	3. Chairfast	3. Poor	
	4. Stuporous	4. Absence of Control	4. Immobile	4. Bedfast		
	5. Unconscious					

Pressure Sore Risk Assessment Medication Profile

Medication	Dosage	*Frequency	Route	Date Begun	Date Discontinued

*If PRN record pattern past 48 hours

Appendix B: Gosnell Scale *(continued)*

Guidelines for Numerical Rating of the Defined Categories

Rating	1	2	3	4	5
Mental Status: An assessment of one's level of response to his environment.	**Alert:** Oriented to time, place, & person. Responsive to all stimuli, and understands explanations.	**Apathetic:** Lethargic, forgetful, drowsy, passive & dull. Sluggish, depressed. Able to obey simple commands. Possibly disoriented to time.	**Confused:** Partial and/or imtermittent disorientation to TPP. Purposeless response to stimuli. Restless, aggressive, irritable, anxious & may require tranquilizers or sedatives.	**Stuporous:** Total disorientation. Does not respond to name, simple commands, or verbal stimuli.	**Unconscious:** Non-responsive to painful stimuli.
Continence: The amount of bodily control of urination & defecation.	**Fully Controlled:** Total control of urine and feces.	**Usually Controlled:** Incontinent of urine &/or of feces not more often than once q 48 hrs. **OR** has Foley catheter & is incontinent of feces.	**Minimally Controlled:** Incontinent of urine or feces at least once q 24 hrs.	**Absence of Control:** Consistently incontinent of both urine & feces.	
Mobility: The amount and control of movement of one's body.	**Full:** Able to control and move all extremities at will. May require the use of a device but turns, lifts, pulls, balances, and attains sitting position at will.	**Slightly Limited:** Able to control and move all extremities but a degree of limitation is present. Requires assistance of another person to turn, pull, balance &/or attain a sitting position at will but self-initiates movement or request for help to move.	**Very Limited:** Can assist another person who must initiate movement via turning, lifting, pulling, balancing &/or attaining a sitting position (contractures, paralysis may be present).	**Immobile:** Does not assist self in any way to change position. Is unable to change position without assistance. Is completely dependent on others for movement.	
Activity: The ability of an individual to ambulate.	**Ambulatory:** Is able to walk unassisted. Rises from bed unassisted. With the use of a device such as cane or walker is able to ambulate without the assistance of another person.	**Walks with Help:** Able to ambulate with assistance of another person, braces, or crutches. May have limitation of stairs.	**Chairfast:** Ambulates only to a chair, requires assistance to do so **OR** is confined to a wheelchair.	**Bedfast:** Is confined to bed during entire 24 hours of the day.	
Nutrition: The process of food intake.	Eats some food from each basic food category every day and the majority of each meal served **OR** is on tube feeding.	Occasionally refuses a meal or frequently leaves at least half of a meal.	Seldom eats a complete meal and only a few bites of food at a meal.		

Appendix B: Gosnell Scale *(continued)*

	Vital Signs				Diet	24-Hour Fluid Balance		Color	General Skin Appearance			Interventions		
									Moisture	Tempera-ture	Texture			
Date	T	P	R	BP	Diet	Intake	Output	1. Pallor 2. Mottled 3. Pink 4. Ashen 5. Ruddy 6. Cyanotic 7. Jaundice 8. Other	1. Dry 2. Damp 3. Oily 4. Other	1. Cold 2. Cool 3. Warm 4. Hot	1. Smooth 2. Rough 3. Thin/ Trans- parent 4. Scaly 5. Crusty 6. Other	No	Yes	Describe

Vital Signs: The temperature, pulse, respiration and blood pressure to be taken and recorded at the time of every assessment rating.

Skin Appearance: A description of observed skin characteristics: color, moisture, temperature, and texture.

Diet: Record the specific diet order.

24-hour fluid balance: The amount of fluid intake and output during the previous 24-hour period should be recorded.

Interventions: List all devices, measures and/or nursing care activity being used for the purpose of pressure sore prevention.

Medications: List name, dosage, frequency and route for all prescribed medications. If a PRN order, list the pattern for the period since last assessment.

Comments: Use this space to add explanation or further detail regarding any of the previously recorded data, patient condition, etc. *or* Describe anything which you believe to be of importance but not accounted for previously.

NOTE: For any item marked "other" please describe.
If any signs of pressure, etc. on bony prominences or other body parts are observed, please describe in detail the location, color, temperature, moisture, texture, and size and any other pertinent items.

Instrument to Assess Client Risk for Pressure Sores used by permission of Davina Gosnell, RN, PhD.

Appendix C: Braden Scale

Patient's Name _____ Evaluator's Name _____ Date of Assessment _____

	1	2	3	4	
SENSORY PERCEPTION ability to respond meaningfully to pressure-related discomfort	**1. Completely Limited:** Unresponsive (does not moan, flinch, or grasp) to painful stimuli, due to diminished level of consciousness or sedation. OR limited ability to feel pain over most of body surface.	**2. Very Limited:** Responds only to painful stimuli. Cannot communicate discomfort except by moaning or restlessness. OR has a sensory impairment which limits the ability to feel pain or discomfort over 1/2 of body.	**3. Slightly Limited:** Responds to verbal commands, but cannot always communicate discomfort or need to be turned. OR has some sensory impairment which limits ability to feel pain or discomfort in 1 or 2 extremities.	**4. No Impairment:** Responds to verbal commands. Has no sensory deficit which would limit ability to feel or voice pain or discomfort.	
MOISTURE degree to which skin is exposed to moisture	**1. Constantly Moist:** Skin is kept moist almost constantly by perspiration, urine, etc. Dampness is detected every time patient is moved or turned.	**2. Very Moist:** Skin is often but not always moist. Linen must be changed at least once a shift.	**3. Occasionally Moist:** Skin is occasionally moist, requiring an extra linen change approximately once a day.	**4. Rarely Moist:** Skin is usually dry; linen only requires changing at routine intervals.	
ACTIVITY degree of physical activity	**1. Bedfast:** Confined to bed.	**2. Chairfast:** Ability to walk severely limited or nonexistent. Cannot bear own weight and/or must be assisted into chair or wheelchair.	**3. Walks Occasionally:** Walks occasionally during day, but for very short distances, with or without assistance. Spends majority of each shift in bed or chair.	**4. Walks Frequently:** Walks outside the room at least twice a day and inside room at least once every 2 hours during waking hours.	
MOBILITY ability to change and control body position	**1. Completely Immobile:** Does not make even slight changes in body or extremity position without assistance.	**2. Very Limited:** Makes occasional slight changes in body or extremity position but unable to make frequent or significant changes independently.	**3. Slightly Limited:** Makes frequent though slight changes in body or extremity position independently.	**4. No Limitations:** Makes major and frequent changes in position without assistance.	
NUTRITION *usual* food intake pattern	**1. Very Poor:** Never eats a complete meal. Rarely eats more than 1/3 of any food offered. Eats 2 servings or less of protein (meat or dairy products) per day. Takes fluids poorly. Does not take a liquid dietary supplement. OR is NPO and/or maintained on clear liquids or IV's for more than 5 days.	**2. Probably Inadequate:** Rarely eats a complete meal and generally eats only about 1/2 of any food offered. Protein intake includes only 3 servings of meat or dairy products per day. Occasionally will take a dietary supplement. OR receives less than optimum amount of liquid diet or tube feeding.	**3. Adequate:** Eats over half of most meals. Eats a total of 4 servings of protein (meat, dairy products) each day. Occasionally will refuse a meal, but will usually take a supplement if offered. OR is on a tube feeding or TPN regimen which probably meets most of nutritional needs.	**4. Excellent:** Eats most of every meal. Never refuses a meal. Usually eats a total of 4 or more servings of meat and dairy products. Occasionally eats between meals. Does not require supplementation.	
FRICTION AND SHEAR	**1. Problem:** Requires moderate to maximum assistance in moving. Complete lifting without sliding against sheets is impossible. Frequently slides down in bed or chair, requiring frequent repositioning with maximum assistance. Spasticity, contractures or agitation leads to almost constant friction.	**2. Potential Problem:** Moves feebly or requires minimum assistance. During a move skin probably slides to some extent against sheets, chair restraints, or other devices. Maintains relatively good position in chair or bed most of the time but occasionally slides down.	**3. No Apparent Problem:** Moves in bed and in chair independently and has sufficient muscle strength to lift up completely during move. Maintains good position in bed or chair at all times.		
					Total Score

Appendix D: Bates-Jensen Pressure Sore Status Tool

Instructions for Use

General guidelines

Fill out the attached rating sheet to assess a pressure sore's status after reading the definitions and methods of assessment described below. Evaluate once a week and whenever a change occurs in the wound. Rate according to each item by picking the response that best describes the wound and entering that score in the item score column for the appropriate date. When you have rated the pressure sore on all items, determine the total score by adding together the 13 item scores. The *higher* the total score, the more severe the pressure sore status. Plot total score on the Pressure Sore Status Continuum to determine progress.

Specific instructions

1. **Size:** Use ruler to measure the longest and widest aspect of the wound surface in centimeters; multiply length x width.
2. **Depth:** Pick the depth and thickness most appropriate to the wound using these additional descriptions:
   1 = tissues damaged but no break in skin surface
   2 = superficial, abrasion, blister, or shallow crater. Even with, and/or elevated above, skin surface (e.g., hyperplasia)
   3 = deep crater with or without undermining of adjacent tissue
   4 = visualization of tissue layers not possible due to necrosis
   5 = supporting structures include tendon and joint capsule.
3. **Edges:** Use this guide:
   Indistinct, diffuse   = unable to clearly distinguish wound outline
   Attached   = even or flush with wound base; *no* sides or walls present; flat
   Not attached   = sides or walls *are* present; floor or base of wound is deeper than edge
   Rolled under, thickened = soft to firm and flexible to touch
   Hyperkeratosis   = callous-like tissue formation around wound and at edges
   Fibrotic, scarred   = hard, rigid to touch.
4. **Undermining:** Assess by inserting a cotton-tipped applicator under the wound edge; advance it as far as it will go without using undue force; raise the tip of the applicator so it may be seen or felt on the surface of the skin; mark the surface with a pen; measure the distance from the mark on the skin to the edge of the wound. Continue process around the wound. Then use a transparent metric measuring guide with concentric circles divided into four (25%) pie-shaped quadrants to help determine percentage of wound involved.
5. **Necrotic tissue type:** Pick the type of necrotic tissue that is *predominant* in the wound according to color, consistency, and adherence using this guide:
   White/gray nonviable tissue   = may appear prior to wound opening; skin surface is white or gray
   Nonadherent, yellow slough   = thin, mucinous substance; scattered throughout wound bed; easily separated from wound tissue
   Loosely adherent, yellow slough   = thick, stringy clumps of debris; attached to wound tissue
   Adherent, soft, black eschar   = soggy tissue; strongly attached to tissue in center or base of wound
   Firmly adherent, hard and black eschar   = firm, crusty tissue; strongly attached to wound base
   and   edges (like a hard scab).
6. **Necrotic tissue amount:** Use a transparent metric measuring guide with concentric circles divided into four (25%) pie-shaped quadrants to help determine percentage of wound involved.
7. **Exudate type:** Some dressings interact with wound drainage to produce a gel to trap liquid. Before assessing exudate type, gently cleanse wound with normal saline or water. Pick the exudate type that is *predominant* in the wound according to color and consistency, using this guide:
   Bloody   = thin, bright red
   Serosanguineous   = thin, watery pale red to pink
   Serous   = thin, watery clear
   Purulent   = thin or thick, opaque tan to yellow
   Foul purulent   = thick, opaque yellow to green with offensive odor.

Appendix D: Bates-Jensen Pressure Sore Status Tool *(continued)*

8. **Exudate amount:** Use a transparent metric measuring guide with concentric circles divided into four (25%) pie-shaped quadrants to determine percentage of dressing involved with exudate. Use this guide:

   None = wound tissues dry
   Scant = wound tissues moist; no measurable exudate
   Small = wound tissues wet; moisture evenly distributed in wound; drainage involves ≤25% dressing
   Moderate = wound tissues saturated; drainage may or may not be evenly distributed in wound; drainage involves >25% to ≤75% dressing
   Large = wound tissues bathed in fluid; drainage freely expressed; may or may not be evenly distributed in wound; drainage involves >75% of dressing.

9. **Skin color surrounding wound:** Assess tissues within 4 cm of wound edge. Dark-skinned persons show the colors "bright red" and "dark red" as a deepening of normal ethnic skin color or a purple hue. As healing occurs in dark-skinned persons, the new skin is pink and may never darken.

10. **Peripheral tissue edema:** Assess tissues within 4 cm of wound edge. Nonpitting edema appears as skin that is shiny and taut. Identify pitting edema by firmly pressing a finger down into the tissues and waiting for 5 seconds; on release of pressure, tissues fail to resume previous position and an indentation appears. Crepitus is accumulation of air or gas in tissues. Use a transparent metric measuring guide to determine how far edema extends beyond wound.

11. **Peripheral tissue induration:** Assess tissues within 4 cm of wound edge. Induration is abnormal firmness of tissues with margins. Assess by gently pinching the tissues. Induration results in an inability to pinch the tissues. Use a transparent metric measuring guide with concentric circles divided into four (25%) pie-shaped quadrants to determine percentage of wound and area involved.

12. **Granulation tissue:** Granulation tissue is the growth of small blood vessels and connective tissue to fill in full-thickness wounds. Tissue is healthy when bright, beefy red, shiny and granular with a velvety appearance. Poor vascular supply appears as pale pink or balanced to dull, dusky red.

13. **Epithelialization:** Epithelialization is the process of epidermal resurfacing and appears as pink or red skin. In partial-thickness wounds, it can occur throughout the wound bed as well as from the wound edges. In full-thickness wounds it occurs from the edges only. Use a transparent metric measuring guide with concentric circles divided into four (25%) pie-shaped quadrants to help determine percentage of wound involved and to measure the distance the epithelial tissue extends into the wound.

Pressure sore status tool   Name _____

Complete the rating sheet to assess pressure sore status.
Evaluate each item by picking the response that best
describes the wound and entering the score in the item score
column for the appropriate date.

Location: Anatomic site. Circle, identify right (R) or left (L)
        and use "X" to mark site on body diagrams:
   ___Sacrum and coccyx   ___Lateral ankle
   ___Trochanter   ___Medial ankle
   ___Ischial tuberosity ___Heel
   ___Other site

Shape: Overall wound pattern; assess by observing perimeter
      and depth. Circle and *date* appropriate description:
   ___Irregular   ___Linear or elongated
   ___Round or oval   ___Bowl or boat
   ___Square or rectangle   ___Butterfly
   ___Other shape

Appendix D: Bates-Jensen Pressure Sore Status Tool *(continued)*

Item	Assessment	Date Score	Date Score	Date Score
1. Size	1 = Length x width <4 cm^2 2 = Length x width 4 to 16 cm^2 3 = Length x width 16.1 to 36 cm^2 4 = Length x width 36.1 to 80 cm^2 5 = Length x width >80 cm^2			
2. Depth	1 = Nonblanchable erythema on intact skin 2 = Partial-thickness skin loss involving epidermis and/or dermis 3 = Full-thickness skin loss involving damage or necrosis of subcutaneous tissue; may extend down to but not through underlying fascia; and/or mixed partial and full thickness and/or tissue layers obscured by granulation tissue 4 = Obscured by necrosis 5 = Full-thickness skin loss with extensive destruction, tissue necrosis or damage to muscle, bone or supporting structure			
3. Edges	1 = Indistinct, diffuse, none clearly visible 2 = Distinct, outline clearly visible, attached, even with wound base 3 = Well-defined, not attached to wound base 4 = Well-defined, not attached to base, rolled under, thickened 5 = Well-defined, fibrotic, scarred or hyperkeratotic			
4. Undermining	1 = Undermining <2 cm in any area 2 = Undermining 2 to 4 cm involving <50% wound margins 3 = Undermining 2 to 4 cm involving >50% wound margins 4 = Undermining >4 cm in any area 5 = Tunneling and/or sinus tract formation			
5. Necrotic tissue type	1 = None visible 2 = White or gray nonviable tissue and/or nonadherent yellow slough 3 = Loosely adherent yellow slough 4 = Adherent, soft black eschar 5 = Firmly adherent, hard, black eschar			
6. Necrotic tissue amount	1 = None visible 2 = <25% of wound bed covered 3 = 25% to 50% of wound covered 4 = >50% and <75% of wound covered 5 = 75% to 100% of wound covered			
7. Exudate type	1 = None or bloody 2 = Serosanguineous: thin, watery, pale red or pink 3 = Serous: thin, watery, clear 4 = Purulent: thin or thick, opaque, tan or yellow 5 = Foul purulent: thick, opaque, yellow or green with odor			
8. Exudate amount	1 = None 2 = Scant 3 = Small 4 = Moderate 5 = Large			

Appendix D: Bates-Jensen Pressure Sore Status Tool *(continued)*

Item	Assessment	Date Score	Date Score	Date Score
9. Skin color surrounding wound	1 = Pink or normal for ethnic group 2 = Bright red and/or blanches to touch 3 = White or gray pallor or hypopigmented 4 = Dark red or purple and/or nonblanchable 5 = Black or hyperpigmented			
10. Peripheral tissue edema	1 = Minimal swelling around wound 2 = Nonpitting edema extends <4 cm around wound 3 = Nonpitting edema extends ≥4 cm around wound 4 = Pitting edema extends <4 cm around wound 5 = Crepitus and/or pitting edema extends ≥4 cm			
11. Peripheral tissue induration	1 = Minimal firmness around wound 2 = Induration <2 cm around wound 3 = Induration 2 to 4 cm extending <50% around wound 4 = Induration 2 to 4 cm extending ≥50% around wound 5 = Induration >4 cm in any area			
12. Granulation tissue	1 = Skin intact or partial thickness wound 2 = Bright, beefy red; 75% to 100% of wound filled and/or tissue overgrowth 3 = Bright, beefy red; <75% and >25% of wound filled 4 = Pink and/or dull, dusky red and/or fills ≤25% of wound 5 = No granulation tissue present			
13. Epithelialization	1 = 100% wound covered; surface intact 2 = 75% to <100% wound covered and/or epithelial tissue extends >0.5 cm into wound bed 3 = 50% to <75% wound covered and/or epithelial tissue extends to <0.5 cm into wound bed 4 = 25% to <50% wound covered 5 = <25% wound covered			
Total Score				
Signature				

Pressure sore status continuum

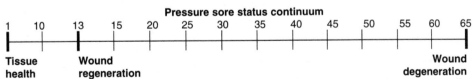

```
1    10   13   15   20   25   30   35   40   45   50   55   60   65
├────┼────┼────┼────┼────┼────┼────┼────┼────┼────┼────┼────┼────┤
```

Tissue   Wound   Wound
health   regeneration   degeneration

Plot the total score on the Pressure Sore Status Continuum by putting an "X" on the line and the date beneath the line. Plot multiple scores with their dates to see, at a glance, if regeneration or degeneration of the wound is occurring.

Appendix E: Pressure Ulcer Flow Chart

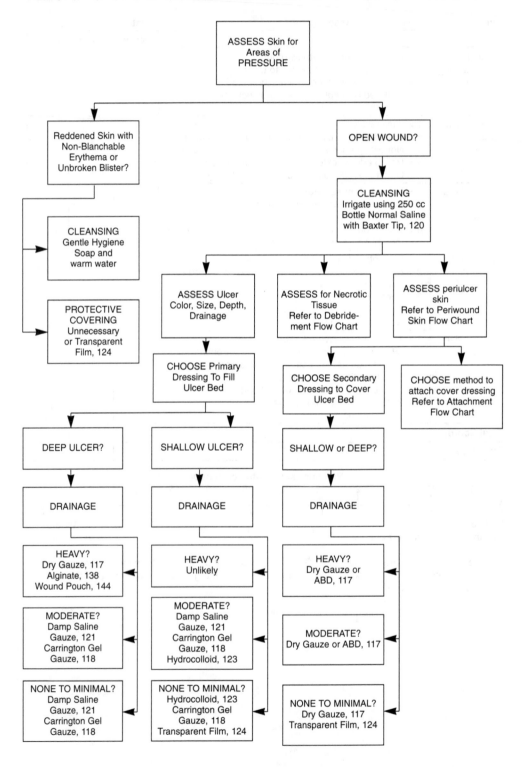

Appendix F: Leg Ulcer Flow Chart

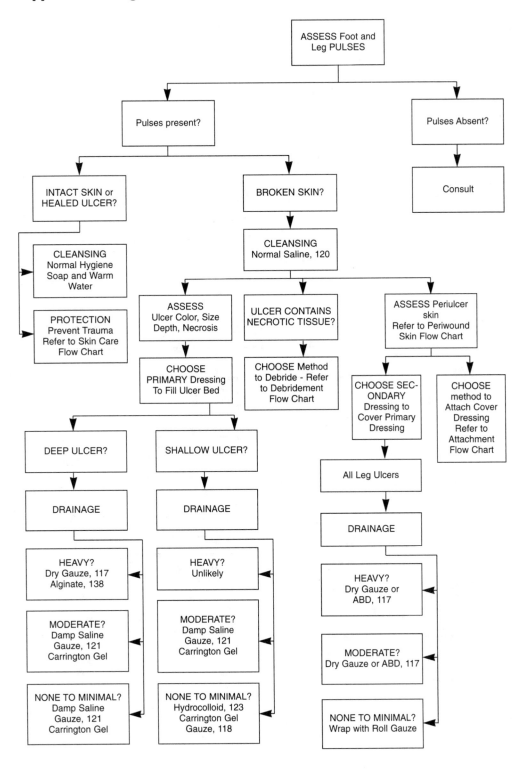

Appendix G: Surgical Wound Flow Chart

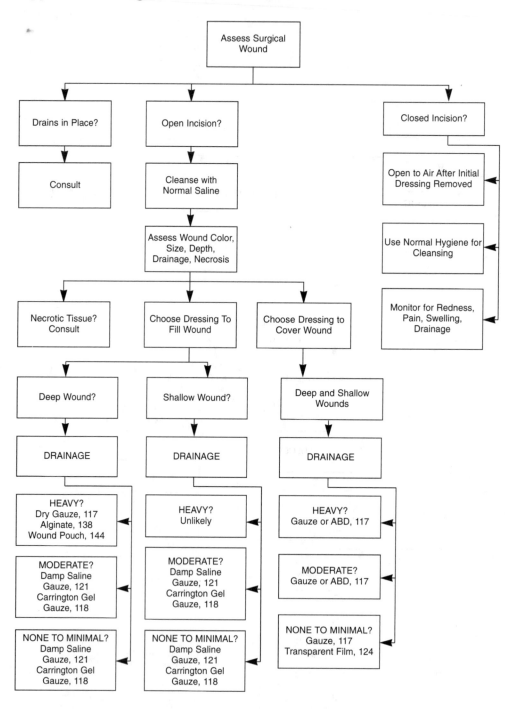

Appendix H: Peri-wound Skin Flow Chart

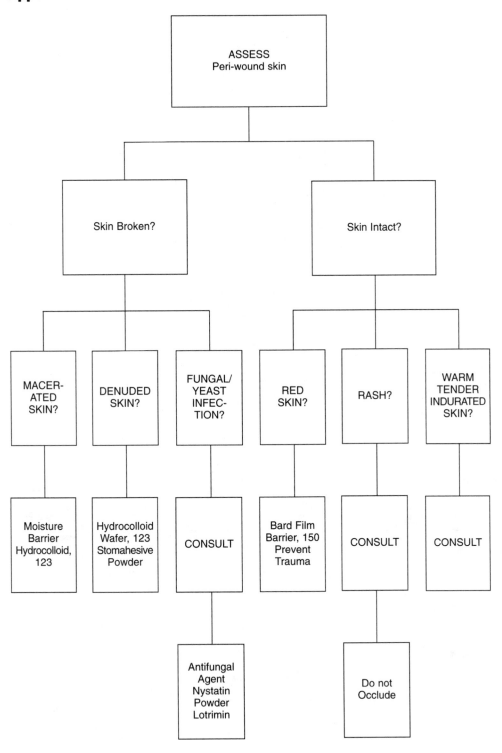

Appendix I: Dressing Attachment Flow Chart

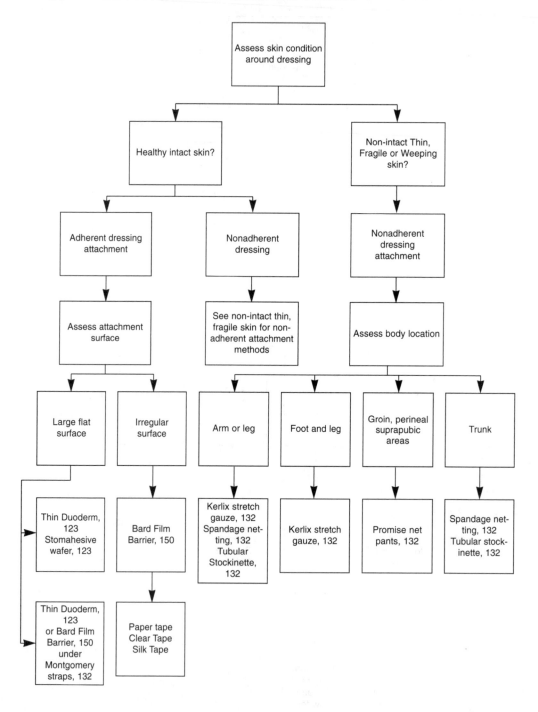

Appendix J: Debridement Flow Chart

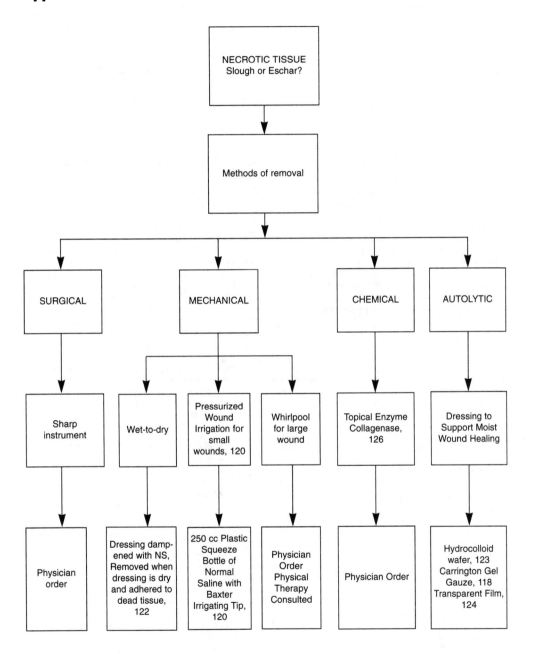

Appendix K: Nursing Admission Data Base

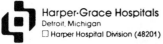

Harper-Grace Hospitals
Detroit, Michigan
☐ Harper Hospital Division (48201)

NURSING ADMISSION DATA BASE

PRESSURE ULCERS:

A CASE STUDY

DATE __4-14-90__ TIME __1700__

ADMITTED VIA:
☐ Ambulatory ☐ Wheelchair ■ Stretcher

ADMITTED FROM: ■ Home
☐ Emergency Room ☐ Nursing Facility
☐ Other _____

INFORMATION GIVEN BY: ☐ Patient
■ Family Member ☐ Friend
☐ Unable to Take History - Patient Unresponsive/
Not Accompanied by Family or Friend

ORIENTATION TO ROOM: – To daughter
■ Visiting Hours ■ Use of Phones
■ Call Light System ■ Operation of Bed and
(Bedside/Bath) Side Rails

REASON FOR ADMISSION AND EXPECTED TREATMENT: _____

__Dehydration__

__Sacral Pressure Ulcer__

CURRENT MEDICATIONS, SUPPLEMENTS, NON-PRESCRIPTION DRUGS

NAME	DOSE	LAST DOSE	FREQUENCY
Dyazide	25 mg	8 am	BID
Motrin	400mg	12 noon	q 12°

ALLERGENS: (DRUGS, FOODS, TAPES, DYES, OTHERS)

ALLERGEN	SYMPTOMS
Penicillin	Rash

■ Correct ID Band
Height __5'2"__ Weight __100__ Pulse __100__
Respirations __16__ Temperature __97°__
BP __100/68__ ☐ Sitting ☐ Lying
Physician/PA __Dr. Ray Jowes__ notified of admission

SUBJECTIVE DATA:
NUTRITIONAL/METABOLIC PATTERN:
Diet __Isocal 250 md q 6°__
Weight: ☐ No Problems
☐ Gain ■ Loss How Much __8/b__
History Of: ☐ No Problems ☐ Anorexia
☐ Nausea ☐ Vomiting ☐ Dysphagia
Skin: ☐ No Problems ■ Healing Problems
☐ Other _____

RESPIRATION/CIRCULATION PATTERN:
Respiratory: ■ No Problems
☐ Shortness of Breath
  ☐ Without Exercise
  ☐ With Exercise
☐ Cough ☐ Sputum
Sleeps on __2__ Pillows
Circulation: ■ No Problems ☐ Chest Pain
☐ Pedal Edema ☐ Pacemaker ☐ Rate _____
☐ Other _____

ELIMINATION PATTERN:
Bowel Habits: ☐ No Problems Last BM __This a.m.__
■ Soft/Formed ☐ Constipated
☐ Diarrhea ■ Incontinence
Bladder Habits: ☐ No Problems
☐ Urgency ■ Frequency
☐ Dysuria ☐ Hematuria
■ Incontinence ☐ Self Cath
☐ Other _____

OBJECTIVE DATA:
NUTRITIONAL/METABOLIC PATTERN:
Oral Mucosa: ■ Healthy
Color __Pink__
Lesions __None__
Dentures: ■ Upper ■ Lower ■ With Patient
Tubes __Gastrostomy__
Skin Integrity: ☐ Intact
■ Other __Ulcerated area over sacrum__

RESPIRATION/CIRCULATION PATTERN:
Breath Sounds __Shallow – no rales or rhonchi__

☐ Use of Accessory Muscles
Cough: ☐ Yes ■ No Productive: ☐ Yes ☐ No
Sputum Color _____
Apical Rate __90__ Rhythm: ■ Regular ☐ Irregular
Pedal Edema ☐ Present ■ Absent
Pedal Pulses ■ Present ☐ Absent
Tubes/Catheter Site _____

ELIMINATION PATTERN:
Abdomen: ■ Soft ☐ Firm
☐ Distended If yes, Girth _____ cm
■ Bowel Sounds Present
☐ Bowel Sounds Absent
☐ Ostomies/Tubes/Urinary Devices _____

300950 (3/90)

Appendix K: Nursing Admission Data Base *(continued)*

ACTIVITY/EXERCISE PATTERN:
Energy Level: ☐ No Problems
    ■ Tires Easily   ☐ High Energy
Able to: ☐ Feed Self   ☐ With Assistance
☐ Bathe Self   ☐ With Assistance
☐ Ambulate   ☐ Climb Stairs   ☐ With Assistance
Aids: ☐ None   ☐ Walker   ☐ Wheelchair
☐ Cane   ☐ Oxygen   ☐ Bedside Commode
☐ Hospital Bed   ☐ Other: _____
DME Company _____
Other _____

COGNITIVE/PERCEPTUAL PATTERN:
Hearing: ■ Normal   ☐ Impaired
☐ Left Ear   ☐ Right Ear   ☐ Aid   ☐ With Patient
Vision: ☐ Normal   ■ Impaired
    ☐ Glasses   ☐ Contacts   ■ With Patient
Communication Problem: ☐ No   ■ Yes
  <u>Minimal interaction</u>
Discomfort/Pain: ■ No   ☐ Yes
Where? _____
How do you manage your pain? _____
_____
Other _____

SLEEP/REST PATTERN:
Difficulty Sleeping: ■ No   ☐ Yes
Sleeping Medication: ■ No   ☐ Yes

ROLE/RELATIONSHIP PATTERN:
Who lives at home with you? <u>daughter</u>
_____
Support System (Close Friend/Family Member)
<u>daughter</u>_____
Phone Number: _____

Who is able to help you with care at home? _____
_____
Other _____

SEXUALITY/REPRODUCTIVE PATTERN:
LMP (If applicable) _____

COPING/STRESS TOLERANCE PATTERN:
Do you have concerns regrarding your
hospitalization?
☐ No   ☐ Yes
_____
Use of Alcohol: ■ No   ☐ Yes _____
    Smoking ■ No   ☐ Yes _____
    Drugs ■ No   ☐ Yes _____

ACTIVITY/EXERCISE PATTERN:
ROM: ☐ Full   ■ Other
Balance and Gait: ☐ Steady   ☐ Unsteady
Hand Grasps: ⟨Weakness⟩ Paralysis ■ Right ☐ Left ☐ WNL
Leg Muscles: Weakness/⟨Paralysis⟩ ■ Right ☐ Left ☐ WNL
Other <u>Not ambulatory</u>

COGNITIVE/PERCEPTUAL PATTERN:
Level of Consciousness: ☐ Alert
■ Responds to Pain   ☐ No Response – Upper extremities
Oriented To: ☐ Person   ☐ Place   ☐ Time Unable to assess
Pupils: ■ Equal   ■ Reactive
☐ Other _____
Cognition: ☐ Able to Follow Simple Commands
☐ Responds Appropriately to Questions
    ■ Unable to Follow Commands
Other <u>Responds to name by turning toward speaker</u>

DISCHARGE PLANNING ASSESSMENT:
Services pre-hospitalization ■ None
☐ Home Care If Yes, Agency _____
    Last Visit (Date) _____
☐ Meal Service   ☐ Chore Service
☐ Other _____
Environmental: ■ No Problems
☐ Architectural Barriers in Home   ☐ None
☐ Bathroom Not on First Level
☐ Bed Not on First Level   ☐ Stairs in Home
☐ Stairs to Enter Home   ☐ Other _____
Transportation: ■ No Problems
☐ Transport to Appointments   ☐ Clinic/M.D. Appointment
☐ ROC   ☐ Other _____
Financial: ■ No Problems   ☐ Unable to Obtain Medications
☐ Assist with Insurance
☐ Other _____
Teaching Needs Prior to Discharge:
☐ Disease Process   ☐ Medications
☐ ADL Training   ■ Treatments
■ Equipment/Supplies   ☐ Long Term Venous Catheter
☐ Diet   ☐ Other _____
Barriers to Teaching: _____

DISCHARGE PLAN:
Goal: Discharge: ☐ Home, Self-Care per Patient
    ■ Home, Care Provided by Significant Other
    ■ Support Needed by Home Care Agency
    ☐ Extended Care Facility
    ☐ Dependent on Response to Treatment
    ☐ Equipment
    ☐ Community Resources _____
Other _____
Referral Needed _____

General Comments: <u>Daughter has been caring for patient at home. Expressed concern that</u>
<u>she is now faced with the possibility that she may be unable to continue</u>
<u>care</u>

_____
R Callasandro RN   4/14/90
Clinical Nurse Signature/Date

M Tilmer RN, CT, CVS   4/14/90
Reviewed by Case Manager Signature/Date

Appendix K: Nursing Admission Data Base *(continued)*

Harper-Grace Hospitals
Detroit, Michigan

☐ Harper Hospital Division (48201)
☐ Grace Hospital Division (48235)

Care, Inida

PROGRESS NOTES

| 1700 | Impaired Tissue Integrity (Pressure Ulcer) |

O: 76 year old very pale female admitted from home. Cared for by daughter. Responds to name. Does not move trunk or rt. lower extremity when asked to do so. Moves arms and head when requested to do so. Fed per gastrostomy tube. Took small amounts of fluid orally until yesterday. Is incontinent of stool and urine. Skin over entire body is dry and scaly. Has necrotic pressure ulcer (sacral area) that is covered with dry gauze dressing. Dressing was difficult to remove because it was sticking to wound. Daughter indicates that she cleansed wound with soap and water and replaced gauze daily. Ulcer base measures 3.0 cm x 5.0 cm.

A: Impaired Tissue Intregrity: Stage III pressure ulcer RT immobility, incontinence, and inadequate nutritional status.

P: Consult ET nurse for wound care regimen. Consult social worker to assist with decision making regarding post-hospital placement.

K. Callasortu, RN 7/4/9

300270 Rev. 11/79

Appendix L: Nursing Care Plan

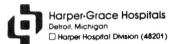

Harper·Grace Hospitals
Detroit, Michigan
☐ Harper Hospital Division (48201)

NURSING CARE PLAN

Care, Inida

NURSING DIAGNOSIS ☒	COLLABORATIVE PROBLEM ☐	DATE: 4-15-90	INITIALS: RC

Impaired tissue intregity: Stage III Pressure Ulcer RT prolonged pressure from immobility, incontinence and malnutrition/dehydration.

MEASURABLE GOALS/EXPECTED OUTCOMES:	INITIATED		REVISED	
	DATE	INITIALS	DATE	INITIALS
1. Ulcer base will decrease in size and wound will be free of necrotic tissue prior to discharge.				
2. Patient will increase fluid intake to 2000 cc/day by taking H20 per gastrostomy tube.				
3. Daughter will verbalize pressure ulcer prevention strategies.				
4. Daughter will demonstrate local wound care.				

MEASURABLE GOALS/EXPECTED OUTCOMES SET WITH PATIENT/FAMILY ☒ YES   ☐ NO

IF NO, EXPLAIN

INITIATED		DELETED		INTERVENTIONS
DATE	INITIALS	DATE	INITIALS	
				1) Measure ulcer base and record q Tuesday.
				2) Assess status of ulcer base and surrounding tissue every day and record.
				3) Use Sof-Care bed cushion for pressure relief. Do hand check q shift and reinflate prn.
				4) Turn q 2 hr. Use turning clock to remind about correct body position.
				5) Use Bard Protective Barrier Film on buttock and skin area exposed to urine and stool.
				6) Cleanse ulcer base with normal saline using a 35 cc syringe and a 19 G angiocatheter for correct irrigation pressure.
				7) Fill wound bed with Bard absorption drsg. Cover with ABD.
				8) Teach daughter signs & symptoms of dehydration & importance of fluid intake.
				9) Have daughter demonstrate measuring & giving water per G-tube following each tube feeding.
				10) Give pressure ulcer management brochure to daughter.
				11) Review relationship of nutrition, hydration, incontinence & unrelieved pressure to formation of ulcers.
				12) Have daughter demonstrate local wound care.

RESOLVED DATE:		INITIALS:

SUMMARY IF UNRESOLVED AT DISCHARGE:

INITIALS	SIGNATURE & TITLE	INITIALS	SIGNATURE & TITLE	INITIALS	SIGNATURE & TITLE	INITIALS	SIGNATURE & TITLE
RC	R. Caci...						

300826 (3/90)

Appendix M: Nursing Shift Assessment

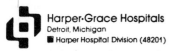

Harper·Grace Hospitals
Detroit, Michigan
■ Harper Hospital Division (48201)

Care, Inida

NURSING SHIFT ASSESSMENT

CODE: LOC = LEVEL OF CONSCIOUSNESS   + = POSITIVE
　　　　NA = NOT APPLICABLE   − = NEGATIVE
　　　　NP = NO PROBLEM   x = TIMES

INITIAL ASSESSMENT	2300-0700	0700-1500	1500-2300
NUTRITION/ METABOLIC PATTERN	Skin: ☐ NP ☐ Edema ■ Pressure Areas: _Sacral_ Other: _____	Skin: ☐ NP ☐ Edema ■ Pressure Areas: _Sacral_ Other: _____	Skin: ☐ NP ☐ Edema ■ Pressure Areas: _Sacral_ Other: _____
RESPIRATION/ CIRCULATION PATTERN	Breath Sounds: ■ Normal ☐ Abnormal _____ ☐ NA Cough: ☐ YES ■ NO ☐ Productive ☐ Non-productive Peripheral Pulses: ☐ NA ■ + ☐ − Other: _____	Breath Sounds: ■ Normal ☐ Abnormal _____ ☐ NA Cough: ☐ YES ■ NO ☐ Productive ☐ Non-productive Peripheral Pulses: ☐ NA ■ + ☐ − Other: _____	Breath Sounds: ■ Normal ☐ Abnormal _____ ☐ NA Cough: ☐ YES ■ NO ☐ Productive ☐ Non-productive Peripheral Pulses: ☑ NA ■ + ☐ − Other: _____
ELIMINATION PATTERN	☐ Nausea ☐ Vomiting ■ Diarrhea ☐ NP Abdomen: ☐ Distended ■ Non-Distended Bowel Sounds: ■ + ☐ − ☐ NA Other: _____	☐ Nausea ☐ Vomiting ■ Diarrhea ☐ NP Abdomen: ☐ Distended ■ Non-Distended Bowel Sounds: ■ + ☐ − ☐ NA Other: _____	☐ Nausea ☐ Vomiting ■ Diarrhea ☐ NP Abdomen: ☐ Distended ■ Non-Distended Bowel Sounds: ■ + ☐ − ☐ NA Other: _____
COGNITIVE/ PERCEPTUAL PATTERN	LOC: ☐ Person ☐ Place ☐ Time Responds appropriately to questions: ☐ Yes ■ No Discomfort: ☐ + ■ − Type: _____ Location: _____ Other: _____	LOC: ☐ Person ☐ Place ☐ Time Responds appropriately to questions: ☐ Yes ■ No Discomfort: ☐ + ■ − Type: _____ Location: _____ Other: _____	LOC: ☐ Person ☐ Place ☐ Time Responds appropriately to questions: ☐ Yes ■ No Discomfort: ☐ + ■ − Type: _____ Location: _____ Other: _____
ONGOING ASSESSMENT	Time:	Time:	Time:
HEALTH PERCEPTION/ HEALTH MANAGEMENT PATTERN	Safety: Siderails x _4_ ☐ Equipment _____ ☐ Restraints _____ ☐ Special Precautions _____ Other: _____	Safety: Siderails x _4_ ☐ Equipment _____ ☐ Restraints _____ ☐ Special Precautions _____ Other: _____	Safety: Siderails x _4_ ☐ Equipment _____ ☐ Restraints _____ ☐ Special Precautions _____ Other: _____
NUTRITION/ METABOLIC PATTERN	Supplement/Tube Feeding _Isocal 250 cc x 1_ ☐ NPO Other _G-tube_	Diet _Isocal 250 ml x 2_ Breakfast: ☐ 100% ☐ 75% ☐ 50% ☐ 25% ☐ Refused ☐ NPO Lunch: ☐ 100% ☐ 75% ☐ 50% ☐ 25% ☐ Refused ☐ NPO Supplement _____ Other: _G-tube_	Diet _Isocal 250 cc x 1_ Dinner: ☐ 100% ☐ 75% ☐ 50% ☐ 25% ☐ Refused ☐ NPO Supplement _____ Other: _G-Tube_
ELIMINATION PATTERN	Bowel Movement X _3_ ■ Incontinent of stool Urine: ☐ NP ■ Incontinent of Urine Devices _____ Other: _____	Bowel Movement X _1_ ■ Incontinent of stool Urine: ☐ NP ■ Incontinent of Urine Devices _____ Other: _____	Bowel Movement X _1_ ☐ Incontinent of stool Urine: ☐ NP ■ Incontinent of Urine Devices _____ Other: _____
ACTIVITY/EXERCISE PATTERN	Hygiene: ■ Complete ☐ Partial ☐ Self-Care ☐ NA Skin Products _____ Mouth Care _x 1_ Ambulated x _____ Chair x _____ ■ Bedrest Positioned x _3_ Other: _____	Hygiene: ■ Complete ☐ Partial ☐ Self-Care ☐ NA Skin Products _____ Mouth Care _x 2_ Ambulated x _____ Chair x _____ ■ Bedrest Positioned x _6_ Other: _____	Hygiene: ■ Complete ☐ Partial ☐ Self-Care ☐ NA Skin Products _____ Mouth Care _x 1_ Ambulated x _____ Chair x _____ ■ Bedrest Positioned x _4_ Other: _____
SLEEP/REST PATTERN	☐ Restless ■ Sleeping at Intervals ☐ Awake ☐ None Other: _____	☐ Restless ☐ Sleeping at Intervals ■ Awake ☐ None Other: _____	☐ Restless ■ Sleeping at Intervals ☐ Awake ☐ None Other: _____
SIGNATURE & TITLE			

300955 (3/90)

Appendix N: Discharge Instruction Sheet

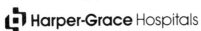

Harper-Grace Hospitals

Detroit, Michigan
Harper Hospital Division
Grace Hospital Division

Care, Inida

DISCHARGE INSTRUCTION SHEET

Follow-Up Care	Make an appointment to see Dr. ___Jones___ When: ___1 week in office___ Please call office for time 773 - 9024
Activities	Resume usual activities: ☐Yes ☐No Specific limitations: Bedrest with side rails up. Turn every 2 hours. Use lift or 2 assistants to get into chair daily.
Diet	Type of diet: ☐Regular ☒Modified, specify Isocal 250 ml / G-tube 5 X per day Printed instructions given: ☑Yes ☐No Instructions: Flush G- Tube with 100 cc H$_2$O after tube feeding

Medications	Special Instructions ☐None
Vitamin C 500 mg	2 X per day – Crush. Pour into syringe barrel connected to feeding tube. Fill with water and allow to run in.
Kaopectate 30 ml	Give after each loose BM - no more than 6 doses in 24hr
Motrin 400 mg	Give q 6 hours

Physician Signature ___C. Th— M. D.___   Date ___4 - 28 - 90___

Special Instructions (i.e. equipment / supplies / treatments)	G - tube Foley catheter Use pressure relieving device when in chair.

[ ] HOME CARE AGENCY: ___Renaissance Health Care___   Date of Visit: ___4 - 29- 90___

[ ] EQUIPMENT SUPPLIER: _____   Delivery Date: _____

I have been instructed and understand the above information.

Signature ___S____ ___   Date ___4 - 28 - 90___
                    Patient or Patient Representative

Signature of Nurse ___K Cll— RN___   Date ___4 - 28 - 90___

3/88
301410

WHITE COPY: Patient   YELLOW COPY: Medical Records

Appendix O: Pressure Ulcer Care Plan

PRESSURE ULCERS: PREVENTION AND CARE

CARE PLAN: to be filled in by the nurse or doctor and
information explained to the caregiver,
patient and/or family.

1. **Turning Schedule - Use the "Turn Clock"** every two hours during waking hours.
   Left hip _____ to ___ Right hip
   Mini shifts ____ - move arms and legs - turn slightly -support back with pillows
   Keep off back _____ _____

2. **Times for dressing changes**
   Sacral/ tailbone area daily in a. m.
   _____ _____

3. **Wash hands**

4. **Get supplies together**
   Normal saline Travase ointment Barrier film packet
   Irrigation set Bard Absorption Dressing Gauze squares Outer dressing pad
   Paper tape

5. **Remove old dressing and throw away in plastic trash bag**

6. **Wash hands**

7. **Wear "hospital gloves"**

8. **Clean or rinse ulcer with:**
   Normal Saline _____ _____
   Use gauze squares to dry skin around ulcer

9. **Rinse again with:**
   Apply small amount of Travase ointment to yellow area and ulcer using gloved finger

10. **Cover or fill with:**
    Use Bard Absorption Dressing to fill ulcer. Cover with large pad dressing.
    _____ _____

11. **Tape or wrap dressing with:** _____ _____
    Use Barrier film to wipe skin around ulcer. Allow Barrier film to dry.
    Apply paper tape.

12. **Throw gloves away in plastic trash bag**

13. **Wash hands**

14. **Special supplies**

15. **Extra foods or vitamins**
    vit C 500 mg 2 X day (Crush and pour into syringe barrel connected to feeding
    tube. Fill syringe with water and allow to run through. Give extra water to
    rinse syringe.)

M. Palmer RN ET

Nurses signature

Sharon Nay

Patient/family signature

Appendix P: Continuing Patient Care Form

CONTINUING PATIENT CARE FORM (Side 1)

Patient Last Name First Name	TO: Agency Name and Address
Care, Inida	Renaissance Health Care

Address for Care City or Twp.	FROM: Hospital, Clinic, E.C.F. & Address
1111 Brush Detroit, MI 48202 Phone 745 - 1357	Harper Hospital

Patient's Address, if not same as above Phone	Referral Date Reported by:
NA	Agency 1st Visit 4-29-90 Reported to: Date

Complete Birth Date Sex Marital Status	Hospital for Drugs or Services
8 -16 -14 M (F) S M (W) D Sep	Harper HOspital

Responsible Relative or Friend Sharon Myer	Medicare No. 363 00 7000D
daughter 745 - 1357 Relationship Phone	Medicaid No.

Hospital Case No. Room No. Admission 4-14-90	Blue Cross No.
363 00 7001 V 624 Discharge 4 - 28 - 90	Other Ins: (Give Name)

II. REPORT BY PHYSICIAN

Diagnoses: List Primary First and Date of Onset
Sepsis with dehydration.
Sacral pressure ulcer.

Surgery Performed (Type and Date)
Debride. Press. Ulcer. (4-15-90)
Removal and replacement of G tube

Complications:
none

Rehabilitation or Treatment Goal:
Clean granulating ulcer.
No new skin breakdown.

Prognosis   Good ☐   Fair ☒   Guarded ☐   Poor ☐
Patient Informed of Diagnosis   Yes ☒   No ☐
Family Informed of Diagnosis   Yes ☒   No ☐

Brief Medical History:
Rheumatoid arthritis with deteriorating
mental status.

Date and Place of Physician's Next Visit:
Home ☐   Office ☐   Clinic ☒   E.C.F. ☐

MEDICAL ORDERS AND PLAN OF TREATMENT

Minimum Number of Hosp. Days Saved ☐

Diet (Specify) Isocal 250ml / G- Tube 5 X per day. Follow with 100cc water.

Dressings or Treatment (Specify) Change sacral dressing daily. Flush with normal saline. Apply absorption dressing.

Catheter ☒   Size 14foley **Frequency of Change** 1 X mo **Irrigation Solution** _____ **Amount** _____ **Frequency** _____

Enema (Specify) Replace gastrostomy tube (#18) every month.

Medications: Kaopectate 30 ml after each loose BM. Not to exceed 6 doses in 24 hours.
Travase Oint. sparingly to necrotic area in sacral ulcer daily.
Vitamin C 500 mg. BID crushed and given through G- tube
Motrin 400 mg - give every 6 hours through G tube

Specify Therapeutic Exercise Program
Range of Motion - extremities 6 times per day.
Turn, reposition every 2 hours. Use 30° laterally inclined position.

Activity Allowance:
Chair sit daily with pressure relieving cushion - no longer than 30 minutes.

Patient Uses: Prostheses ☐   Brace ☐   Walker ☐   Wheelchair ☒   Cane ☐   Other Vascular Boots

Physical Therapy ☐   Occupational Therapy ☐   Social Service ☐   Speech ☐   Evaluate Need for Home Health Aide ☒

Teaching Patient or Family RN
Teach use of Vascular Boots, incontinent products to protect perirectal area.
Dressing changes to sacral area and around feeding tube. Review use of Sof-Care
Bed Cushion and importance of turning.

I certify that the above patient is under my care and requires the above Home Health Services because he is confined to his home. These professional services are to be provided on an intermittent basis and the established plan contained in the record will be reviewed by me at least every two months. These services are needed to treat all of the conditions for which the patient was treated during the related in-patient hospital or post-hospital extended care facility approved stay.

Date Physician's Signature	Address	Phone Signed by Resident
K JONES MD		S. Thom M.D

Form #300560

Appendix P: Continuing Patient Care Form (continued)

CONTINUING PATIENT CARE FORM   (Side 2)

III. HOSPITAL NURSE'S ASSESSMENT: Reason For Referral? Altered tissue integrity
related to immobility, incontinence, and pressure as evidenced by sacral ulcer, ulcer
arough G-tube and slightly red but intact perirectal area.

Activity Limitations:		Activities of Daily Living:		Vital Signs with Ranges & Dates:
Ambulatory	☐	Independent	☐	TPR 98ax 100 22
Ambulatory with assistance	☐	Needs Assistance	☐	BP 100/50
Confined to Bed ☒ Chair ☒		Unable to do	☒	WT 94 lb

Mental State:
Alert ☐   Depressed ☐
Apathetic ☒   Disoriented ☐
Confused ☒   Other _____

Incontinence:

	None	Partial	Complete	
Bowel	☐	☐	☒	Loose stool. LL Base atelect
Bladder	☐	☐	☒	Foley cath. resolved.

X-Ray: Findings & Dates

Disabilities and Impairments:
Mentality	☐	Amputation	☐
Speech	☐	Paralysis	☐
Hearing	☐	Contractures	☐
Vision	☐	Decubitﬁ	☑
Sensation	☐		

In-Hospital Teaching:
Bowel Training _____
Bladder Training _____
Colostomy Care _____
Insulin Administration _____
Modified Diet Instruction ☐
Copy of Diet to Patient ☐
Copy of Diet to Agency ☐
Other Dressings= sacral
    ulcer and around G tube.

Laboratory: Findings & Dates
Hb.   9.5
B.S.   105
BUN
Culture
Serology

Other Significant Findings:
Serum albumin 2.5

Allergies:
  NKA

Special Problems and Other Narrative: Sacral ulcer - yellow slough approx 2 x 3 cm in undermined
area. Ulcerated pressure area from G tube bumper - 1cm each side feeding tube.
G tube replacement #18 in place. Sof-Care with tire pump adapter for inflation.
Hand check q 8 hours. Daughter has assisted with dressing changes x 2.

Diagram to Show Location, Size, Extent, etc., of Wound, Stoma, Burn, Decubitﬁ Graft or Other Affected Area.
Undermining from 12 to 5 oclock .
4x6 cm
2cm deep
3 cm deep in undermined area with yellow slough.
Wound base - major area clean and granulating.
Wound margin - free of eschar.
Drainage - small to moderate sero-sanguinous.
Surrounding tissue decreased redness- no induration or swelling.
TREATMENT PLAN FOR DAILY DRESSING CHANGE:
-Flush with normal saline to remove debris and old Absorption Dressing
-Apply small amount of Travase Ointment to yellow slough
-Fill ulcer with Bard Absorption Dressing including undermined area.
-Apply liquid barrier film to intact skin around ulcer.
-Allow barrier film to dry.
-Cover with ABD and picture frame with paper tape over dried barrier film.

Signature _____ RN   Title _____

IV. REPORT OF SPECIAL HOSPITAL SERVICES: Dietitian, Physical Therapist, Social Worker, etc.
TREATMENT PLAN FOR G TUBE:
    Ulcer area - 1 cm each side of G tube - 1 cm deep
    Change Stomahesive dressing q 3 days of prn leakage'
    Remove wafer and clean ulcers with normal saline. Pat skin dry.
    Fill ulcer crater with Stomahesive paste.
ulcers
    Cut hole in 4 x 4 wafer and fit around G tube over ulcers.
    Picture frame with paper tape.
    Reistablish pressure on G-tube disc to prevent feeding / GI contents from
        leaking around G tube.
                        (Call if there are any questions - 555-1234)
            Signature _____ Title CNS

INDEX

f refers to a figure; t, to a table.

f refers to a figure; t, to a table.

f refers to a figure; t, to a table.

W-X-Y-Z